Immunological and Inflammatory Disorders of the Central Nervous System

Immunological and Inflammatory Disorders of the Central Nervous System

Edited by

Neil Scolding, MRCP PhD
University Lecturer and Honorary Consultant Neurologist,
University of Cambridge Neurology Unit, Addenbrooke's
Hospital, Cambridge, UK

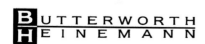

OXFORD   AUCKLAND   BOSTON   JOHANNESBURG   MELBOURNE   NEW DELHI

Butterworth-Heinemann
Linacre House, Jordan Hill, Oxford OX2 8DP
225 Wildwood Avenue, Woburn, MA 01801-2041
A division of Reed Educational and Professional Publishing Ltd

Ⓡ A member of the Reed Elsevier plc group

First published 1999

British Library Cataloguing in Publication Data

A catalogue record for this book is available from the British Library

Library of Congress Cataloguing in Publication Data

A catalogue record for this book is available from the Library of Congress

ISBN 0 7506 2357 8

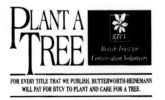

FOR EVERY TITLE THAT WE PUBLISH, BUTTERWORTH-HEINEMANN
WILL PAY FOR BTCV TO PLANT AND CARE FOR A TREE.

Typeset by Bath Typesetting
Printed and bound by MPG Books Ltd, Bodmin, Cornwall

Contents

Preface   vii

List of contributors   viii

Chapter 1   Immune responses and the nervous system   1
             Alasdair Coles and Neil Scolding

Chapter 2   Multiple sclerosis   21
             Neil Scolding

Chapter 3   Inflammatory demyelinating disease (II): syndromes
             and disorders related to multiple sclerosis   74
             Neil Scolding

Chapter 4   Current and future therapies for multiple sclerosis   93
             David C. Wraith

Chapter 5   Paraneoplastic disorders of the central nervous system   118
             Neil Scolding

Chapter 6   Stiff man syndrome   139
             Neil Scolding

Chapter 7   Neurological complications of rheumatological and
             connective tissue disorders   147
             Neil Scolding

Chapter 8   Organ-specific autoimmune and inflammatory disease
             and the central nervous system   181
             Neil Scolding

Chapter 9   Sarcoidosis and the central nervous system   193
             John Zajicek

Chapter 10   Cerebral vasculitis   210
             Neil Scolding

Index   258

Preface

Professor Martin Raff, a most senior figure in glial cell biology, having been asked to contribute to some neuroimmunological meeting, or book, or organization, is widely quoted as declining with the encouraging words "'Neuroimmunology'? There's no such thing!". Many years ago, a general physician, not noted for his humility, bestowed upon the editor this general advice: "you don't want to do neurology, Schofield. Waste of time! Only two disorders – steroid-responsive and steroid-unresponsive. Do something interesting".

The neurological physician, faced perhaps with a patient suffering a subacutely progressive cerebellar syndrome and a raised ESR, and wondering whether this might be vasculitis, or paraneoplasia, or just 'funny' multiple sclerosis, may find little direction or assistance in conventional neurological texts. The experimental immunologist, interested in autoimmunity to neural elements and wishing to enquire into the clinical relevance of his field, will often find himself in a similar position.

So this is a small book which, overlooking peripheral nerves and muscles and their junction, fails to cover half of an uninteresting clinical specialty which has a non-existent biological basis. I hope very much that it may nevertheless be of interest and of use, both to neurologists, and to scientists interested in clinical immunoneurobiology.

I hope too that Edward, Peter, Wilf and Emma, and Charlotte, find the product to be worth the encouragement they have steadfastly given to the producer and the production.

List of contributors

Alasdair Coles, MRCP, PhD
Specialist Registrar, Neurology Unit, University of Cambridge, Cambridge, UK

Neil Scolding, MRCP, PhD
University Lecturer and Honorary Consultant Neurologist, University of Cambridge Neurology Unit, Addenbrooke's Hospital, Cambridge, UK

David C. Wraith, BSc, PhD
Professor of Experimental Pathology, Department of Pathology and Microbiology, University of Bristol, Bristol, UK

John Zajicek, MA, MRCP, PhD
Consultant Neurologist, Honorary Senior Lecturer, Derryford Hospital, Plymouth, UK

Chapter 1

Immune responses and the nervous system

Alasdair Coles and Neil Scolding

Introduction	1
Immune responses in the central nervous system	3
Tolerance and autoimmunity in the nervous system	8
Therapeutic strategies in autoimmune disease	13
References	16

Introduction

For many years it was thought that the central nervous system (CNS) was inaccessible to the immune system. This concept of 'immune privilege' originated from four entirely disparate historical observations. The first was Ehrlich's finding that parenterally administered aniline dyes stained almost all body tissues except the CNS (Ehrlich, 1885); from this arose the concept of the blood–brain barrier, physiologically separating central nervous tissue from the systemic circulation and – it was later argued – from systemic immune responses. The second observation concerned transplantation: mouse sarcoma tissue was found not to be rejected following implantation into rat brain (Murphy and Sturm, 1923), implying that the CNS was exempt from the immunological processes responsible for graft rejection. The absence in the brain of direct lymphatic drainage – and by implication of circulating lymphocytes – depriving the CNS of an apparently essential requirement for immune response generation (Sabin, 1916), provided a third powerful argument in favour of immune isolation. Finally, and much later, normal nervous tissue was reported not to express major histocompatibility complex (MHC) antigens (Ediden, 1972), exempting the brain from participation in cell mediated immune reactions.

Notwithstanding these objections to the immunocompetence of the nervous system, it was paradoxically this site where adverse immune reactions were first recognized. Pasteur's 1885 rabies virus vaccine precipitated, in a small number of recipients, a neuroparalytic illness that was later found to constitute an autoimmune hypersensitivity reaction; and experimental allergic encephalomyelitis (EAE) in monkeys, an acute disseminated CNS inflammatory disorder precipitated by inoculation with nervous tissue, was described by Rivers and his associates in 1933. These observations, as well as the usually favourable outcome of infectious encephalitides and the brisk cerebrospinal fluid (CSF) pleocytosis which commonly accompanies brain infection, indicate that immune responses can and must be generated within the brain.

The role of the immune system in the CNS is, as elsewhere in the body, to protect the host against infections and perhaps also neoplasia. The three critical steps in this protection are first *identification* of the invading microbe

Antigen specific immune response

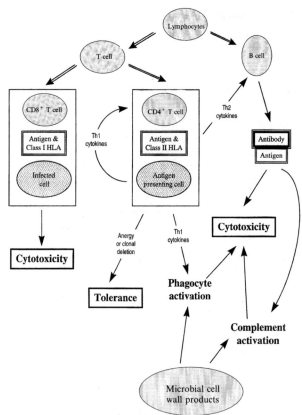

Antigen non-specific immune response

Figure 1.1 A simplified overview of immune responses.

or tumour cell, then its *clearance* and, finally, *memory* for the pathogen so that the immune system is equipped to defend against repeated infections. The task of identifying foreign tissue requires the ability to distinguish *self* from *non-self* accurately; inappropriate recognition of self as non-self leads to autoimmune disease, whereas misidentification of a microbe as self leads to unchallenged infection. Clearance of an infection needs to be efficient but restrained to the target alone; an excessive immune response, such as in tuberculoid leprosy or tuberculosis, may cause as much damage as the precipitating infection. To achieve effective targeted clearance of a pathogen without causing harm, the immune system is composed of a network of regulatory processes. One way to conceptualize the components of the immune response is to consider the *antigen-specific* and *antigen non-specific* immune responses (Figure 1.1).

Immune responses in the central nervous system

The antigen-specific immune response

The specificity of the recognition of pathogens by the immune system rests on the interaction of antibodies and lymphocyte receptors with specific molecular components (usually peptides) of the pathogen, termed *antigens*. The huge diversity of antigen specificity required by the immune system is generated by a sequence of random events in the generation of the proteins that make up the antibodies and lymphocyte receptors. For instance, immunoglobulin mRNA is transcribed randomly from one each of 51 *variable*, 27 *diversity* and six *joining* gene segments. This recombination of genes generates thousands of possible antigen-binding sites, that are further increased in number by mistakes in the recombination process. Then, when B cells encounter antigen, their binding specificity is increased by a Darwinian selection process within the germinal centres of lymph nodes. Here there is a high rate of somatic point mutations, and antibodies that bind tightly to antigen survive preferentially. Once B cells have encountered antigen, they proliferate and differentiate into antibody-producing *plasma cells* or *memory cells* that respond rapidly on re-exposure to the same antigen.

T cells only recognize antigen when presented in the grooves of *human leukocyte antigen* (HLA) proteins. They recognize the antigen–HLA complex through the T cell receptor (TCR) whose diverse antigen specificities are probably generated in a similar way to that of antibodies. HLA molecules come in two forms: *Class I* and *Class II*, which are associated with $CD8^+$ and $CD4^+$ T cells, respectively. Nearly all cells in the body express Class I HLA protein, which binds antigen from pathogens that replicate within the cytoplasm of cells principally viruses. The antigen–Class I complex is recognized by $CD8^+$ T cells, which are predominantly cytotoxic and destroy the infected cell.

In contrast, $CD4^+$ lymphocytes recognize antigens only when bound to HLA Class II proteins, which are expressed on a select group of cells and which bind peptides derived from proteins degraded in intracellular vesicles. The outcome of antigen recognition by $CD4^+$ cells is a central determinant of the immune response and is mediated by the secretion of cytokines, which are soluble peptides that signal immune responses between cells in a paracrine way. Several responses are possible, e.g.

- The $CD4^+$ T cell may secrete cytokines that promote B cell proliferation and antibody production. Antibody then binds the antigen; this interaction then recruits and focuses the non-antigen-specific immune attack such as complement, as well as stimulating antibody-dependent cytotoxicity. In this context, the T *helper* (T_h) cell is providing *help* to B cells. In truth, B cells and T cells are mutually dependent, and the classical distinction between the humoral and cellular components of the immune system is proving increasingly unhelpful.
- Cytokines may be released that activate microglia and also expand the T cell population. As activated microglia may present antigen to T cells, this sets up a positive feedback loop of antigen presentation and T cell expansion. Also activated microglia, as part of the non-antigen-specific

immune response (see below), may mediate cell death by antibody-targeted phagocytosis and cytotoxicity.

- In certain cases (see below) the T cell may secrete no cytokines on antigen recognition and so not generate an immune response. This response is termed *anergy* and is one form of immune *tolerance*.
- Alternatively, there may be no T cell that recognizes the antigen–Class II complex. The immune system is thus blind to that particular antigen and no response is made. This form of tolerance is achieved by *clonal deletion*, discussed below.

The CD4$^+$ T cell is therefore the principal arbitrator of the immune response to a specific antigen, and the mechanisms of its antigen recognition and cytokine secretion have attracted enormous attention. It has become clear that the formation of the *trimolecular complex* (Class II HLA–antigen–TCR) alone is insufficient to activate T cells. The binding of additional *co-stimulatory* molecules is also required (Figure 1.2), such as lymphocyte function-associated antigen (LFA)-1 and intercellular adhesion molecule (ICAM)-1 (Simmons *et al.*, 1987). Without such co-stimulation, antigen recognition does not generate an immune response; this is one mechanism for clonal anergy. CTLA-4 is expressed on the surface of activated T cells and competes with CD28 to bind the B7 family of receptors. Its function may be to terminate T cell activation, e.g. preventing CD28 binding it ameliorates EAE (Khoury *et al.*, 1995).

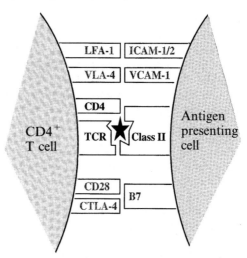

Figure 1.2 Co-stimulation of the interaction between the CD4$^+$ lymphocyte and the antigen-presenting cell.

There are two important exceptions to this scheme of T cell activation. First, *superantigens* have been discovered. These are microbial products that bind to the non-antigen specific ('outside') of the TCR and thus activate a whole class of T cells rather than one clone, the implications of which are discussed below. Secondly, T cells have been found that use the γ and δ

chains in their TCR in contrast to the usual α and β chains. These $\gamma\delta$ *T cells* recognize antigen without HLA class restriction and release interferon (IFN)-γ on microbial stimulation.

CD4$^+$ lymphocyte phenotypes: the T$_h$1/2 paradigm

In a pivotal study, Mosmann showed that the response of murine CD4$^+$ T cells to antigen may be categorized on the basis of the induced cytokine secretion. 'T$_h$1' cells secrete interleukin (IL)-12, tumour necrosis factor (TNF)-β and IFN-γ, which activate macrophages; 'T$_h$2' cells promote B lymphocyte responses through the release of IL-4 and IL-10 (Mosmann *et al.*, 1986). To a certain extent, each class of cytokines antagonizes the other and so the outcome of any immune response depends upon the balance between the two phenotypes. 'T$_h$0' cells secrete few cytokines and are considered to be uncommitted lymphocytes. Human CD4$^+$ lymphocytes show similar, but not identical, phenotypes to those in the mouse (reviewed in Romagnani *et al.*, 1997). For instance, the expression of IL-6, IL-10 and IL-13 is less restricted than in the mouse, and individual T cells may secrete T$_h$1 and T$_h$2 cytokines equally. There are now putative surface markers of human T$_h$1 and T$_h$2 phenotypes: LAG-3 (Annunziato *et al.*, 1996) and CD30 (Del Prete *et al.*, 1995), respectively.

The factors controlling differentiation of CD4$^+$ cells into these phenotypes remain controversial. The identity of the antigen-presenting cell may be important: macrophages and dendritic cells favouring T$_h$1 differentiation, and B cells promoting T$_h$2 (Gajewski *et al.*, 1991). Other determinants of phenotype are the co-stimulatory molecules expressed on the antigen-presenting cell, such as the two forms of B7 which interact with CD28 on the T cell: administration of an antibody against B7.1 at immunization in an EAE model resulted in the generation of T$_h$2 clones which on transfer prevented induction of disease, while anti-B7.2 increased disease severity (Kuchroo *et al.*, 1995). The local cytokine environment also helps determine T$_h$ differentiation. *In vitro,* IL-12 can promote the differentiation of allergen-specific T$_h$0 or T$_h$2 cells to T$_h$1, and the neutralization of IL-12 in bulk culture causes tuberculin-specific cells to shift from T$_h$1 to T$_h$2 (Manetti *et al.*, 1993, 1994). IL-10 and IL-4 (perhaps from mast cells or other T cells) promotes a T$_h$2 response.

The balance between CD4$^+$ lymphocyte phenotypes is critical to the pathogenesis of infectious and autoimmune disease. A classical example comes from studies of the susceptibility of mice to infection by *Leishmania major*. Mouse strains that raised a T$_h$1 response were protected against disease (or even developed a delayed-type hypersensitivity reaction), whereas T$_h$2 strains succumbed to the disease (Heinzel *et al.*, 1989). Experimental allergic encephalomyelitis is suppressed by anti-IFN-γ antibodies (Lublin *et al.*, 1993) and IL-4. In contrast, its recovery phase is associated with increased IL-10 and transforming growth factor (TGF)-β production, implying a switch to a T$_h$2 response (Kennedy *et al.*, 1992). Therefore, EAE has been labelled a 'T$_h$1 disease'. Not all studies are compatible with this idea. For instance, knocking out the IFN-γ gene of the BALB/c mice abolishes its normal resistance to EAE (Krakowski and Owens, 1996). An example of T$_h$1 cytokines being associated with human autoimmunity comes from a study of diabetic siblings; disease was associated with CD4⁻CD8⁻ cells of a particular TCR that secreted excessive IFN-γ and no IL-4 (Wilson *et al.*, 1998).

The antigen non-specific inflammatory response

One of the main functions of the antigen-specific processes described above is the recruitment of inflammatory mediators. For instance, antibodies bound to antigen may activate the *classical* pathway of *complement*. This group of serum proteins circulates in an inactive form. Activation results in the formation of vasoactive and chemotactic peptides, and terminal membrane attack complexes, which may injure or lyse target cells.

Cells of the *macrophage/monocyte* lineage are present in most tissues, including the brain, where they are represented by the *microglia*. Macrophages, activated by T_h1 cytokines, phagocytose debris and secrete a variety of toxic substances, including free oxygen radicals and TNF-α. As they present antigen to T cells and are activated by T cells, a positive feedback loop promoting T cell responses can be initiated by microglia. In addition, the cytokines secreted by microglia act on local endothelia to recruit further inflammatory and immunologically active cells (Hickey *et al.*, 1991).

As well as being effectors of the antigen-specific immune cells, macrophages and complement may also be activated directly by pathogens. For instance, lipopolysaccharide found on some bacterial cell walls may activate macrophages and the *alternative* pathway of complement is initiated by the non-specific binding of the C3b component to the microbial cell surface. These innate immune responses form a first line of defence against infections, before T cell responses have been activated.

Restrictions to immune responses in the central nervous system

Of the original evidence in favour of the brain as an immunologically inaccessible site, the most telling has been the apparent restriction of immune cells by the blood–brain barrier and the lack of HLA expression within the brain.

The blood–brain barrier is a complex structure composed of a layer of endothelial cells abutting a basement membrane interspersed with pericytes, around which a continuous covering is provided by the extended foot processes of type 1 astrocytes (Juhler and Neuwelt, 1989) and microglial processes. The ultrastructure of this blood vessel : tissue interface differs markedly from that seen elsewhere in the microvasculature in that there are tight junctions between adjacent endothelial cells; these cells have many mitochondria and also lack the vesicles which elsewhere effect transport of proteins into extravascular tissue. Astrocytes are responsible for inducing endothelial cells to form this barrier between the systemic circulation and the CNS (Janzer and Raff, 1987). Whilst highly permeable to water and lipid soluble molecules, the blood–brain barrier prevents the free passage of solutes from the systemic circulation into the CNS. Essential nutrients including glucose and certain amino acids, together with some ions, are transported by specific carrier mechanisms, but the majority of larger polar molecules, including proteins, cannot reach the abluminal surface. The blood–brain barrier therefore normally excludes circulating immune effector molecules, such as immunoglobulin and complement, from the CNS. A similar barrier in the choroid plexus performs a parallel function, separating blood and CSF; this barrier is anatomically situated at the epithelial cell lining of the choroid plexus, not in the choroidal capillary endothelium.

However, *activated* T cells are able to cross the intact blood–brain barrier. In experimental encephalomyelitis, lymphocytes infiltrate the CNS at a very early stage, when the blood–brain barrier remains impermeable to horseradish peroxidase (Simmons *et al.*, 1987) and appears normal both structurally and functionally. Systemic immune responses against antigens not expressed by neural tissue result in the appearance of activated T cells within the CNS (Hickey *et al.*, 1991). The mechanism of lymphocyte passage across the blood–brain barrier is presumably similar to that seen in other organs. First, they are tethered by selectin/glycoprotein interactions on the endothelium, during which lymphocytes roll along the endothelium. Next, they are brought to a halt by binding to other adhesion molecules (especially the integrin and immunoglobulin gene families). Finally, T cell blasts secrete enzymes that degrade endothelial cell basement membranes, this presumably facilitating their passage through the blood–brain barrier (Naparstek *et al.*, 1984).

There are also areas of the CNS where the blood–brain barrier is constitutively incompetent – the hypothalamus, area postrema, periventricular areas, and spinal and cranial nerve roots (Bradbury, 1979; Juhler and Neuwelt, 1989). Thus, lymphocytes are normally present in the brain and indeed in the CSF (Matsui *et al.*, 1990), albeit in low number. Traffic of activated T cells may occur through the CNS, exiting via channels ultimately draining through the cribriform plate into the post-nasal space and thence the cervical lymphatics (Bradbury *et al.*, 1981). This traffic provides the brain with a degree of immune surveillance but at the same time potentially exposes it to immune attack.

Hence the conventional dogma that lymphocytes do not have access to the CNS is no longer tenable. Nor is it true, as originally believed, that Class II HLA is absent from the brain. Specifically, microglia may express Class II MHC molecules (Hayes *et al.*, 1987).

Three subpopulations of CNS macrophage lineage cells are recognized. One population is resident deep in the CNS and probably is relatively inactive immunologically. Another population, found near vessels in human brain (Graeber *et al.*, 1992), expresses Class II. Finally, actively phagocytic macrophages in diseased areas of the CNS may be derived from circulating monocytes (Li *et al.*, 1993). Pathological studies in multiple sclerosis brain show that microglia may be activated in areas that appear otherwise normal (Hayes *et al.*, 1987). Microglia that express Class II are thereby capable of presenting antigen to lymphocytes. *In vitro,* Class I and II MHC products may also be induced on astrocytes and cerebral vascular endothelial cells, but this has not been demonstrated *in vivo.*

Therefore, despite its original designation as an immunologically privileged site, the brain contains the two critical ingredients for an immune response, i.e. T cells and Class II expressing antigen-presenting cells. This said, there are two important restrictions on the range of immune responses that may be generated within the CNS. First, as long as the blood–brain barrier remains intact, only *previously activated* T cells may penetrate into the brain. Secondly, there are (in all probability) no *professional* antigen-presenting cells in the brain. These cells, the classic example of which are the dendritic cells found in lymph nodes, constitutively express Class II *and* all the co-stimulatory molecules necessary to activate naïve lymphocytes. Microglia, even when activated and induced to express Class II, are sufficiently equipped only to present antigen to activated lymphocytes. Professional antigen presentation does take place in the cervical lymphatics; hence the importance of establishing whether CNS antigens and lymphocytes drain there in man as well as animals (Bradbury *et al.*, 1981). The implications of these two restrictions are that, whilst the blood–brain barrier remains intact and if lymphatic drainage is not significant in humans, immune responses in the brain can only be initiated in the periphery. This assertion is supported by the finding that the majority of cells in the inflammatory infiltrate of EAE proliferated *outside* the CNS (Ohmori *et al.*, 1992). This important point clearly has repercussions for the investigation and treatment of CNS autoimmune diseases. Of course, once the blood–brain barrier breaks down, as in multiple sclerosis, naïve lymphocytes may encounter CNS antigens and generate primary immune responses.

One of the persistent enigmas of immune responses in the brain has been how the inflammatory response is terminated. There is little evidence that lymphocytes leave the brain via the vascular, lymphatic or CSF compartments. One alternative possibility is that activated lymphocytes die *in situ* by *apoptosis* – a mechanism by which cells 'commit suicide' when appropriately triggered.

This has been demonstrated *ex vivo* for encephalitogenic rodent T cell lines. Microglia purified from rat brain are capable of antigen presentation to these T cell lines, as a result of which activation pro-inflammatory cytokines are (as expected) released. However, for unknown reasons, IL-2 is not secreted and so lymphocyte proliferation does not follow T cell activation. Rather, apoptosis of the T cell lines is induced (Ford *et al.*, 1996). Thus, microglia support an incomplete and ultimately self-destructive form of T cell activation, tending towards the curtailment of inflammation. Such a mechanism may also regulate autoimmune responses (Bauer *et al.*, 1995). This is suggested by the finding that mice lacking the gene for *Fas*, a cell surface trigger for apoptosis, develop lymphoproliferative disorders and autoimmune diseases.

Tolerance and autoimmunity in the nervous system

"For many years only foreign proteins were considered true antigens." So begins one of Rose and Witebsky's seminal papers on autoimmunity (Witebsky *et al.*, 1957). Although Ehrlich had introduced *horror autotoxicus*, the possibility that the body could generate antibodies against itself, autoimmunity was not demonstrated experimentally until 1956 in three landmark studies of the thyroid. It was shown that rabbits immunized with rabbit thyroid extract in complete Freund's adjuvant developed thyroid autoantibodies and chronic inflammatory destruction of the thyroid gland (Witebsky and Rose, 1956). Then the sera of patients with Hashimoto's thyroiditis were shown to contain precipitating autoantibodies directed against a constituent of normal thyroid extract, ultimately shown to be thyroglobulin (Roitt *et al.*, 1956). Finally, sera of patients with Graves' disease were found to contain a *long acting stimulator*, later identified as an IgG directed against the thyrotropin stimulating hormone receptor, that caused prolonged release of ^{131}I from guinea-pig thyroid (Adams and Purves, 1956).

The implication of the term autoimmunity is that an inappropriate immune response is directed against a normal tissue component and that this directly leads to disease *in the absence of persisting infection*. Microbes may initiate autoimmunity but if this persists during the disease it is inappropriate to term the disease autoimmune. For instance, the pathology of tuberculoid leprosy, which is a delayed-type hypersensitivity reaction, is not dissimilar to the inflammatory infiltrate of multiple sclerosis. Yet in one disease, a microbe can be demonstrated and hence is clearly 'infectious'. Hence the distinction between diseases that are commonly regarded as autoimmune or infectious may only lie in the ability to demonstrate persistent infection. As culture techniques are developed (or, in the case of *Helicobacter pylori*, the significance of previous observations recognized!), it is possible for disease to move from one category to another.

The distinction between autoimmune responses triggered by an infection and inflammation directed against a persistent microbe has been further blurred by a recent study on Theiler's virus-induced demyelination in the mouse (Miller *et al.*, 1997). T cell reactivity against the major encephalito-genic peptides of proteolipid protein and myelin basic protein (MBP) emerged some 40 days after the appearance of T cells against Theiler's virus and 20 days after the onset of clinical disease. There was no evidence for significant molecular mimicry between virus protein and the myelin proteins, suggesting that anti-myelin reactivity emerged through epitope spreading of the primary anti-viral response. Pathogenicity of the (secondary) anti-myelin responses was not demonstrated in this study, but it raises the possibility that a delayed-type hypersensitivity reaction against a persistent microbe may induce secondary true autoimmune disease.

It is illustrative to consider the evidence usually cited for multiple sclerosis as an autoimmune disease:

1. *Acute multiple sclerosis lesions are similar to those seen in EAE which is an autoimmune process.* However, no models of EAE accurately mimic the clinical course of multiple sclerosis and not all have demyelination. Furthermore, infection with Theiler's virus induces demyelinating plaques in the CNS.
2. *Multiple sclerosis is associated epidemiologically with specific HLA-DR Class II molecules.* The implication is that a particular self-antigen binds to this Class II molecule and activates an autoaggressive T cell clone. However, HLA associations are seen in some infections (Gaston, 1994).
3. *Immunosuppressants such as IFN-β have a therapeutic effect in multiple sclerosis.* However, IFN-α is efficacious in hepatitis C infection.

Hence these observations offer at best circumstantial evidence for an autoimmune process. More rigorous criteria for an autoimmune disease are

Witebsky's postulates which were modelled on Koch's postulates: (i) there must be an autoantibody or self-reactive T cell, which (ii) corresponds to a self-antigen; (iii) an analogous immune response must be induced in experimental animals which then (iv) develop a similar disease. None of these criteria are adequately fulfilled in multiple sclerosis. Anti-myelin responses exist in patients with multiple sclerosis but they are found in equal frequency amongst controls (Pette *et al.*, 1990; van Noort *et al.*, 1993) and no definite autoantigen has emerged. Although EAE is certainly an auto-immune disease, none of the various EAE models are sufficiently faithful models of multiple sclerosis to satisfy the final criterion. Thus multiple sclerosis does not fulfil strict criteria for an autoimmune disease. It is important not to overlook this point, despite the circumstantial evidence for an autoimmune cause, the lack of evidence for an infection and the therapeutic effect of immunosuppression.

Thymic tolerance and clonal deletion

Autoimmunity must involve the breakdown of the normal mechanisms of self-tolerance. The term 'tolerance' is used in different ways in the immunological literature. In this work, the word is defined to mean immunological unresponsiveness to an antigen.

The classic experiments of Peter Medawar and colleagues in the 1950s showed that the murine immune system did not respond to antigens encountered during neonatal life. If CBA mice were injected with cells from A mice *in utero*, then as adults they accepted skin grafts from the A strain but not from other strains (AU) (Billingham *et al.*, 1953). In other words, antigen-specific tolerance had been acquired. Miller subsequently demon-strated that neonatal thymectomy of mice led to prolonged lymphocyte depletion and acceptance of skin grafts of another strain, thus showing the importance of the thymus gland for neonatal tolerization (Miller, 1961).

Immature T cells, migrating from bone marrow to the thymus, lack rearranged TCRs and CD4 or CD8 receptors. The first step in their differentiation is the expression of both CD4 and CD8 on their surface. MHC is expressed on thymic epithelial cells and $CD4^+CD8^+$ thymocytes that bind with low affinity to self-MHC differentiate into $CD4^+CD8^-$ or $CD4^-CD8^+$ cells. By this *positive selection* MHC restriction is achieved. Following this there is *negative selection* of T cells that bind with high affinity to complexes of MHC and self-antigen that are expressed on thymic stromal cells. This eliminates autoreactive clones (termed *clonal deletion*) and is an important mechanism of self-tolerance.

However, clonal deletion is not completely efficient. For instance, some brain antigens that are expressed in the thymic medulla have corresponding autoreactive T cell clones capable of inducing CNS inflammation if activated (Wekerle *et al.*, 1996). Hence there are additional *peripheral* mechanisms of tolerance.

Mechanisms of peripheral (thymic independent) tolerance

Any disruption of the requirements for T cell activation may induce tolerance. This *clonal ignorance* usually arises in health because the antigen is at very low concentration or anatomically inaccessible. Nonetheless such clones represent a potential source of autoreactive cells. This was demonstrated by an elegant experiment in which double transgenic mice were generated that expressed (i) the lymphocytic choriomeningitis viral (LCMV) glycoprotein in the β islet cells of the pancreas, and (ii) a TCR specific for LCMV and H-2D^b (Ohashi et al., 1991). No response was mounted against the 'foreign pancreas', presumably because the glycoprotein had not been presented to the transgenic TCR in sufficient concentration. However, when the mice were infected with LCMV, in high concentration and correctly co-stimulated, naïve T cells were then stimulated and raised against the LCMV glycoprotein, resulting in inflammatory destruction of the pancreas.

Alternatively, antigens that are present in high concentration may induce a second form of non-deletional tolerance, *anergy*, if there is insufficient co-stimulation to the TCR-antigen-MHC binding (Harding et al., 1992).

A final mechanism of tolerance is active inhibition of an activated T cell clone by *suppressor T cells*. In a classic demonstration of suppression, spleen cells from an animal that had received a high dose of sheep red blood cells inhibited the antibody response of another animal against red blood cells. This effect was abolished by T cell depletion of the spleen cells (Gershon and Kondo, 1971). Rocken has described *immune deviation*, where the cytokine phenotype of an immune response is reversed, as another 'dimension of tolerance' (Rocken and Shevach, 1996). However, such $T_h1/2$ switching does not generate an *unresponsive* immune system, merely one that responds in a different way to an antigen and so does not fulfil the above definition of tolerance.

Potentially autoaggressive mechanisms in health

An important conceptual advance in autoimmunity since Witebsky's postulates has been the recognition that there exist in health several constitutive autoreactive processes. For instance 'natural antibodies', produced principally by CD5$^+$ B cells, react with low affinity to multiple specificities including many self and bacterial antigens (Wing, 1995). Their V genes are in germline configuration. Their biological function may be to act as a first defence against microbes or to clear tissue damage. In mice and perhaps humans, there is a parallel group of CD3$^+$ CD4$^-$CD8$^-$ T cells that carry the B cell surface antigen B220 and react strongly with self-T cells (Asano et al., 1988). The role of these cells in autoimmune disease is unknown.

There are T cells directed against normal tissue antigens which are presumably suppressed in health but which may become self-destructive in appropriate conditions. This was shown in the marmoset where siblings share a placenta allowing adoptive transfer of T cell populations without an alloresponse. Myelin basic protein-reactive T cells present in healthy marmosets were isolated by limiting dilution and then transferred to naïve animals, with adjuvant stimulation from *Bordetella pertussis* toxin. This produced EAE, demonstrating that autoreactive cells in healthy animals can mediate autoimmune disease (Genain et al., 1994).

One mechanism for suppression of such autoreactive T cell clones is the presence of T cells directed against self TCRs responsible for recognizing autoantigens. For example, a MBP-specific T cell clone was isolated from a healthy donor and its TCR genes sequenced. Two peptides generated from these sequences were recognized by four cytotoxic T cell clones from the same donor (Saruhan Direskeneli *et al.*, 1993). From observations such as these has grown the concept that there is an *anti-idiotypic network* that suppresses autoreactive T cells in health.

Mechanisms of autoimmunity

From the section above, it is clear that in health there is a balance between regulation and autoimmunity. This may be disrupted and autoimmunity *initiated*, following which regulatory mechanisms tend to restore self-tolerance unless autoimmunity is *maintained* by a secondary process.

Autoimmunity may be *initiated* in three ways. Firstly, a self-antigen may be modified and appear as foreign; in this way α-methyl dopa induces an autoimmune haemolytic anaemia. Secondly, ignorant clones may be 'educated'. Microbes may cross-react with self-antigens to which the immune system is ignorant, perhaps because the epitope is at low concentration. A cross-reacting microbe, present in greater numbers than the original antigen, is able to activate and prime T cells. Once so primed, the original antigen is sufficient to perpetuate the inflammation (hence the 'autoimmune diabetes' of Ohashi *et al.*'s viral transgene model mentioned above).

Another example, of relevance to multiple sclerosis, is the demonstration that a hepatitis virus polymerase peptide shares six consecutive amino acids with the encephalitogenic site of rabbit MBP. In rabbits immunized with this viral peptide *peripherally* there was a mononuclear cell infiltrate in the brain, resembling EAE (Fujinami and Oldstone, 1985). One hundred and twenty-nine *molecular mimics* of the immunodominant MBP peptide have been identified theoretically and then tested *in vitro* with seven MBP-reactive T cell clones: seven viral and one bacterial peptides activated three of these clones (Wucherpfennig and Strominger, 1995).

A third mechanism of autoimmunity is the removal of suppression of autoreactive processes. For instance, microbes might cross-react with idiotope and so disrupt the anti-idiotypic network in favour of immunity. *Superantigens* bind to parts of the Class II–TCR complex that are not antigen specific, and so may activate ignorant clones and induce autoimmunity. For instance, staphylococcal enterotoxin B activates cells carrying the $V_\beta 8$ TCR, which in certain mice strains is the TCR family that engages MBP to cause EAE. Thus, during clinical remission from this model of EAE, staphylococcal enterotoxin B induced relapses of disease (Brocke *et al.*, 1993). The interpretation was that autoaggressive T cell clones had been reactivated, which does not accord with the same group's demonstration that staphylococcal enterotoxin B induces anergy *in vitro* in T cells using $V_\beta 8$ TCR (Gaur *et al.*, 1993). Infection may break tolerance in other ways. For example, adult mice exposed to repeated injections of staphylococcus enterotoxin B become *anergic*; $CD4^+$ T cells from such mice failed to secrete any cytokines in response to staphylococcus enterotoxin B *in vitro*. But infection with the nematode *Nippostrogylus brasiliensis* broke this state of tolerance and staphylococcus enterotoxin B-reactive clones not only proliferated but also released substantial IL-2 and IL-4 (Rocken *et al.*, 1992).

The normal regulatory mechanisms of the immune response should restore self-tolerance after the initiation of autoimmunity. Thus, in many models of EAE, animals become resistant to induction of a second round of disease. Therefore the *maintenance* of autoimmune disease must require either multiple rounds of autoimmunity to different self-antigens, or a single autoimmune response that is perpetuated by defective regulation. For instance, removal of $CD8^+$ T cells from mice by monoclonal antibody depletion does not alter the recovery from the first round of MBP-induced EAE, but does abolish the normal resistance to subsequent disease induction (Jiang *et al.*, 1992). Another form of altered immune regulation is an abnormal cytokine response. For example, the lupus syndrome induced by mercuric chloride is driven by the secretion of excessive T_h2 cytokines (Ochel *et al.*, 1991).

It seems that the majority of autoimmune processes are driven by T cellular processes. Important exceptions are the anti-acetylcholine receptor antibody of myasthenia gravis and antibodies against epithelial adhesion molecules in the bullous skin diseases. In the CNS, the pathogenicity of autoantibodies, such as those associated with the paraneoplastic syndromes or stiff man syndrome (see Chapters 5 and 6) is not as clearly established.

Therapeutic strategies in autoimmune disease

Discussion of the mechanisms of autoimmunity leads naturally to consideration of rational approaches to disrupt autoimmunity, a theme that will be taken up in Chapter 4. Conventional immunosuppressant drugs, such as steroids, cyclophosphamide or azathioprine, incapacitate a broad range of immune components. Although the autoimmune process may thus be modulated, it is at the cost of widespread immune dysfunction. However, the ideal treatment of autoimmune disease is specifically to abrogate the abnormal immune response, leaving the immune system competent to deal with infections. In other words, the goal of therapy is to restore antigen-specific self-tolerance. The most appropriate strategy depends largely on whether the causative autoantigen is known. In the vast majority of human diseases, the driving autoantigen remains unknown, which hinders the goal of antigen-specific tolerance.

Tolerance regimes that identify an antigen

In experimental conditions, repeated exposure to an antigen induces tolerance. For example, in EAE in SJL/J mice, repeated doses of intravenous antigen induce anergy and so prevent the disease (Racke *et al.*, 1996). Feeding low doses of MBP to the Lewis rat protects against EAE, and is associated with increased numbers of MBP-reactive cells secreting T_h2 cytokines and TGF-β (Chen *et al.*, 1995). Such experiments lead to therapeutic studies in patients with multiple sclerosis using oral myelin, which have been largely disappointing (see Chapter 4). Another strategy to induce tolerance is to eliminate the effectors required to mediate autoreactivity. This is the logic behind vaccinating animals with TCR components believed to be involved in autoantigen processing. In EAE, pathogenic T cells have restricted use of the TCR. For instance, in rat MBP-induced EAE in the PL/J mouse, the $V_\beta 8.2$ variable region is most commonly used by encephalitogenic T cells and 'vaccination' with DNA encoding this region ameliorates disease and shifts the cytokine profile of responding cells to a $T_h 2$ pattern (Waisman et al., 1996). This strategy has been translated to humans by vaccinating patients against their own irradiated MBP-specific T cells (see Chapter 4 for further details).

An elegant series of experiments demonstrates the requirements for tolerance induction where the antigen is known (Lanoue et al., 1997). This group initially used mice that were double transgenics for (i) the TCR that recognizes influenza haemagglutinin presented by $I\text{-}E^d$ and (ii) haemagglutinin expressed under the $Ig\kappa$ promoter. Under these conditions most cells carrying the transgenic TCR were deleted, but a few remained in the periphery in a state of anergy. Mature $CD4^+$ cells from mice transgenic only for the TCR were transferred into the double transgenic and thus exposed to high concentration of antigen; most were deleted and the remainder became anergic. In contrast, single doses of antigen given orally, intraperitoneally or intravenously failed to induce tolerance. However, when $CD4^+$ cells were first depleted by 60–70% using a monoclonal antibody, and then mice were injected intravenously with the antigen, responding cell numbers were reduced and they secreted less IFN-γ; 14 days later they recovered responsiveness. However, prolonged unresponsiveness could be achieved by repeated antigen administration after $CD4^+$ depletion. A $T_h 2$ pattern of cytokine secretion was not seen. The implication from this study is that exogenous antigen may induce tolerance by deletion and anergy, provided co-stimulation through CD4 is withdrawn.

An important limitation of all these approaches is that they require knowledge of the driving autoantigen which, as mentioned above, is far from the case in most autoimmune diseases of the nervous system. One attractive solution to this problem is 'bystander suppression' of pathogenic immune response by generating a $T_h 2$- or TGF-β-secreting cell towards an antigen that is physically close to the real autoantigen. In multiple sclerosis, for instance, this might mean generating an immunosuppressive response against one or more components of myelin and oligodendrocytes.

Suppression of pro-inflammatory cytokines

A direct approach to the treatment of diseases driven by $T_h 1$ cytokines is to suppress pro-inflammatory cytokines. For instance, rheumatoid arthritis has been treated with a monoclonal anti-TNF-α. While TNF-α is suppressed, so too are serum levels of IL-6 and the adhesion molecules, E-selectin and ICAM-1, and there is an associated clinical improvement (Paleolog et al., 1996). However, once the antibody treatment is stopped, both inflammatory markers and disease activity return to pre-treatment levels. Similarly, EAE can be temporarily suppressed by TGF-β (Racke et al., 1991).

There are three problems with such approaches. First, cytokines have a plethora of actions, many beneficial, which are all non-specifically suppressed, to potential disadvantage. For instance, there is a raised incidence of anti-nuclear antibodies after anti-TNF-α treatment in rheumatoid arthritis (M. Feldmann, personal communication). Secondly, when treatment is withdrawn, the inflammatory activity returns. Thirdly, post-translational control of cytokines, which normally act in low concentrations and as paracrine messengers, requires high antibody levels to neutralize biological activity. Preferably, a permanent change should be induced in immune reactivity to the autoantigen, either by restoring tolerance or switching the cytokine response. The advantage of this approach is that, once the immune system is 're-educated', disease suppression should be maintained indefinitely.

T_h1 to T_h2 phenotype switching

A prediction of the $T_h1/2$ paradigm is that a disease driven by T_h1 cytokines would be ameliorated by deviation of immune responses towards the T_h2 phenotype. A potential mechanism to achieve this switch is for autoantigen presentation to occur in a microenvironment enriched for IL-4, which favours differentiation towards a T_h2 phenotype. This source of the IL-4 need not be antigen specific, e.g. SJL mice that have been preimmunized to produce IL-4 in response to keyhole limpet haemocyanin do not get EAE when challenged with guinea-pig myelin and keyhole limpet haemocyanin in Freund's adjuvant, because the encephalitogenic T cells are deviated towards a T_h2 response (Falcone and Bloom, 1997). Similarly, if exogenous IL-4 is given during the adoptive transfer of T_h1 MBP-reactive T cells, a stable population of T_h2 MBP-reactive T cells is generated, and, although the extent of the cellular infiltrate is unchanged, there is dramatically less TNF-α production and no CNS tissue damage (Racke et al., 1994).

Alternatively, if the autoantigen were presented by B cells, a T_h2-dominated response also follows. If animals are pre-treated with an encephalitogenic MBP peptide covalently linked to mouse anti-rat immunoglobulin, MBP induced EAE is suppressed. The expression of IFN-γ in lymph node cells is reduced and IL-4 increased (Saoudi et al., 1995).

It is naïve to assume, however, that an up-regulation of T_h2 cytokines would be without problems, as Hauser's group has demonstrated in a primate EAE model induced by myelin oligodendrocyte glycoprotein (MOG). Here, the normal T_h1 response against MOG was successfully deviated towards a T_h2 response. This abolished the acute phase of the disease, as predicted. Unexpectedly, however, a pronounced antibody-mediated anti-MOG response was made some time later and severe demyelination resulted (Genain et al., 1996). Similarly worrying was the result of oral administration of ovalbumin in a murine model of insulin-dependent diabetes mellitus, where transgenic mice express ovalbumin under the insulin promoter. $CD4^+$-mediated autoimmunity was suppressed by 'oral tolerance', but cytotoxic $CD8^+$ cells were generated which exacerbated the disease (Blanas et al., 1996).

In conclusion, switching antigen-specific responses from T_h1 to T_h2 is superficially attractive, but may be hazardous because one form of autoimmunity is potentially being traded for another, as Hauser's group has demonstrated. Ideally, the autoreactive responses should be rendered unresponsive, i.e. tolerant.

Antigen-specific tolerance to unknown autoantigens

In most autoimmune disease of the nervous system, the driving autoantigen is unknown. So ideally a treatment is required that makes no assumptions about the provoking antigen and yet induces antigen-specific tolerance. Such a strategy seems paradoxical at first, but has support from a series of animal experiments where tolerance to allografts is induced by monoclonal antibodies directed against T cells.

In the 1980s it was shown that prolonged antigen-specific tolerance was induced in mice if foreign antigen was presented at the same time as a depleting or even non-depleting anti-CD4 monoclonal antibody (Benjamin and Waldmann, 1986; Benjamin et al., 1988). Transplantation tolerance to minor MHC mismatched skin grafts in athymic mice was achieved with non-depleting anti-CD4 and -CD8 monoclonal antibodies (Qin et al., 1990). However, tolerance to major MHC mismatched skin grafts was only achieved by depleting $CD4^+$ and $CD8^+$ cells followed by antibodies that block these receptors (Cobbold et al., 1990). Once such tolerance was induced, it was unaffected by the transfusion of normal lymphocytes (Qin et al., 1993). Indeed the naïve cells then acquired tolerance themselves with retained antigen specificity.

These experiments were repeated in mice transgenic for human $CD2^+$. Tolerance to skin grafts was generated and naïve T cells (non-transgenic) were then transferred. If host T cells were depleted immediately, by anti-CD2 antibody, a skin graft was rejected. If, however, tolerant and naïve cells were allowed to co-exist for 2 weeks before host cell depletion, tolerance persisted. In such mice, with only 'second-generation' tolerant cells present, tolerance was still maintained despite a further infusion of naïve lymphocytes. These observations implied that tolerance was actively transferred from tolerant to naïve cells in an 'infectious' way. This transfer of tolerance was uninfluenced by anti-IL-4 antibody (Chen et al., 1996), but was dependent on the continued presence of the driving antigen; if tolerant cells were 'parked' in T cell-depleted mice without a graft, they lost tolerance after about 6 months (Scully et al., 1994).

In this way, therefore, a short pulse of antigen non-specific therapy sets up a sequence of events leading to the perpetuation of antigen-specific tolerance. This strategy has been used to justify the use of the humanized monoclonal antibody, Campath-1H, in the treatment of multiple sclerosis (Moreau et al., 1994). *Antigen-specific* tolerance is achieved by timing treatment to coincide with active disease, when the autoantigen is presumably being presented to the autoaggressive lymphocytes.

References

Adams, D. D. and Purves, H. D. (1956) Abnormal responses in the assay of thyrotropin. *Proc. Univ. Otago. Med. School*, **34**, 11.

Annunziato, F., Manetti, R., Tomasevic, I., Guidizi, M. G., Biagiotti, R., Gianno, V., et al. (1996) Expression and release of LAG-3-encoded protein by human $CD4^+$ T cells are associated with IFN-gamma production. *FASEB J.*, **10**, 769–776.

Asano, T., Tomooka, S., Serushago, B. A., Himeno, K. and Nomoto, K. (1988) A new T cell subset expressing B220 and CD4 in *lpr* mice: defects in the response to mitogens and in the production of IL-2. *Clin. Exp. Immunol.*, **74**, 36–40.

Bauer, J., Wekerle, H. and Lassmann, H. (1995) Apoptosis in brain-specific autoimmune disease. *Curr. Opin. Immunol.*, **7**, 839–843.

Benjamin, R. J. and Waldmann, H. (1986) Induction of tolerance by monoclonal antibody therapy. *Nature*, **320**, 449–451.

Benjamin, R. J., Qin, S. X., Wise, M. P., Cobbold, S. P. and Waldmann, H. (1988) Mechanisms of monoclonal antibody-facilitated tolerance induction: a possible role for the CD4 (L3T4) and CD11a (LFA-1) molecules in self–non-self discrimination. *Eur. J. Immunol.*, **18**, 1079–1088.

Billingham, R. E., Brent, L. and Medawar, P. B. (1953) 'Actively acquired tolerance' of foreign cells. *Nature*, **172**, 603–606.

Blanas, E., Carbone, F. R., Allison, J., Miller, J. F. and Heath, W. R. (1996) Induction of autoimmune diabetes by oral administration of autoantigen. *Science*, **274**, 1707–1709.

Bradbury, M. (1979) *The Concept of the Blood–Brain Barrier.* New York: John Wiley.

Bradbury, M. W., Cserr, H. F. and Westrop, R. J. (1981) Drainage of cerebral interstitial fluid into deep cervical lymph of the rabbit. *Am. J. Physiol.*, **240**, F329–F336.

Brocke, S., Gaur, A., Piercy, C., Gautam, A., Gijbels, K., Fathman, C. G., *et al.* (1993) Induction of relapsing paralysis in experimental autoimmune encephalomyelitis by bacterial superantigen. *Nature*, **365**, 642–644.

Chen, F. Q., Okamura, K., Sato, K., Kuroda, T., Mizokami, T., Fujikawa, M., *et al.* (1996) Reversible primary hypothyroidism with blocking or stimulating type TSH binding inhibitor immunoglobulin following recombinant interferon-alpha therapy in patients with pre-existing thyroid disorders. *Clin. Endocrinol. Oxf.*, **45**, 207–214.

Chen, Y., Inobe, J. I. and Weiner, H. L. (1995) Induction of oral tolerance to myelin basic protein in CD8-depleted mice: both CD4[+] and CD8[+] cells mediate active suppression. *J. Immunol.*, **155**, 910–916.

Cobbold, S. P., Martin, G. and Waldmann, H. (1990) The induction of skin graft tolerance in major histocompatibility complex-mismatched or primed recipients: primed T cells can be tolerized in the periphery with anti-CD4 and anti-CD8 antibodies. *Eur. J. Immunol.*, **20**, 2747–2755.

Del Prete, G., De Carli, M., Almerigogna, F., Daniel, C. K., D'Elios, M. M., Zancuoghi, G., *et al.* (1995) Preferential expression of CD30 by human CD4[+] T cells producing T_h2-type cytokines. *FASEB J.*, **9**, 81–86.

Ediden, M. (1972) *Transplantation Antigens*, pp. 125–140. New York: Academic Press.

Ehrlich, P. (1885) *Das Sauerstaff-Bedurfniss des Organesmus.* Berlin: Hiorschwald.

Falcone, M. and Bloom, B. R. (1997) A T helper cell 2 (T_h2) immune response against non-self antigens modifies the cytokine profile of autoimmune T cells and protects against experimental allergic encephalomyelitis. *J. Exp. Med.*, **185**, 901–907.

Ford, A. L., Foulcher, E., Lemckert, F. A. and Sedgwick, J. D. (1996) Microglia induce CD4 T lymphocyte final effector function and death. *J. Exp. Med.*, **184**, 1737–1745.

Fujinami, R. S. and Oldstone, M. B. (1985) Amino acid homology between the encephalitogenic site of myelin basic protein and virus: mechanism for autoimmunity. *Science*, **230**, 1043–1045.

Gajewski, T. F., Pinnas, M., Wong, T. and Fitch, F. W. (1991) Murine T_h1 and T_h2 clones proliferate optimally in response to distinct antigen-presenting cell populations. *J. Immunol.*, **146**, 1750–1758.

Gaston, J. S. (1994) The role of infection in inflammatory arthritis. *Quart. J. Med.*, **87**, 647–651.

Gaur, A., Fathman, C. G., Steinman, L. and Brocke, S. (1993) SEB induced anergy: modulation of immune response to T cell determinants of myoglobin and myelin basic protein. *J. Immunol.*, **150**, 3062–3069.

Genain, C. P., Lee Parritz, D., Nguyen, M. H., Massacesi, L., Joshi, N., Ferrante, R., *et al.* (1994) In healthy primates, circulating autoreactive T cells mediate autoimmune disease {see comments}. *J. Clin. Invest.*, **94**, 1339–1345.

Genain, C. P., Abel, K., Belmar, N., Villinger, F., Rosenberg, D. P., Linington, C., *et al.* (1996) Late complications of immune deviation therapy in a nonhuman primate. *Science*, **274**, 2054–2057.

Gershon, R. K. and Kondo, K. (1971) Infectious immunological tolerance. *Immunology*, **21**, 903–914.

Graeber, M. B., Streit, W. J., Buringer, D., Sparks, D. L. and Kreutzberg, G. W. (1992) Ultrastructural location of major histocompatibility complex (MHC) class II positive perivascular cells in histologically normal human brain. *J. Neuropathol. Exp. Neurol.*, **51**, 303–311.

Harding, F. A., McArthur, J. G., Gross, J. A., Raulet, D. H. and Allison, J. P. (1992) CD28-mediated signalling co-stimulates murine T cells and prevents induction of anergy in T-cell clones. *Nature*, **356**, 607–609.

Hayes, G. M., Woodroofe, M. N. and Cuzner, M. L. (1987) Microglia are the major cell type expressing MHC class II in human white matter. *J. Neurol. Sci.*, **80**, 25–37.

Heinzel, F. P., Sadick, M. D., Holaday, B. J., Coffman, R. L. and Locksley, R. M. (1989) Reciprocal expression of interferon gamma or interleukin 4 during the resolution or progression of murine leishmaniasis. Evidence for expansion of distinct helper T cell subsets. *J. Exp. Med.*, **169**, 59–72.

Hickey, W. F., Hsu, B. L. and Kimura, H. (1991) T-lymphocyte entry into the central nervous system. *J. Neurosci. Res.*, **28**, 254–260.

Janzer, R. C. and Raff, M. C. (1987) Astrocytes induce blood–brain barrier properties in endothelial cells. *Nature*, **325**, 253–257.

Jiang, H., Zhang, S. I. and Pernis, B. (1992) Role of CD8$^+$ T cells in murine experimental allergic encephalomyelitis. *Science*, **256**, 1213–1215.

Juhler, M. and Neuwelt, E. A. (1989) The blood–brain barrier and the immune system. In *Implications of the Blood–Brain Barrier and its Manipulation* (Neuwelt, E. A., ed.). New York: Plenum Press.

Kennedy, M. K., Torrance, D. S., Picha, K. S. and Mohler, K. M. (1992) Analysis of cytokine mRNA expression in the central nervous system of mice with experimental autoimmune encephalomyelitis reveals that IL-10 mRNA expression correlates with recovery. *J. Immunol.*, **149**, 2496–2505.

Khoury, S. J., Akalin, E., Chandraker, A., Turka, L. A., Linsley, P. S., Sayegh, M. H., *et al.* (1995) CD28-B7 costimulatory blockade by CTLA4Ig prevents actively induced experimental autoimmune encephalomyelitis and inhibits T_h1 but spares T_h2 cytokines in the central nervous system. *J. Immunol.*, **155**, 4521–4524.

Krakowski, M. and Owens, T. (1996) Interferon-gamma confers resistance to experimental allergic encephalomyelitis. *Eur. J. Immunol.*, **26**, 1641–1646.

Kuchroo, V. K., Das, M. P., Brown, J. A., Ranger, A. M., Zamvil, S. S., Sobel, R. A., *et al.* (1995) B7-1 and B7-2 costimulatory molecules activate differentially the T_h1/T_h2 developmental pathways: application to autoimmune disease therapy. *Cell*, **80**, 707–718.

Lanoue, A., Bona, C., von Boehmer, H. and Sarukhan, A. (1997) Conditions that induce tolerance in mature CD4$^+$ T cells. *J. Exp. Med.*, **185**, 405–414.

Li, H., Newcombe, J., Groome, N. P. and Cuzner, M. L. (1993) Characterization and distribution of phagocytic macrophages in multiple sclerosis plaques. *Neuropathol. Appl. Neurobiol.*, **19**, 214–223.

Lublin, F. D., Knobler, R. L., Kalman, B., Goldhaber, M., Marini, J., Perrault, M., *et al.* (1993) Monoclonal anti-gamma interferon antibodies enhance experimental allergic encephalomyelitis. *Autoimmunity*, **16**, 267–274.

Manetti, R., Parronchi, P., Giudizi, M. G., Piccinni, M. P., Maggi, E., Trinchieri, G., *et al.* (1993) Natural killer cell stimulatory factor (interleukin 12 {IL-12}) induces T helper type 1 (T_h1)-specific immune responses and inhibits the development of IL-4-producing T_h cells. *J. Exp. Med.*, **177**, 1199–1204.

Manetti, R., Gerosa, F., Giudizi, M. G., Biagiotti, R., Parronchi, P., Piccinni, M. P., *et al.* (1994) Interleukin 12 induces stable priming for interferon gamma (IFN-gamma) production during differentiation of human T helper (T_h) cells and transient IFN-gamma production in established T_h2 cell clones. *J. Exp. Med.*, **179**, 1273–1283.

Matsui, M., Mori, K. J. and Saida, T. (1990) Cellular immunoregulatory mechanisms in the central nervous system: characterization of noninflammatory and inflammatory cerebrospinal fluid lymphocytes. *Ann. Neurol.*, **27**, 647–651.

Miller, J. F. (1961) Immunological function of the thymus. *Lancet*, **ii**, 748–749.

Miller, S. D., Vanderglut, C. L., Begolka, W. S., Pao, W., Yauch, R. L., Neville, K., *et al.* (1997) Persistent infection with Theiler's virus leads to CNS autoimmunity via epitope spreading. *Nat. Med.*, **3**, 1133–1136.

Moreau, T., Thorpe, J., Miller, D., Moseley, I., Hale, G., Waldmann, H., *et al.* (1994) Preliminary evidence from magnetic resonance imaging for reduction in disease activity after lymphocyte depletion in multiple sclerosis {published erratum appears in *Lancet* **344**(8920), 486}. *Lancet*, **344**, 298–301.

Mosmann, T. R., Cherwinski, H., Bond, M. W., Giedlin, M. A. and Coffman, R. L. (1986) Two types of murine helper T cell clone. I. Definition according to profiles of lymphokine activities and secreted proteins. *J. Immunol.*, **136**, 2348–2357.

Murphy, J. B. and Sturm, E. (1923) Conditions determining the transplantation of tissues in the brain. *J. Exp. Med.*, **39**, 183–197.

Naparstek, Y., Cohen, I. R., Fuks, Z. and Vlodavsky, I. (1984) Activated T lymphocytes produce a matrix-degrading heparin sulphate endoglycosidase. *Nature*, **310**, 241–244.

Ochel, M., Vohr, H. W., Pfeiffer, C. and Gleichmann, E. (1991) IL-4 is required for the IgE and IgG1 increase and IgG1 autoantibody formation in mice treated with mercuric chloride. *J. Immunol.*, **146**, 3006–3011.

Ohashi, P. S., Oehen, S., Buerki, K., Pircher, H., Ohashi, C. T., Odermatt, B., *et al.* (1991) Ablation of 'tolerance' and induction of diabetes by virus infection in viral antigen transgenic mice. *Cell*, **65**, 305–317.

Ohmori, K., Hong, Y., Fujiwara, M. and Matsumoto, Y. (1992) *In situ* demonstration of proliferating cells in the rat central nervous system during experimental autoimmune encephalomyelitis. *Lab. Invest.*, **66**, 54–62.

Paleolog, E. M., Hunt, M., Elliott, M. J., Feldmann, M., Maini, R. N. and Woody, J. N. (1996) Deactivation of vascular endothelium by monoclonal anti-tumor necrosis factor alpha antibody in rheumatoid arthritis. *Arthritis Rheum.*, **39**, 1082–1091.

Pette, M., Fujita, K., Kitze, B., Whitaker, J. N., Albert, E., Kappos, L., *et al.* (1990) Myelin basic protein-specific T lymphocyte lines from MS patients and healthy individuals. *Neurology*, **40**, 1770–1776.

Qin, S., Cobbold, S. P., Pope, H., Elliott, J., Kioussis, D., Davies, J. and Waldmann, H. (1993) 'Infectious' transplantation tolerance. *Science*, **259**, 974–977.

Qin, S. X., Wise, M., Cobbold, S. P., Leong, L., Kong, Y. C., Parnes, J. R., *et al.* (1990) Induction of tolerance in peripheral T cells with monoclonal antibodies. *Eur. J. Immunol.*, **20**, 2737–2745.

Racke, M. K., Dhib Jalbut, S., Cannella, B., Albert, P. S., Raine, C. S. and McFarlin, D. E. (1991) Prevention and treatment of chronic relapsing experimental allergic encephalomyelitis by transforming growth factor-beta 1. *J. Immunol.*, **146**, 3012–3017.

Racke, M. K., Bonomo, A., Scott, D. E., Cannella, B., Levine, A., Raine, C. S., *et al.* (1994) Cytokine-induced immune deviation as a therapy for inflammatory autoimmune disease. *J. Exp. Med.*, **180**, 1961–1966.

Racke, M. K., Critchfield, J. M., Quigley, L., Cannella, B., Raine, C. S., McFarland, H., *et al.* (1996) Intravenous antigen administration as a therapy for autoimmune demyelinating disease. *Ann. Neurol.*, **39**, 46–56.

Rocken, M. and Shevach, E. M. (1996) Immune deviation the third dimension of nondeletional T cell tolerance. *Immunol. Rev.*, **149**, 175–194.

Rocken, M., Urban, J. F. and Shevach, E. M. (1992) Infection breaks T-cell tolerance. *Nature*, **359**, 79–82.

Roitt, I., Doniach, D., Campbell, P. N. and Hudson, R. V. (1956) Autoantibodies in Hashimoto's Disease (lymphadenoid goitre). *Lancet*, **ii**, 820–821.

Sabin, F. R. (1916) The origin and development of the lymphatic system. *Johns Hopkins Hosp. Rep.*, **17**, 347–440.

Saoudi, A., Simmonds, S., Huitinga, I. and Mason, D. (1995) Prevention of experimental allergic encephalomyelitis in rats by targeting autoantigen to B cells: evidence that the protective mechanism depends on changes in the cytokine response and migratory properties of the autoantigen-specific T cells. *J. Exp. Med.*, **182**, 335–344.

Saruhan Direskeneli, G., Weber, F., Meinl, E., Pette, M., Giegerich, G., Hinkkanen, A., *et al.* (1993) Human T cell autoimmunity against myelin basic protein: CD4$^+$ cells recognizing epitopes of the T cell receptor beta chain from a myelin basic protein-specific T cell clone. *Eur. J. Immunol.*, **23**, 530–536.

Scully, R., Qin, S., Cobbold, S. and Waldmann, H. (1994) Mechanisms in CD4 antibody-mediated transplantation tolerance: kinetics of induction, antigen dependency and role of regulatory T cells. *Eur. J. Immunol.*, **24**, 2383–2392.

Simmons, R. D., Buzbee, T. M., Linthicum, D. S., Mandy, W. J., Chen, G. and Wang, C. (1987) Simultaneous visualization of vascular permeability change and leukocyte egress in the central nervous system during autoimmune encephalomyelitis. *Acta Neuropathol. Berl.*, **74**, 191–193.

van Noort, J. M., van Sechel, A., Boon, J., Boersma, W. J., Polman, C. H. and Lucas, C. J. (1993) Minor myelin proteins can be major targets for peripheral blood T cells from both multiple sclerosis patients and healthy subjects. *J. Neuroimmunol.*, **46**, 67–72.

Waisman, A., Ruiz, P. J., Hirschberg, D. L., Gelman, A., Oksenberg, J. R., Brocke, S., *et al.* (1996) Suppressive vaccination with DNA encoding a variable region gene of the T-cell receptor prevents autoimmune encephalomyelitis and activates T_h2 immunity {see comments}. *Nat. Med.*, **2**, 899–905.

Wekerle, H., Bradl, M., Linington, C., Kaab, G. and Kojima, K. (1996) The shaping of the brain-specific T lymphocyte repertoire in the thymus. *Immunol. Rev.*, 231–243.

Wilson, S. B., Kent, S. C., Patton, K. T., Orban, T., Jackson, R. A., Exley, M. A., *et al.* (1998) Extreme T_h1 bias of invariant Va24JaQ T cells in type 1 diabetes. *Nature*, **391**, 177–181.

Wing, M. G. (1995) The molecular basis for a polyspecific antibody {editorial}. *Clin. Exp. Immunol.*, **99**, 313–315.

Witebsky, E., Rose, N. R., Terplan, K., Paine, J. R. and Egan, R. W. (1957) Chronic thyroiditis and autoimmunization. *J. Am. Med. Ass.*, **164**, 1439–1447.

Witebsky, E. and Rose, N. R. (1956) Studies on organ specificity: IV. Production of rabbit thyroid antibodies in rabbit. *J. Immunol.*, **76**, 408–416.

Wucherpfennig, K. W. and Strominger, J. L. (1995) Molecular mimicry in T cell-mediated autoimmunity: viral peptides activate human T cell clones specific for myelin basic protein. *Cell*, **80**, 695–705.

Chapter 2

Multiple sclerosis

Neil Scolding

Introduction: the nature of the problem	21
The clinical features of multiple sclerosis	22
Pathophysiology	24
Diagnosis	28
Symptomatic treatment of multiple sclerosis	29
The cause of multiple sclerosis	32
The process of inflammatory demyelination	35
A summary: the pathogenesis of multiple sclerosis	53
Future approaches to treating multiple sclerosis:	
immunomodulation and repair	54
The repair of demyelinated lesions	55
References	58

Introduction: the nature of the problem

Multiple sclerosis, with a prevalence of 50–150 per 100 000, affects approximately 80 000 people in the UK; 300 000 in the USA (Compston, 1997). It is characterized clinically by the classical relapsing–remitting course, each relapse representing an acute or subacute self-limiting episode of focal neurological disturbance. The pathological substrate for each episode is the inflammatory demyelinating lesion, wherein circumscribed perivascular oedema and inflammation disrupts conduction in myelinated axons in the central nervous system (CNS). Imaging studies show, and histopathological studies have confirmed, that any part of the brain can be affected, but certain white matter tracts are particularly (and thus far inexplicably) susceptible, resulting in characteristic and recognizable clinical patterns – these, together with the relapsing course, result in a unique neurological picture. By no means all patients conform to this classical pattern, however, and a substantial variability in the impact and severity of disease expression is found. Contrary to the prevalent perception of multiple sclerosis as a universally devastating disease, a substantial proportion of patients – 30% or more – do not develop severe disability even after 15 years of disease (Confavreux *et al.*, 1980; Weinshenker and Ebers, 1987). Nevertheless, in many patients, the initially sporadic and often rather benign phase of the disease gives way to a steady and relentless accumulation of increasing disability and handicap – secondary progressive multiple sclerosis. Until very recently, no therapeutic agents were available which could usefully influence the course of the disease, but a number of approaches to treatment currently under assessment are generating increasing optimism.

The clinical features of multiple sclerosis

Multiple sclerosis affects women more commonly than men, with a ratio of approximately 2:1. It presents in 80–90% of cases (Poser, 1978) with an acute or subacute episode of focal neurological disturbance, progressing to a peak over a period of hours to a few days, then spontaneously remitting (after perhaps a week or so) over the next few weeks. Recovery is typically near-complete, regardless of the exhibition of any treatment.

A variety of presentations may be seen. Sub-acute sensory loss in the limbs – an arm, one or both legs – is one of the commoner, accounting for approximately 20% of cases (Matthews, 1991a). Whilst often mild and occasionally ignored (only emerging as an historical feature during a later, presenting episode), the more completely deafferented upper limb, resulting from an inflammatory lesion in the region of the cervical dorsal root entry zone, is profoundly disabling – the so-called useless limb of Oppenheim. Acute optic neuritis is the presenting feature in 18–20% of cases (Matthews, 1991a); monocular visual impairment is accompanied by pain on eye movement. Impaired colour perception, either as a symptom or a sign disclosed by Isihara Plate testing, may be an early clue. A brainstem or cerebellar disturbance is the first feature in 10% of cases, causing complex eye movement disorders (classically the internuclear ophthalmoplegia – with impaired adduction of the lateral-gazing eye and horizontal nystagmus in the opposite abducting eye, from a lesion sited in the peculiarly vulnerable medial longitudinal fasciculus), and ataxia of speech, limb movement and/or gait. That proportion of cases presenting with isolated weakness of one or more limbs (whether of spinal, brainstem or hemispheric origin) varies significantly between different surveys, from 12 to 40% (McAlpine *et al.*, 1955; Matthews, 1991a). Rarer but well-recognized presentations include a hemiparesis, isolated incontinence, bulbar disturbances and even movement disorders (see Figure 2.1). Neuropsychological or neuropsychiatric abnormalities are increasingly recognized (Kujala *et al.*, 1997), though rarely in early disease. To complete the picture, paroxysmal symptoms may herald disease in perhaps 2% of patients, occurring at some point during the course of disease in around 5% (Matthews, 1991b). Sensory phenomena (principally trigeminal neuralgia), dysarthria and ataxia, and tonic spasms (abrupt involuntary posturing of one (usually upper) limb) all may occur. (Neither Lhermitte's sign, nor Uthoff's phenomenon (see below) are conventionally considered as part of the spectrum of paroxysmal disorders of multiple sclerosis.)

Often there are no subsequent episodes, so that the crucial diagnostic criteria of clinical dissemination of lesions in both time and space are not met, and a diagnosis of multiple sclerosis cannot be made – although the same pathological process is probably responsible (for obvious reasons rather difficult to prove). 'An episode of inflammation' may be offered by way of explanation to the patient. More commonly, further relapses do occur and a relapsing–remitting pattern becomes established. Overall, 25–40% of patients suffer their first relapse within 12 months of the first episode. The proportion varies with the nature of the initial site: over the 5 year period following the first symptom, approximately 40% of patients with optic neuritis, 50% of those with an initial brainstem disturbance and 35%

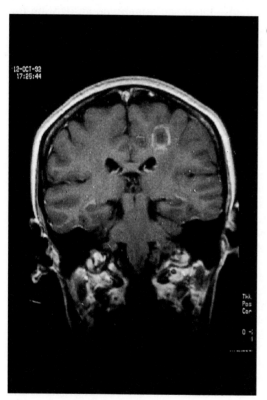

A happy man or woman is a better thing to find than a five-pound note. He or she is a radiating focus of goodwill.

(a)

(b)

Figure 2.1 Micrographia in multiple sclerosis. In addition to the conventional and common clinical features, almost any neurological symptom or sign may more rarely be seen in multiple sclerosis. This female patient developed micrographia as the principal manifestation of an acute relapse (a). Magnetic resonance imaging scanning showed the (enhancing) responsible lesion to be situated in the left parietal cortex (b). After intravenous methylprednisolone, the patient's handwriting returned to normal (c).

(c)

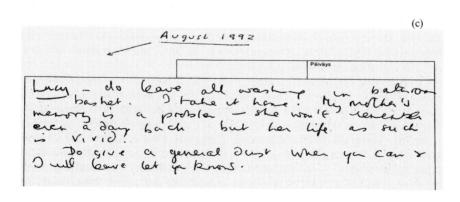

of those with a spinal cord presentation will relapse and acquire a clinical diagnosis of multiple sclerosis (Morrissey *et al.*, 1993). Not surprisingly, increasing rates of conversion to multiple sclerosis are found with increasing duration of follow up, e.g. in the case of optic neuritis, the figure by 12 years is 55% (Francis *et al.*, 1987).

In 10–20% of cases, no relapsing–remitting phase is ever apparent, and the onset and subsequent course is one of steadily accumulating neurological disability is witnessed from the onset – primary progressive multiple sclerosis. This proportion significantly increases with age – 40–60% of patients presenting over the age of 40 exhibiting a primary progressive course (Weinshenker *et al.*, 1989). There is a significant body of evidence indicating that this may represent a rather different disease process and should be considered separately, not only in prognostication, but in underlying disease mechanisms and immune therapy (Thompson *et al.*, 1997). Most patients with more conventional episodic disease eventually also develop a non-remitting progressive course (25% by 2 years; 50% by 10 years; 60% by 12 years) – secondary progressive multiple sclerosis.

Pathophysiology

At the heart of this complex disease lies a single cell type, the oligodendrocyte and its extension, the myelin sheath. First described only 80 years ago by the Spanish neurobiologist del Rio Hortega (Rio Hortega, 1921), a student of Cajal, the oligodendrocyte is the glial cell responsible for both the initial synthesis and (importantly) the subsequent life-long maintenance of myelin in the CNS (Figure 2.2). Compact myelin consists of a dynamic, metabolically active membrane wrapped spirally many times around axons to form a segmented sheath. This is interrupted periodically along the course of the axon at the (unmyelinated) nodes of Ranvier, areas where electrical resistance is low and depolarization is facilitated.

In myelinated axons, the action potential induced by depolarization at one node of Ranvier generates electrical currents which in turn trigger depolarization not along the immediately contiguous myelinated (and insulated) internode, but preferentially at the next node of Ranvier; saltatory conduction is considerably more rapid than continuous propagation of the nerve impulse. In demyelinating diseases, saltatory conduction is disrupted: conduction block in some fibres results in a reduced (overall) amplitude of an impulse, while slowed conduction in partially demyelinated fibres contributes towards the diminished velocity of impulse transmission (McDonald and Sears, 1970; Smith, 1996). Depending on the anatomical site and severity, this may precipitate neurological disturbance.

Considerable progress in dissecting the precise pathophysiological changes responsible for these conduction abnormalities has been made in studies of optic neuritis, exploiting the unique opportunities offered by inflammatory demyelination at this site to correlate gadolinium-enhanced magnetic resonance imaging (MRI), electrophysiological abnormalities and clinical symptoms and signs (Youl *et al.*, 1991). Here, and it is assumed similarly in other acute lesions, both inflammation (with oedema) and demyelination produce conduction block, which is responsible for acute impairment of

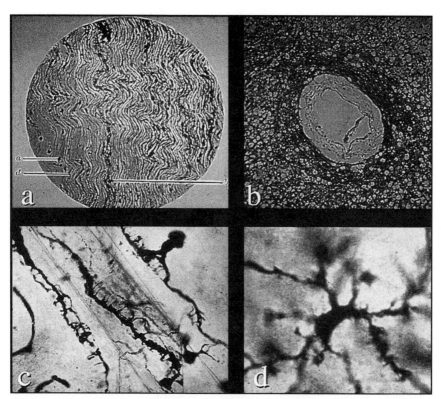

Figure 2.2 The key elements of multiple sclerosis. Within the first two decades of this century, the principal histopathological changes in multiple sclerosis, and the two key glial cell types underlying disease processes, had been clearly described. Dawson depicted the scar-like demyelinated plaque (a) and identified its ultimate origin, the perivascular inflammatory cuff (b). Meanwhile, del Rio Hortega discovered both the oligodendrocyte (c), the immunological target in multiple sclerosis and (d) the microglia, the central nervous system immune effector cell playing a fundamental role in generating local inflammatory (demyelinating) responses.

vision, or other symptoms elsewhere (see Figure 2.3). The resolution of inflammation allows conduction block to improve with subsequent restoration of vision. Demyelination persists, causing the characteristically persistent delay or slowing of conduction which, however, is often asymptomatic (although subtle abnormalities may be apparent on testing).

The acute resolution of symptoms therefore owes more to the resolution of oedema and inflammation than to myelin repair, at least in the optic nerve (McDonald, 1996). Demyelinated fibres can re-attain the capacity for functionally useful conduction, probably as a result of reactive rearrangement of sodium channels, previously clustered at the nodal region, into a more diffuse distribution along the axon (Waxman, 1997). There is some evidence that continuing inflammation impedes this redistribution (Rivera-Quinones *et al.*, 1998). Alternatively, it may be that conduction block at least partially results from functional myelin disturbance, rather than anatomical demyelination (McDonald, 1994); compression (from oedema) or soluble mediators associated with inflammation, such as

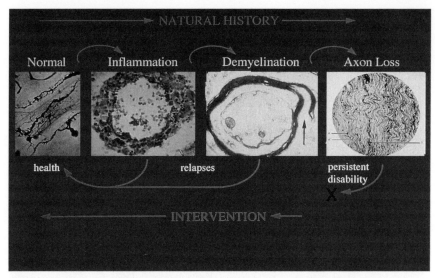

Figure 2.3 Disease processes in multiple sclerosis. This much simplified cartoon is presented only to help illustrate the relationship between pathological processes in multiple sclerosis and clinical course, and more particularly to indicate one possible reason for the very modest effects of even the most powerful therapeutic suppressors of immune and inflammatory responses. Neither persisting demyelination nor axon loss, two major components of the underlying pathophysiology, are targeted by such treatments. (It must be emphasized, however, that a number of assumptions in this model lack definitive evidence, as discussed in more detail in the text. Thus, while it is likely (as shown) that both inflammation and demyelination contribute to the functional deficits characterizing acute relapses in multiple sclerosis, axonal loss as the substrate for persistent disability is yet to be proven; many data suggest demyelination is in fact a sufficient and indeed important cause. Also, the mechanism of axon loss is in fact unknown – here it is shown as a component of chronic disease which follows axon loss; others have suggested axon loss occurs in acute inflammatory lesions.)

complement or tumour necrosis factor (TNF), might be responsible, and resolution of either would therefore allow the rapid restoration of conduction. Remyelination (which is seen pathologically; see below) is more likely to be a slower process accounting for the later clinical and electrophysiological improvements (more common, at least in optic neuritis, in children). Whilst well-established formation of compact myelin may be necessary to secure normal conduction (Smith *et al.*, 1979), it should be mentioned that glial ensheathment alone can restore nerve conduction (Smith *et al.*, 1982).

Fragile conduction in previously damaged pathways may be responsible for a number of characteristic symptoms in patients with multiple sclerosis. Rasminsky (1973) has shown that a small rise in temperature (0.5°C) may result in conduction blocked in demyelinated fibres, reversed when the temperature falls. It is suggested that this accounts for the Uhtoff phenomenon, in which a hot bath or shower, or physical exertion, temporarily impedes conduction in previously inflamed pathways, precipitating the transient re-emergence or exacerbation of symptoms – visual deterioration in a patient with previous optic neuritis would be a common example.

Patients receiving the T cell-depleting monoclonal antibody (Campath-1H) experience an acute effect within hours of the first dose, attributed to the massive release of cytokines (Moreau *et al.*, 1994, 1996), and this is accompanied by a similarly temporary, often severe, recrudescence of one or more of their previous symptoms; this again may reflect the vulnerability of previously affected pathways to further insult, though here the mechanism remains obscure, as artificially inducing a simple rise in temperature alone fails to mimic the antibody effect.

The more acutely transient symptoms are also often associated with clear precipitants. Perhaps the commonest is Lhermitte's sign, a sudden electrical or shock-like sensation radiating from the neck downwards, triggered by neck flexion. Classical paroxysmal symptoms – trigeminal neuralgia, paroxysmal dysarthria and/or ataxia, and tonic spasms – can be spontaneous, but may have specific motor or sensory triggers. Ephaptic (side-to-side) transmission of electrical impulses between adjacent demyelinated axons, which certainly occurs in the spinal roots of dystrophic mice (Rasminsky, 1980), was suggested as a possible pathophysiological substrate for such phenomena. It now appears more likely, however, that the ectopic generation of discharges in demyelinated axons, either spontaneously or following mechanical triggers, explains these symptoms (Smith and McDonald, 1982; Felts *et al.*, 1995). Spontaneous muscle twitching, myokymia, which particularly affects facial and peri-ocular muscles in multiple sclerosis, probably has a similar origin.

Ultimately, in many patients, permanent functional loss occurs, perhaps following repeated episodes of inflammation at the same site (Prineas *et al.*, 1984). It is increasingly recognized that a failure of remyelination *per se* may not provide an adequate or at least complete pathophysiological explanation for this. Persistently demyelinated fibres can conduct, and it is suggested that axonal loss, increasing with disease progression (Raine, 1983), contributes significantly to chronic disability in multiple sclerosis (Davie *et al.*, 1995; De Stefano *et al.*, 1995). There is abundant histopathological evidence for axon loss in chronic multiple sclerosis (see below) and more recent pathological studies show axon damage also in acute inflammatory (demyelinating) lesions. However, *functionally* important loss of axons in acute relapses would, of course, be very difficult to reconcile with the usual remitting clinical course of such episodes (see Figure 2.3). Electrophysiological investigations have also long provided clear evidence that impairment of conduction – through functional or structural disturbance of myelin – is of paramount importance in acute relapse (Smith, 1996; McDonald, 1998).

There are, however, some clinical electrophysiological and imaging data which are at least consistent with increasing axon damage in chronic lesions (Suzuki *et al.*, 1969; Barnes *et al.*, 1991). The amplitude of evoked potentials steadily and progressively diminishes over periods of months to years (Matthews and Small, 1979), and magnetic resonance studies show a progressive loss of brain volume (on serial MRI) (Losseff *et al.*, 1996a, b), and reductions in (axon-specific) *N*-acetylaspartate (NAA) demonstrable by magnetic resonance spectroscopy (MRS) (Davie *et al.*, 1994; De Stefano *et al.*, 1995), findings which correlate significantly with increasing disability.

Whilst it is tempting therefore to assume that chronic axon loss provides the physiological substrate for permanent loss of neurological function (De

Stefano *et al.*, 1995), the case remains to be proven. Matthews commented that the steady decline in amplitude of visual evoked potentials did not correlate with changes in visual acuity (or conduction latency) (Matthews and Small, 1979). Uthoff's phenomenon – the transient deterioration in acute *and chronic* symptoms with fever – provides strong evidence for demyelination, not axon loss, as an important pathophysiological substrate for chronically impaired function (Smith, 1996; McDonald, 1996). Clinical benefit, albeit transient, in chronic stable symptoms following treatment with 4–aminopyridine also implies that demyelination, rather than axon loss, represents a major physiological substrate for long-standing functional impairment (Davis *et al.*, 1995) – though others have suggested that enhanced synaptic transmission in fact underlies the effect of aminopyridine (Felts and Smith, 1994). Finally, in axonal tract injury and regeneration a figure of 85–95% is commonly quoted as the percentage of axons which must be lost before effective function is irrevocably lost (Sabel, 1997) – a figure rarely reached in acute or chronic lesions (Greenfield and King, 1936).

Other explanations may be offered for the loss of brain volume on serial magnetic resonance studies (Losseff *et al.*, 1996a, b) and reductions in (axon-specific) NAA on MRS (Davie *et al.*, 1994; De Stefano *et al.*, 1995). Myelin loss, the resolution of oedema and contraction of acutely hypertrophied astrocytes to form scar tissue – the eponymous sclerosis – might contribute to volume changes. Reductions in MRS NAA signals can be at least partially reversible (De Stefano *et al.*, 1995), raising the possibility that (transient) changes in axon function – not inconceivably the simple consequence upon inflammation or demyelination – rather than in axon numbers, are being registered. Finally, since axons (including, pertinently, retinal ganglion cells) may degenerate as a direct consequence of prolonged electrical silence (Lipton, 1986), it is possible that cause and effect of axon loss have become confused – that axon degeneration is a *consequence* of the persistent functional impairment caused by long-standing demyelination (see Figure 2.3). In Class I MHC-deficient mice infected with Theiler's virus, impaired inflammatory processes have been linked to successful sodium channel redistribution (following extensive demyelination); useful conduction (and function) is restored and there is substantial preservation of axons (RiveraQuinones *et al.*, 1998).

Diagnosis

The diagnosis of multiple sclerosis is a clinical one, resting on the clinical dissemination of lesions in both time and space (as mentioned above) – combined with the absence of any other obvious explanation. A number of investigations may offer supporting evidence, but none may be used as an ultimate arbiter to refute or prove a diagnosis of multiple sclerosis.

Thus, the visual evoked potential is abnormal, usually with delayed conduction, in 50–80% cases (Asselman *et al.*, 1975) indicating one or more episodes of optic neuritis (which may or may not have been manifest symptomatically), and usually remains abnormal, albeit with partial improvement. However, it is non-specific, and may also be abnormal in sarcoidosis, lupus, hereditary ataxias and spastic paraplegias, compression, and B_{12} deficiency. Evoked potentials can also be measured along auditory, somatosensory and motor pathways, and although abnormal conduction may provide paraclinical evidence for dissemination of lesions, these changes again lack specificity.

Spinal fluid examination during an acute episode may reveal the presence of a mild to moderate lymphocyte (more rarely neutrophil) pleocytosis, or a mildly elevated protein level, but these parameters are more often completely normal. However, electrophoretic examination for the presence of oligo-clonal bands of immunoglobulin is extremely sensitive. Properly performed, it is positive in approximately 98% of cases (Lee *et al.*, 1991; Filippini *et al.*, 1994), but this still leaves one case in 50 with a normal result and the analysis also lacks specificity: any other cerebral inflammatory process may yield a positive result, and oligoclonal bands are also reported in a very small proportion of cases of stroke, brain tumour and other disorders, and in 2% of normal healthy individuals.

Magnetic resonance imaging reveals the presence of lesions in both brain, and, with more recent technical modifications, spinal cord and optic nerve (Miller *et al.*, 1998a, b). The periventricular areas and centrum semi-ovale are particularly and conspicuously involved – with no obvious clinical sympto-matology, and gadolinium 'enhancement' allows the detection of acute and new lesions – dynamic imaging studies have indicated that leakage of gadolinium across the damaged blood–brain barrier represents the earliest discernible radiological abnormality during the development of inflamma-tory demyelinating lesions, which has important pathophysiological implications (see above). Sensitivity and specificity again are found wanting – approximately 5% cases have no MRI abnormalities (Filippini *et al.*, 1994), while changes similar to those in multiple sclerosis are also seen in infectious and other inflammatory diseases. Ageing alone is associated with MRI appearances which can be difficult to distinguish from those of multiple sclerosis, although criteria for establishing this distinction have been suggested: the presence of lesions over 6 mm in diameter, immediate proximity to the ventricles and location below the tentorium cerebelli all mitigating in favour of multiple sclerosis (Fazekas *et al.*, 1988).

Poser has laid down diagnostic criteria which have been widely accepted, particularly for the purposes of standardization for research into the epidemiology, genetics and treatment of multiple sclerosis (Poser *et al.*, 1983). These take into account both the reliability of individually described episodes and paraclinical (cerebrospinal fluid (CSF) and MRI) data (Table 2.1).

Symptomatic treatment of multiple sclerosis

Multiple (or disseminated) sclerosis has been familiar to neurologists for well over a century and yet still the search for treatments which dramatically influence the course of the disease continues. Partly this reflects the complexity of the disease process and the inaccessibility of the tissue involved, and an important reason for attempting to understand mechanisms of myelin injury is obviously to predict and design logical strategies for treatment.

Table 2.1 Poser Committee new diagnostic criteria for multiple sclerosis

Category	Number of episodes — Attacks (number)	Number of separate sites involved — Clinical evidence		Paraclinical evidence[a]	CSF OB/ IgG
(A) Clinically definite					
CDMS A1	2	2		–	
CDMS A2	2	1	and	1	
(B) Laboratory-supported definite	2	1	or	1	+
LSDMS B1	1	2		–	+
LSDMS B2	1	1	and	1	+
LSDMS B3					
(C) Clinically probable					
CPMS C1	2	1			
CPMS C2	1	2			
CPMS C3	1	1	and	1	
(D) Laboratory-supported probable	2				+
LSPMS D1					

[a] Paraclinical evidence includes imaging, electrophysiology or urodynamics. The conventional foundation on the criteria of dissemination in time and space is indicated in the (italicized) top row of column group headings.

Steroids in a variety of forms have been used for almost 40 years in multiple sclerosis (Miller and Gibbons, 1953), a large trial in 1970 having shown a significant benefit in approximately two-thirds of the 103 treated patients (Rose *et al.*, 1970). Although corticosteroids have a wide variety of activities modifying immune and inflammatory responses, the principal site of action in multiple sclerosis may be at the level of the blood–brain barrier, reducing vascular permeability, tissue inflammation and oedema (Kesselring *et al.*, 1989).

The preparation most used at present, high-dose intravenous cortico-steroids (e.g. 1 g daily of methylprednisolone for 3 days), accelerates recovery from acute relapses in multiple sclerosis, but does not influence the course of the disease (Durelli *et al.*, 1986; Milligan *et al.*, 1987). Oral methylprednisolone may have an equal effect (Barnes *et al.*, 1997). Steroids may have a small beneficial effect on chronic spasticity (Milligan *et al.*, 1987), but otherwise have little place in treatment outside acute relapse.

A similar benefit – improving the speed, but not the extent, of recovery – was found in a trial of steroids in the treatment of acute optic neuritis (Beck *et al.*, 1992). Additional retrospective analysis of data from this trial indicated that in the case of optic neuritis, steroid treatment might have the further and unexpected beneficial effect of delaying the onset of subsequent neurological events in those patients destined to develop multiple sclerosis (Beck *et al.*, 1993), but this suggested inference has been disputed and clearly requires confirmation: slightly longer term analysis failed to show any sustained benefit in this respect (Beck, 1995).

Conventional immunosuppressive drugs including azathioprine, cyclophosphamide and cyclosporin A have all been used with the aim of retarding progression of the disease. The conventional view has been that the adverse effects of these agents outweigh the modest benefits reported (albeit variably) for all three relatively non-specific immune suppressants (Hughes, 1994). It is, however, increasingly accepted that azathioprine in particular, may offer benefits no less substantial than some of the newer and much vaunted immunotherapeutic agents, and perhaps should be more widely used (Palace and Rothwell, 1997). (It has always been more commonly used in continental Europe than in the UK and USA.) These and more novel therapeutic modalities will be considered in detail in Chapter 4. In the meantime, it should not be forgotten that, particularly in patients who have progressive disease and fixed neurological deficits, symptomatic management potentially offers a far more dramatic impact than either steroids or currently available immune suppressive agents not only upon the sense of well-being, but also on handicap (Thompson, 1996; Kidd and Thompson, 1997).

Urinary frequency, urgency and incontinence are among the most troublesome and distressing complaints, and often respond well to anti-cholinergic treatment. These drugs do, however, carry the risk of inducing retention either acutely, in patients whose symptoms paradoxically reflect a flaccid paretic bladder, or chronically, where a small volume of residual urine is no less attractive to microbes than any other pool of nutrient-rich, heated, stagnant water. At the very least, catheterization to measure residual volume is mandatory before exhibiting anti-cholinergic drugs; some would advocate formal urodynamic studies. In those who poorly tolerate these agents, nocturnal doses alone can help allow a decent night's sleep, perhaps supplemented by sporadic occasion-related diurnal doses. Nocturnal and diurnal nasal anti-diuretic hormone analogues (DDAVP) can also help reduce nocturia (Hilton et al., 1983; Hoverd and Fowler, 1998). Where hesitancy or retention is the principal problem, self-intermittent catheterization is often successful, effected either by the patient, if upper limb function and vision permit, or by partner or attendant. Indwelling catheters are a less satisfactory solution, encumbering, prone to infection and rarely guaranteed not to leak, though superior to nothing at all when circumstances dictate; suprapubic catheterization may be better. Faecal incontinence (Fowler and Henry, 1996), fortunately not common, is as dispiriting to the patient as it is difficult to treat. After excluding constipated impaction with overflow incontinence, most would advocate anti-cholinergics, but these are infrequently of value.

Sexual difficulties are not at all rare. Commonly, psychological factors relating to self-image, depression and confidence are paramount, and libido is rarely improved by sphincter inefficiencies or lingering evidence thereof. Professional counselling and proper nursing and doctoring can go far, but neurological deficits must be more specifically addressed. Loss of perineal sensation cannot be treated; lubricants may improve dyspareunia. Erectile dysfunction may respond to yohimbine or to intracorporeal injection of papaverine. Considerable excitement has surrounded the introduction of the phosphodiesterase inhibitor sildenafil for male impotence (Boolell et al., 1996); it is at the time of writing licensed in the USA but not the UK. Surgically implanted prostheses may be considered.

Spasticity and painful spasms, usually predominant in the lower limbs, commonly respond to baclofen; dantrolene, followed by diazepam are next used (usually in this order); vigabatrin and tizanidine have an increasing role. As mentioned above, pulsed intravenous methylprednisolone can help. Clearly, excluding or treating precipitating factors, including bladder infections, pressure areas etc., precedes pharmacological treatments. In difficult cases, intrathecal baclofen has not (at least yet) gained widespread use; destructive surgery, usually with phenol, is as attractive as destructive surgery ever can be, but has a role (after a trial of block by a reversible local anaesthetic agent). Finally, botulinum toxin is currently under assessment. Fatigue is common, and whilst amantidine and pemoline have been advocated, neither is overwhelmingly valuable.

The profoundly disabling, violent ataxic tremor (rubral tremor) characteristic of chronic severe multiple sclerosis is enormously difficult to treat; drugs (primidone, propranolol, isoniazid) almost invariably fail, and while stereotactic ventrolateral thalamotomy can yield useful results, it carries the risk of severe hemiparesis or dysphasia. Thalamic stimulation may help some movement disorders associated with multiple sclerosis (Whittle *et al.*, 1998).

The potential impact of proper and careful symptomatic treatment in patients with chronic multiple sclerosis cannot be exaggerated.

A definitive disease-modifying treatment for multiple sclerosis might emerge in either of two ways – accidentally, when new (presumably immune active) agents are speculatively presented to the disease, or by design, depending on advances in our understanding of the cause of multiple sclerosis and the nature of the cerebral inflammatory processes which underlie tissue damage (see Figure 2.3). To provide a context in which to consider these possibilities in Chapter 4, it is sensible to pause and briefly review current thinking on the aetiology and the pathogenesis of multiple sclerosis.

The cause of multiple sclerosis

Both genetic and environmental factors contribute to the aetiology of multiple sclerosis, but in both cases, the precise nature of the precipitant remains to be defined (reviewed in (Scolding *et al.*, 1994; Compston, 1997)). Early studies established familial and racial susceptibility to the disease, more recent data establishing that identical twins have a 30% risk of developing the disease, compared to approximately 4% for other siblings (including dizygotic twins) and 2% for the offspring of an affected individual (Compston, 1997). The high concordance rate in monozygotic twins, contrasting with the rate in dizygotes, offers powerful evidence that the genetic contribution is substantial and definite, and yet not absolute – environmental influences are implied by the 70% disconcordance in identical twins. The possibility that shared environmental factors within families might mimic a genetic influence has been addressed in a recent investigation of disease incidence in adoptees and/or their families, and has confirmed the over-riding influence of genetic – rather than shared environmental factors – in family studies (Ebers *et al.*, 1995). Similarly, recurrence risks in families where there is conjugal multiple sclerosis also emphasize genetic rather than environmental influences (Robertson *et al.*, 1997).

Genes

Inheritance is polygenic, most models predicting that at least five or six genes are implicated (Compston, A. 1997; Compston, D., 1997; Sawcer *et al.*, 1997a). An association with the D-related locus of the major histocompatibility complex – specifically, HLA-DR15 (DR2) has reliably been shown, though the contribution is weak: whilst certain alleles within the Class II MHC complex increase susceptibility, none so far identified is necessary and sufficient for the development of multiple sclerosis. Furthermore, some variability is observed in those alleles associating with disease between geographically different populations.

T cell receptor (TCR) genes (whose product interacts with antigen presented by Class II MHC molecules, forming the tri-molecular complex crucial to the development of immune responses) have also been much studied. A consensus is yet to emerge, a variety of conflicting and thus far irreconcilable data having been presented (Fugger *et al.*, 1990; Hillert *et al.*, 1991, 1992); reviewed in Ebers and Sadovnick, (1994) and Sawcer *et al.*, (1997b) which at best implies that any influence is (again) rather weak. Tentative evidence for linkage to the β chain (but not the α) gene of the TCR has been presented (Beall *et al.*, 1993; Wood *et al.*, 1995b).

A third complex of genes involved in immune responses much studied in the context of multiple sclerosis are those determining the structure of immunoglobulins. Again, an association has been suggested (Walter *et al.*, 1991); again, conflicting findings have been published; linkage (to the heavy chain variable region) has been tentatively suggested of late (Wood *et al.*, 1995a). Other genes coding for proteins important in the execution (rather than generation) of immune responses, e.g. complement components and TNF, have also been studied; no convincing association has yet been found.

The search for other candidate genes continues. Structural oligodendrocyte and myelin components are obvious suspects, but a possible association with myelin basic protein (MBP) polymorphisms (Tienari *et al.*, 1992) has not found confirmation in a number of larger studies (Rose *et al.*, 1993; Wood *et al.*, 1994), while a recent search for association with polymorphisms of the highly immunogenic surface protein myelin–oligodendrocyte glycoprotein (MOG; see below) was persuasively negative (Roth *et al.*, 1995).

However, more useful information is now beginning to emerge from the more rational genome screen approach currently employed by a number of groups, wherein a battery of markers spaced with variable regularity throughout the genome is screened against a battery of sibling pairs from informative families. 'First-pass' screens have been completed (Sawcer *et al.*, 1997b) and have highlighted areas of importance, while excluding the possibility of any single gene making a major contribution to the development of multiple sclerosis. The identification of the important genes of influence is expected soon.

Multiple sclerosis and the environment

Early epidemiological studies showed the geographical distribution of the disease to be uneven, an increasing prevalence in both hemispheres being associated with increasing distance from the equator, and an environmental contribution to the aetiology was suggested. Adults migrating from areas of high to low prevalence appeared to take with them their high risk of developing the disease (and *vice versa*), while children adopted the risk of the local population (Dean, 1967). Migration studies have been criticized (Delasnerie and Alperovitch, 1992), often involving relatively small numbers both of migrants and of cases of multiple sclerosis, and often assuming (rather than providing evidence for) genetic homogeneity of the migrating cohort with its 'parent' population. However, further support for the modification of genetic susceptibility by the environment has been offered by the finding that children born in London of West Indian immigrant parents have a risk of developing multiple sclerosis which closely approximates to that of the London native (Elian *et al.*, 1990). These data are consistent with the hypothesis that one or more infective agent(s) acquired in childhood but with a long latent period is important in the aetiology.

The significantly lower prevalence of multiple sclerosis in white populations long-established in South Africa and in Australasia (Kurtzke, 1977), in relation to two genetically comparable populations – the 'parental' group in Northern Europe and a 'control' migratory population in North America – also argue for a significant environmental influence. Finally, reports of multiple sclerosis occurring in epidemics, often associated with the arrival in previously 'unexposed' indigenous populations (with low disease incidence) of a small number of migrants from high disease incidence areas, have also been cited in support of an infectious environmental agent (reviewed in Kurtzke, 1993). A number of statistical and methodological observations have questioned the validity of multiple sclerosis epidemics (Benedikz *et al.*, 1994), despite continuing reports thereof (Sheremata *et al.*, 1985; Kurtzke, 1993).

Laboratory attempts to identify a specific infective agent have been unsuccessful or at least inconsistent, various and continuing reports of associations with specific viruses all subsequently having failed to be confirmed. Much evidence was presented of measles-specific antibodies within oligoclonal spinal fluid immunoglobulins (Norrby, 1978; Salmi *et al.*, 1983); later findings suggested a wide range of viruses were included within the intrathecal immunoglobulin repertoire, including herpes zoster, mumps, influenza and rubella, and that no more than a non-specific polyclonal response was present (Dhib *et al.*, 1990). Modern molecular techniques have now been applied and, recently, reverse transcriptase polymerase chain reaction (PCR) has failed to demonstrate DNA sequences of measles, mumps or rubella viruses in cerebral tissue from multiple sclerosis patients (reviewed in Johnson, 1994). Human T lymphotropic virus (HTLV-1) and the paramyxovirus SV5 (Koprowski *et al.*, 1985; Goswami *et al.*, 1987) have also been implicated, but again both associations were refuted in subsequent studies (McLean and Thompson, 1989; Nishimura *et al.*, 1990). Nevertheless, absence of proof is not proof of absence and it remains the majority view that a genetically determined idiosyncrasy in susceptibility or reaction to one or more viruses represents the cause of multiple sclerosis (Ransohoff *et al.*, 1994), with molecular mimicry – immunological confusion of viral epitopes with target tissue determinants (Wucherpfennig and Strominger, 1995) – as the most favoured mechanism. Herpes-6 viruses and novel retroviruses are more recent candidates (Sola *et al.*, 1993; Nielsen *et al.*, 1997; Perron *et al.*, 1997; Soldan *et al.*, 1997); though again may not stand up to close inspection (Mayne *et al.* 1988).

Clearly, until substantial progress is made in the identification of genes and putative viruses, attempts either to cure or to prevent multiple sclerosis cannot be made (although the data concerning disease incidence in families may clearly be exploited to identify a target or 'at-risk' population in whom pre-symptomatic treatment strategies might be justified and appropriate). In the meantime, therapeutic energy must continue to be directed towards interrupting the disease process; rational approaches depend in turn on an understanding of the biology of the disorder, and the mechanisms responsible for tissue damage in multiple sclerosis.

The process of inflammatory demyelination

Quite how putative viruses combine with defective genes to precipitate immune attack against myelin and oligodendrocyte damage remains unknown, but considerable progress has been made in recent years in determining which components of the immune response are implicated, and how they interact to cause inflammatory demyelination though – here too, many details remain to be fully defined. Before considering mechanisms, however, it is of course necessary first to describe the nature of tissue damage in multiple sclerosis.

The histopathology of multiple sclerosis

The demyelinating lesion in multiple sclerosis has a number of key pathological features which help define the disease; most were recognized in early descriptions, and are well-described in Dawson's remarkable and now classic pathological study of 1916, '*On The Histology of Disseminated Sclerosis*' (Dawson, 1916).

(i) The most important is *primary demyelination*, i.e. loss of myelin with relative preservation of other elements in affected areas. "The change in the myelin sheath must be looked upon as the most constant, the most uniform, and ... has all the features of a primary degeneration..." (Dawson, 1916). This crucial feature helps distinguish multiple sclerosis from other disorders where myelin loss occurs in the context of non-specific destruction of axons, glia, myelin and vascular elements, as in acute haemorrhagic encephalo-myelitis (see Chapter 3). It might also be mentioned in passing that primary demyelination also distinguishes multiple sclerosis from the majority of animal models (experimental allergic encephalomyelitis (EAE) in its various guises), where again tissue damage is less selective, emphasizing their limitations.

It has for many years also been established that oligodendrocytes (as well as myelin) are absent in chronic plaques, but the fate of these cells in acute lesions has remained a matter of some uncertainty and indeed controversy. Evidence for very early oligodendrocyte loss in lesions, rapidly followed by repopulation by oligodendrocyte lineage cells, was presented; others described increased, decreased or unchanged numbers (Prineas, 1975; Raine *et al.*, 1981a; Prineas *et al.*, 1989; Raine, 1997). This inconsistency, which depended to some extent on the precise age and stage of lesions studied and the criteria using for this staging, fuelled considerable speculation as to whether disease processes in multiple sclerosis were targeted on oligoden-drocytes or myelin – though many have preferred simply to consider multiple sclerosis a disease of the (functionally single) *oligodendrocyte–myelin unit*, and the spread of immune responses in the course of the disease (see below) also diminishes the importance of the argument.

A more recent suggestion – and potential resolution of previously discrepant histopathological findings – is that fundamental distinctions in disease processes may in fact be drawn depending on the pattern of oligodendrogliopathy in multiple sclerosis, re-kindling the possibility of significant disease heterogeneity. It is proposed that in different lesions, different pathological patterns of inflammation and demyelination are distinguishable. All combinations appear possible: demyelination with oligodendrocyte preservation; simultaneous destruction of both myelin and oligodendrocytes; selective death or injury of oligodendrocytes with secondary demyelination; and primary demyelination followed by secondary oligodendrocyte loss (Lucchinetti *et al.*, 1996). Axon damage also features in certain types of destructive lesion. Clearly the implied subdivision of multiple sclerosis into a number of separate phenotypes has important ramifications for cause, prognosis and indeed treatment – already, evidence of a similar genetic heterogeneity is also emerging (Sawcer and Compston, personal communication).

(ii) The changes of inflammation and primary demyelination occur in *discrete focal lesions*, as indeed suggested by the clinical features. The latter also reflect the commonest anatomical sites for these lesions in pathological studies: the optic nerves, the brainstemand cerebellum, and the spinal cord; these are now demonstrable *in vivo* using MRI, which also reveals one further commonly affected site unaccompanied by marked or obvious clinical manifestations – the periventricular white matter.

(iii) The tendency for lesions to occur around blood vessels was recognized long ago by Dawson (1916). He described cellular elements migrating from vessels in these areas which would now be described as *perivascular inflammatory lesions*, with macrophages and lymphocytes forming a cuff around blood vessels (Figure 2.2).

More sophisticated analysis of the extensive acute perivascular cuffs demonstrates a predominance of T lymphocytes and macrophages (Raine, 1994b; Sobel, 1995). Amongst the T cells, both CD4$^+$ and CD8$^+$ subpopulations are represented, with little agreement in the literature on which predominate (Booss *et al.*, 1983; Sobel, 1989). Interleukin (IL)-2 receptor expression by a proportion of lymphocytes confirms their activated state (Bellamy *et al.*, 1985), but detailed studies of cytokine and adhesion molecule expression by infiltrating inflammatory cells in multiple sclerosis has failed to provide any evidence for patterns unique to multiple sclerosis (Raine, 1994a). A smaller number of $\gamma\delta$ T cells are also found. B lymphocytes are present both within acute lesions and in the perivascular spaces, and persistent intrathecal antibody synthesis reflects sustained activation of mature plasma cells within the CNS and results in the appearance of oligoclonal bands of immunoglobulin in CSF.

(iv) The presence of numerous macrophages and monocytes within lesions again was demonstrated by Dawson, though Babinski's illustrations a

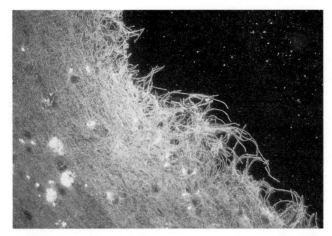

Figure 2.4 Astrocytosis in multiple sclerosis. A dense network of GFAP-positive astrocytes in a chronic multiple sclerosis lesion is shown. Although classically viewed as one of the villains of the piece, astrocytes in fact play a number of contrasting roles in the development of lesions. Acutely reactive astrocytes represent a source of important growth factors for oligodendrocytes and are likely therefore to have a positive influence, encouraging functionally useful repair by remyelinating oligodendrocytes; non-reactive astrocytes in the chronic scar have a no less important role in damage limitation, effecting secondary repair by scar formation but so producing an environment no longer conducive to myelin repair.

generation earlier had clearly shown that phagocytic cells adhere to and ingest myelin along medullated axon bundles. Later electron microscopic studies helped definitively to define the role of these cells – now thought to represent a mixture of infiltrating circulating monocytes and activated parenchymal microglia (the resident CNS macrophage population) – in binding to (opsonized) myelin sheaths and stripping away myelin lamellae to leave denuded axons.

(v) Dawson also recognized at least two distinct pathological stages of the disease: the early or acute lesion, with inflammatory cell infiltration but little loss of myelin, and the later chronic lesion, characterized by demyelination and loss of oligodendrocytes, with little or no persisting inflammation and, importantly and again characteristically, a pronounced astrocytosis (Figure 2.4). These features constitute another key pathological feature of multiple sclerosis, the classical *chronic plaque* or scar.

(vi) Dawson noted a sixth pathological feature reflecting the clinical course of the disease, i.e. that lesions of various stages are identifiable at different sites in the same patient – pathological evidence for *dissemination in time*.

(vii) Damage to axons is clearly described in Charcot's accounts of the microscopic basis of the disorder (Charcot, 1868), while in his monograph (Dawson, 1916) also repeatedly draws attention to such loss – "...(in some lesions)... the persisting axon cylinders are fewer and show more evident indications of a previous involvement". However, these and other authors repeatedly emphasised the primacy of myelin damage and the relative sparing of axons – so-called *dissociation axomyélinique*.

Subsequent accounts of the histopathology of multiple sclerosis have continued to emphasise the primary nature of demyelination, whilst also noting the occurrence of axonal changes and loss (Greenfield and King,

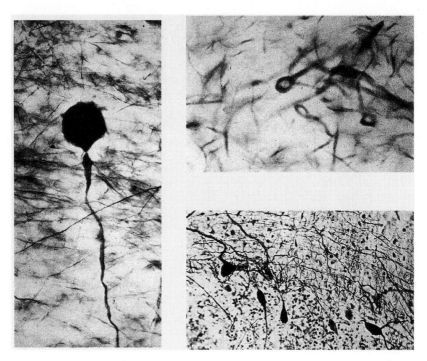

Figure 2.5 Axon fragmentation and loss in multiple sclerosis. Over 60 years ago, Greenfield and King quantified axon loss in multiple sclerosis, illustrating frequent axon end bulbs in cortical lesions (Greenfield and King, 1936).

1936; Lumsden, 1955; Peters, 1968; Raine and Cross, 1989; Allen, 1991; Barnes *et al.*, 1991; Ozawa *et al.*, 1994). Greenfield and King formally quantified axon damage (Figure 2.5), studying over 125 plaques from 13 cases and found less than 10% to show severe reductions, i.e. to 15–20% normal density, in the number of axon fibres (Greenfield and King, 1936). Interestingly, these authors also described fragmented axons within plaques, together with 'retraction balls' or end bulbs. Initial accounts of the ultrastructure of multiple sclerosis also noted axonal changes (Suzuki *et al.*, 1969), while Raine provided electron microscopic images of axon spheroids within lesions two decades ago (Raine *et al.*, 1981a). Pathological studies of both acute and chronic animal models of multiple sclerosis included descriptions of axon loss (Raine, 1983; Raine and Cross, 1989). In 1974, fundoscopic observation provided direct evidence of neuronal loss in the retinal nerve fibre layer of patients with previous optic neuritis (Frisen and Hoyt, 1974).

Axon damage in acute lesions has more recently been reported (Ferguson *et al.*, 1997; Trapp *et al.*, 1998), although (as mentioned above) substantial and functionally relevant loss seems unlikely to explain the pathophysiology of acute episodes in relapsing–remitting multiple sclerosis (Scolding and Franklin, 1998).

(viii) A final and important pathological observation only relatively recently recognized is the occurrence of substantial but often abortive remyelination in the early stages of acute inflammatory damage (Perier and Gregoire, 1965; Prineas and Connell, 1979; Prineas et al., 1993; Raine and Wu, 1993). In these lesions, injury, removal, repair and replacement of myelin are all apparent (Prineas et al., 1984), the latter perhaps depending on inward migration of oligodendrocyte progenitor cells (Prineas et al., 1989). Developmental patterns of myelination events may be recapitulated (Raine et al., 1981b; Capello et al., 1997).

Dawson's findings clearly confirmed the *inflammatory* nature of tissue damage in multiple sclerosis, while the specificity of the demyelinating process – wherein oligodendrocytes and myelin are selectively injured, astrocytes and neurones, at least in the early stages, being spared – bears witness to the role of the *immune* system in recruiting, harnessing, targeting and controlling the inflammatory effectors. Before describing how the immune and inflammatory systems cooperate to generate these pathological changes, it may be timely to review briefly the immunological abnormalities found in multiple sclerosis, particularly those of cellular immune function – not least since these have been intensively studied in the last few decades, and the findings to emerge have at least in part precipitated the simplistic but ubiquitous description in the 1970s of multiple sclerosis as a 'T cell-mediated disease', a notion which invites, if not deconstruction, then modest qualification.

Immunological abnormalities: T cells and multiple sclerosis

Several separate lines of experimental evidence accounted for the 'T cell disease' epithet (Raine, 1991; Wucherpfennig, 1994). These included:

1. Apparent similarities between multiple sclerosis and EAE (Paterson and Day, 1981), which may be induced solely by inoculation with activated T cells (Ben et al., 1981; Zamvil and Steinman, 1990).
2. The presence of activated lymphocytes in lesions.
3. Fluctuations in peripheral T cell phenotype and function during the course of multiple sclerosis (Waksman and Reynolds, 1984; Calder et al., 1989).
4. The association of susceptibility with genes controlling cellular immune responses.
5. The presence of T cells reactive against myelin antigens in samples from some patients with multiple sclerosis (Olsson et al., 1990, 1992; Wucherpfennig et al., 1991).

However, whilst bearing witness to the necessary contribution of T lymphocytes to inflammatory demyelination, these observations provide no direct evidence that myelin-specific T lymphocytes are themselves responsible or sufficient for oligodendrocyte damage and demyelination in multiple sclerosis.

Experimental allergic encephalomyelitis and multiple sclerosis
Direct extrapolation from EAE to multiple sclerosis carries some hazards. Although there are obvious similarities between EAE and human inflammatory demyelinating disease, significant differences must not be overlooked, and most notable among these is the consistently observed lack

of primary demyelination found in histopathological studies of many forms EAE (Linington *et al.*, 1988), including experimental disease passively transferred solely by encephalitogenic activated T cells. Here, substantial myelin loss occurs only when humoral mechanisms are recruited by the availability of anti-myelin antibodies (Linington *et al.*, 1988). It is perhaps to our understanding of basic mechanisms of immunity in relation to the CNS that the true contribution of EAE lies.

Lymphocytes and the oligodendrocyte–myelin unit

Activated lymphocytes are present in lesions, but only a very small proportion is likely to be directly involved. They are likely to play a more important role in the initiation and amplification of local immune and inflammatory responses than in directly mediating tissue damage. Other effectors – B lymphocytes, complement, antibodies and activated macrophages – are also present in substantial numbers.

CNS lesions from patients with multiple sclerosis do not, upon extraction and culture, yield T lymphocytes reactive against myelin antigens, in marked contrast with affected CNS tissue in post viral encephalomyelitis (Hafler *et al.*, 1987). Furthermore, oligodendrocytes do not in health or disease express MHC molecules necessary for direct interactions with T cells (Hayes *et al.*, 1987; Hayashi *et al.*, 1988; Calder *et al.*, 1989), and it is difficult to explain how T cells could direct macrophages or microglia against myelin without invoking opsonising antibody or activated complement fragments. MBP – the single most commonly studied antigen in T cell specificity studies and in EAE is not expressed or exposed on the oligodendrocyte surface (Poduslo and Braun, 1975; Omlin *et al.*, 1982). Finally, demyelination occurs in areas devoid of lymphocytes (Prineas, 1985).

Notwithstanding these observations, there are direct mechanisms by which it is argued that lymphocytes may at least contribute to oligodendrocyte and myelin injury. As mentioned above, the lesions of multiple sclerosis contain small numbers of γδ T lymphocytes, where they have been described in close relation with heat shock protein (HSP)-expressing oligodendrocytes (Selmaj *et al.*, 1992); *in vitro* evidence of cytotoxicity of human γδ T cells to human oligodendrocytes has been offered (Freedman *et al.*, 1997). Similarly, expression of *fas*, a cell surface receptor important in signalling cell death pathways, by oligodendrocytes in multiple sclerosis lesions, and of the death-inducing *fas* ligand by infiltrating lymphocytes, suggest means of lymphocyte-mediated oligodendrocyte injury – human oligodendrocyte *in vitro* express *fas*, and are lysed when exposed to *fas* ligand (D'Souza *et al.*, 1996a). Microglia in lesions also express *fas* ligand, and are therefore likely to contribute to glial injury by these and multiple other mechanisms, while antibodies and complement probably also play a role (Storch *et al.*, 1998; Scolding *et al.*, 1989b): as discussed in more detail below, oligodendrocytes are likely to be damaged by numerous separate or inter-related pathways, perhaps one facet of disease heterogeneity in multiple sclerosis (Lucchinetti *et al.*, 1996).

Lymphocyte function

Fluctuations in T cell function in multiple sclerosis have long been studied, and undoubtedly provide additional evidence for a disorder of immunity in multiple sclerosis. Circulating T lymphocytes fluctuate in both phenotype and function (Antel *et al.*, 1979; Compston and Hughes, 1984; Morimoto *et al.*, 1987), and mononuclear cell products including a variety of cytokine and soluble lymphocyte receptors, have also been studied. Some evidence suggests that various of these changes correlate with the clinical course of the disease. However, conflicting data abound, some carefully executed studies showing no differences at all either between patients and controls, or within patients during clinical exacerbations, when measuring lymphocyte surface activation markers (e.g. Crockard *et al.*, 1988), lymphocyte adhesion markers (Giovannoni *et al.*, 1997) or soluble peptides (IL-2, IL-2 receptor (Gallo *et al.*, 1991)). Furthermore, dynamic MRI studies indicate that many new lesions in multiple sclerosis patients are clinically silent; the consequent poor correlation between pathological activity in multiple sclerosis, as indirectly suggested by MRI, and clinical expression of disease, casts serious doubt on the *primary* significance of any studies attempting to relate biochemical or immunological indices to clinical relapse or progression.

However, evidence for defective non-specific suppressor T cell function is more consistent (Antel *et al.*, 1989), and may account for the presence of enhanced cellular and humoral immune responses in multiple sclerosis (Waksman and Reynolds, 1984; Chofflon *et al.*, 1989; Stinissen *et al.*, 1997), and it is tempting to suggest that a generalized defect in immune suppression lowers the threshold for T cell activation and provides a permissive environment for autoimmune disturbances.

The great majority of mononuclear cells present in the spinal fluid of patients with multiple sclerosis are T cells, $CD4^+$ cells outnumbering $CD8^+$ by approximately $2:1$ (Raine, 1994b). This is a higher ratio than that found in blood, but does not differ from that found in CSF samples from healthy controls (Kuroda and Shibasaki, 1987; Hedlund *et al.*, 1989). Similarly, a lower percentage of $CD45RA^+$ cells (thought to be naïve ($CD4^+$) T cells) is found in CSF from patients with multiple sclerosis compared to blood, but these findings also obtain in normal CSF samples (Hedlund *et al.*, 1989). Accordingly, the proportion of cells which are $CD45RO^+$ and/or $CD29^+$ (memory T cells) is elevated in CSF. Measured by any of a variety of markers, the proportion of activated T cells is consistently increased in CSF from patients with multiple sclerosis, but also from patients with other inflammatory diseases. CSF levels of IL-2 and of TNF are also elevated in multiple sclerosis (Gallo *et al.*, 1991; Sharief and Hentges, 1991; Sharief and Thompson, 1993).

Genes: HLA and multiple sclerosis
The genetic contribution to the cause of multiple sclerosis has been described above. Whilst again supporting an immunological basis for the disease, the genetic evidence is by no means powerful enough to prove that T lymphocytes are necessary and sufficient for the development of disease. Immunoglobulin heavy chain polymorphisms are also probably associated and the recent genome screens point to the involvement of additional loci.

T cell reactivity in multiple sclerosis: a target antigen?
Considerable effort has been expended in elucidating T cell (and B cell) reactivities in multiple sclerosis in attempts to identify a so-called 'multiple

sclerosis antigen'. The absence (thus far), after many years' study, of any single, consistently identifiable antibody or T cell specificity (in conspicuous contrast with, for example, myasthenia gravis) suggests that these efforts may have been misplaced, and some explanation for this is now beginning to emerge.

There are numerous and often conflicting reports of increased numbers of resting or stimulatable circulating T cells specific for MBP, proteolipid protein (PLP), myelin-associated glycoprotein (MAG) and MOG; some studies suggest changes specific to multiple sclerosis, others show no differences between patients and controls. However, using single cell cultures to evaluate cytokine release by lymphocytes in response to antigen, increased reactivity of T cells from patients with multiple sclerosis to various myelin antigens has been reported (Olsson et al., 1990; Sun et al., 1991); furthermore, the difference in these responses between healthy controls and patients with multiple sclerosis is more apparent in studies of CSF lymphocytes (Sun et al., 1991a, b; Soderstrom et al., 1993, 1994). Zhang et al. (1993) and Chou et al. (1992) also report greater IL-2 and/or IL-4 responsive MBP- and PLP-reactive T cells in CSF and/or blood from patients with multiple sclerosis; increased reactivity towards MOG and MAG has also been found (Olsson et al., 1990; Sun et al., 1991a, b; Olsson, 1992).

The question of whether TCR gene utilization is restricted in multiple sclerosis also remains unresolved. Restricted TCR V_β usage in EAE both in mice and rats appears to occur (Acha et al., 1989), and evidence suggesting biased engagement of TCR V_α and V_β in multiple sclerosis has been presented. However, more generalized TCR V_α and V_β gene usage is increasingly reported (e.g. Joshi et al., 1993) – and the position in EAE appears less clear, since diverse V_β gene usage has also been reported in murine EAE (Bell et al., 1993).

Many studies implicate both humoral and cellular immune responses to almost the entire range of known oligodendrocyte and myelin antigens in the pathogenesis of tissue damage in multiple sclerosis. However, consistent evidence for a single specific B or T cell reactivity, common to all patients with disease, is glaringly conspicuous by its absence.

Thus it may be seen that, while many lines of evidence implicate T cells, none truly indicates that multiple sclerosis is an exclusively T cell-mediated disease. It is an interesting parallel that the probable genetic association of multiple sclerosis with immunoglobulin heavy chain polymorphisms, even in conjunction with the almost universal presence of oligoclonal immuno-globulin bands, the presence of B cells in lesions, and variable antibody responses to oligodendrocyte–myelin antigens, has never precipitated any widespread proposal that multiple sclerosis is a B cell or antibody-mediated disorder.

In summary, T lymphocytes are undeniably important, but in this and indeed all normal and autoimmune reactions, it is essentially artificial – albeit occasionally helpful as a reductionist approach – to consider T and B cell mechanisms as separate entities. Each is wholly dependent on the other and no disease can properly be designated a T cell or an antibody-mediated disorder.

The current model, described below, confers upon the T cell the crucial but more defined and restricted role of initiating the disease process, both historically (in the peripheral immune system) and, at the time of CNS disease onset, by opening the blood–brain barrier, setting up an inflammatory focus, and creating the conditions necessary not only for oligodendrocyte and myelin damage, but also for the maintenance, propagation and amplification of oligodendrocyte–myelin specific immune responses, humoral and cellular.

The development of tissue damage in multiple sclerosis

Inconstant immune specificities, with reactivities to numerous myelin antigens, differing between patients with multiple sclerosis, or not differing from healthy controls, are difficult to reconcile with pathological and other evidence supporting not just an immune pathogenesis but, at least in the initial stages, highly targeted damage to the oligodendrocyte–myelin unit. Furthermore, any hypothetical account of tissue damage must also accommodate the fact that the target of this putative autoimmune process has traditionally been viewed as beyond the range of the immune system. Despite these difficulties, a coherent picture of the sequence of events culminating in demyelination is emerging which, while incomplete, can accommodate many of the complicated findings described above (Scolding *et al.*, 1994).

A useful starting point is immune privilege in the CNS (Barker and Billingham, 1977). This concept arose from a number of observations, starting with Ehrlich's finding that parenterally administered aniline dyes stained virtually all body tissues except the brain (Ehrlich, 1885). From this the idea of the blood–brain barrier was developed, physiologically separating central nervous tissue from the systemic circulation and – it was later argued – from systemic immune responses. The absence of rejection of mouse tissue transplants into rat brain (Murphy and Sturm, 1923), and the lack of direct lymphatic drainage and thus (it was thought) of circulating lymphocytes, depriving the CNS of an apparently essential requirement for the generation of immune responses (Sabin, 1916), consolidated this concept of the brain as immunologically naïve (see Chapter 1).

Although it has subsequently emerged that CNS transplants may be rejected (Sabin, 1916; Sloan *et al.*, 1991), that normal brain does contain a small population of passaging lymphocytes (Sabin, 1916; Matsui *et al.*, 1990) and may have its own lymphatic drainage (Bradbury *et al.*, 1981; Cserr and Knopf, 1992; Bradbury, 1993), the blood–brain barrier nevertheless affords significant protection to cerebral tissue, including oligodendrocytes and myelin, from immune mediators. It is therefore equally clear that two independent structural units – the blood–brain barrier and the oligodendrocyte–myelin complex – must each be disrupted in the full evolution of an inflammatory demyelinating focus within the brain. These elements of the development of tissue damage are likely to have separate mechanisms and may be considered separately (Scolding *et al.*, 1989, 1994).

The blood–brain barrier and brain inflammation
The blood–brain barrier is a complex structure composed of a layer of endothelial cells abutting a basement membrane interspersed with pericytes, around which a continuous covering is provided by extended glial cell foot

processes (the glia limitans (Bradbury, 1993; Selmaj, 1996)). It has recently been shown that microglial foot processes contribute significantly (up to 13%) to the glia limitans (Lassmann *et al.*, 1991a), though the majority is provided by astrocytes. The astrocyte role in barrier function is not structural, but in the induction of a barrier phenotype in endothelial cells (Janzer and Raff, 1987), which become linked by tight junctions, equip themselves with numerous mitochondria, and do not develop the fenestrations and pinocytotic vesicles which elsewhere effect transport of proteins into extravascular tissue.

Historically, the first indication that blood–brain barrier damage represented an important factor in myelin injury was provided by Dawson (1916), who proposed that "the disposition of the areas (of demyelination) in close relation to the blood vessels has led to the supposition that these play an important role in the genesis of the areas" (Dawson, 1916). Noting dilatation and engorgement of blood vessels in the early stages of disease, he concluded that "there is an abnormal permeability . . . by which an increased transudation of toxic lymph is made possible". The close relationship of demyelinated areas to blood vessels has repeatedly been confirmed (Lumsden, 1951; Fog, 1965; Adams, 1975).

Studies of EAE in rats have indicated that there is a close temporal relationship between the development of blood–brain barrier permeability and the onset of neurological signs (Oldendorf and Towner, 1974; Daniel *et al.*, 1983), and suppression of blood–brain barrier permeability (using an α_1-adrenergic antagonist, prazocin) protects against EAE (Goldmuntz *et al.*, 1986). In multiple sclerosis, dynamic MRI studies further support the primary role of impaired barrier function in the development of inflammatory demyelinating lesions – leakage of gadolinium–DTPA across the blood–brain barrier is the earliest identifiable change in the development of new lesions and occurs before the appearance of T_2-weighted white matter abnormalities which arise from increased tissue water content and correspond histologically to demyelination and scar formation (Koopmans *et al.*, 1989b; Hawkins *et al.*, 1990; Kermode *et al.*, 1990; Harris *et al.*, 1991).

Finally, ophthalmologic and fluorescein angiographic examination of the retinal vasculature demonstrates active retinal vein leakage and perivenous mononuclear cell cuffing in 25% of patients with optic neuritis and multiple sclerosis (Lightman *et al.*, 1987; Graham *et al.*, 1989). The absence of myelin in the retina indicates that vascular damage cannot be secondary to myelin injury – which inference is corroborated by the absence of blood–brain barrier damage in experimental animals after cuprizone-induced demyelination (Bakker and Ludwin, 1987). Later histopathological studies have confirmed and further characterized the blood–brain barrier changes found in acute and early lesions of multiple sclerosis (Gay and Esiri, 1991).

Lymphocyte–endothelial cell interactions
Several lines of evidence having shown blood–brain barrier damage to be the earliest event in the development of inflammatory demyelination, the mechanism responsible for this change can now be considered. A variety of pathological processes can induce blood–brain barrier breakdown (Greenwood, 1991). The absence of leukocytoclastic change distinguishes the pathological process in multiple sclerosis from vasculitides (Prineas,

1985); destruction of endothelial cells is difficult to demonstrate (Brown, 1978; Lassmann, 1983; Lassmann et al., 1994). In EAE, more subtle changes account for the loss of blood–brain barrier integrity, with increased energy-dependent trans-endothelial vesicular transport, and partial, reversible relaxation of endothelial tight junctions (Hirano et al., 1970; Claudio et al., 1989, 1990; Hawkins et al., 1990, 1991); a similar increase in endothelial vesicular transport has been described in multiple sclerosis (Brown, 1978).

Studies of the relationship between lymphocytes and the blood–brain barrier suggest how these functional changes might occur (Raine et al., 1990; Cross et al., 1991; Cross and Raine, 1991; Raine, 1991). It has become clear that the normal blood–brain barrier is not completely impermeable to lymphocytes and there is in health a small but continuous lymphocyte traffic into the brain (Matsui et al., 1990; Hickey et al., 1991). Passage across the blood–brain barrier depends solely on the lymphocyte activation state and not on antigen specificity. Small numbers of lymphocytes are therefore identifiable in normal brain and CSF (Matsui et al., 1990), and they may leave the CNS via channels ultimately draining into cervical lymphatics (Bradbury et al., 1981; Cserr and Knopf, 1992). This traffic is thought to afford the CNS a limited degree of immune surveillance.

The presence of clathrin-coated pits on endothelial cells interacting with adherent lymphocytes (Raine et al., 1990) suggests that specific receptor-ligand interactions represent the first stage of lymphocyte entry into the CNS (Goldstein et al., 1979). Cell adhesion molecules are the most likely candidates for mediating this lymphocyte–endothelial interaction (Lassmann et al., 1991b; Raine, 1994a; Cannella and Raine, 1995; Hartung et al., 1995). Endothelial cells constitutively display a variety of adhesion molecules, including intercellular adhesion molecule (ICAM)-1, lymphocyte function-associated antigen (LFA)-3, CD44, CD9 and very late antigen (VLA)-6. Intercellular adhesion molecule-1 binds avidly to the LFA-1 receptor on activated lymphocytes; the ligand for LFA-3 (CD2) is also exclusively distributed on T cells. Once adhesion is established, lymphocytes extend pseudopodia into the substance of endothelial cells close to (but not involving) tight junctions. Penetration is facilitated by lymphocyte-derived heparin sulphate endoglycosidase (Naparstek et al., 1984) and (previously) activated lymphocytes thus gain entry to the CNS parenchyma.

In inflammatory demyelinating disease, lymphocyte entry into the CNS is substantially increased, but only a very small proportion of infiltrating T cells is specific for oligodendrocyte–myelin antigens; the great majority is non-specific (Cross et al., 1990). This was directly demonstrated first in EAE, but lymphocytes recovered from lesions in post-mortem studies of patients with multiple sclerosis provide similar data: of 57 T cell clones generated from plaques, together with several hundred from CSF, none was specific for either of the major myelin antigens MBP and PLP (Hafler et al., 1987).

The critical initiating event in inflammatory demyelinating disease is therefore likely to be the specific interaction of a very small population of activated T lymphocytes, which have entered the CNS as part of normal T cell traffic, with target antigen encountered within the parenchyma (Scolding et al., 1989; Cross et al., 1991; Raine, 1991; Scolding et al., 1994). In the case of EAE, this antigen may comprise various peptides of MBP or PLP; in multiple sclerosis, the hypothetical target antigen(s) is (are) as yet unidentified. It is an important aspect of this hypothetical model, however, that the initial (and initiating) stage of T cell activation towards oligodendrocyte/myelin antigens, i.e. sensitization, is peripheral, not central: molecular mimicry or superantigen-related mechanisms are commonly invoked (Brock *et al.*, 1994; Wucherpfennig and Strominger, 1995). Substantial amplification of non-specific activated T cell passage through the blood–brain barrier follows and probably depends on this crucial T cell–oligodendrocyte–myelin antigen interaction (Cross *et al.*, 1991a; Cannella *et al.*, 1990, 1991; Raine, 1991).

Antigen presentation to activated lymphocytes must occur in the context of Class II MHC molecules on the surface of antigen-presenting cells. Since only microglia appear capable of constitutively expressing Class II antigen (Vass *et al.*, 1986; Hayes *et al.*, 1987), it may be inferred that these cells represent the principal antigen-presenting cell in inflammatory demyelination. Consistent with the suggestion that priming and activation of the infiltrating T cell has occurred peripherally are recent observations that microglia may act only as non-professional antigen-presenting cells (Sedgwick, 1997); indeed, some evidence now indicates that a regulatory role, stimulating apoptotic cell death in partially activated lymphocytes, is an important consequence of T cell interactions within the CNS (Ford *et al.*, 1996).

In multiple sclerosis, pro-inflammatory effects appear, however, to hold sway. Specific interactions between infiltrating, previously activated T lymphocyte and antigen-presenting microglia triggers the local release of cytokines synthesized by both cell types and these have the effect of amplifying local immune and inflammatory responses (see Lassmann *et al.*, 1991).

The development of the inflammatory lesion
A variety of cytokines has been identified immunocytochemically at the active edge of lesions in both multiple sclerosis and EAE, including interferon-γ, IL-2 and transforming growth factor-α (Selmaj *et al.*, 1991a; Navikas and Link, 1996; Merrill and Benveniste, 1996), all of which can activate endothelia and increase adhesion molecule expression and lymphocyte adherence. Local cytokine release up-regulates the constitutively expressed endothelial cell adhesion molecules ICAM-1 and LFA-3, and also induces new adhesion molecules including the classical addressin MECA-325 and VCAM-1 (see Yednock *et al.*, 1992), facilitating the further entry of circulating T cells.

Histopathological studies of the early stages of EAE confirm the increased expression of cell-adhesion molecules on endothelial surfaces within lesions, up-regulation of which correlates with increased T cell infiltration (Cannella *et al.*, 1991) and exacerbation of disease (Cannella *et al.*, 1990); furthermore, the entry of lymphocytes into the CNS in EAE can be blocked by treating rats with antibody directed against the lymphocyte ligand for VCAM-1, $\alpha_1\beta_1$ integrin (Yednock *et al.*, 1992), or against inducing cytokines such as TNF-α (Ruddle *et al.*, 1990; Selmaj *et al.*, 1991b); both manoeuvres prevent clinical disease. In multiple sclerosis, activated endothelial cells are found within lesions, with up-regulation of endothelial cell adhesion molecules (Ruddle *et al.*, 1990; Sobel *et al.*, 1990; Selmaj *et al.*, 1991b; Raine, 1994a; Cannella and

Raine, 1995; Navikas and Link, 1996). The pattern of adhesion molecule and activation markers is not different to that found in other inflammatory diseases (Raine, 1994a) – but the model described thus far may be representative of the initial stages of any CNS-specific immune reaction, and a lack of unique changes in multiple sclerosis is to be anticipated.

As well as recruiting T cells into lesions, local release of cytokines is likely to affect the integrity of the blood-brain barrier for soluble immune mediators (Martin et al., 1988; Brett et al., 1989). In EAE, breakdown of the blood–brain barrier to soluble molecules closely follows leukocyte entry into the CNS parenchyma (Simmons et al., 1987); subtle alterations in endothelial cells in the immediate vicinity of T lymphocytes are wholly supportive of a T cell effect mediated by cytokines (Claudio et al., 1989). Vesicular transport in endothelial cells and vascular permeability both increase in response to cytokines (Ellison et al., 1990; Simmons and Willenborg, 1990); these may also alter astrocyte function, and disturb their role in generating and maintaining barrier properties in endothelial cells (Vidovic et al., 1990; Greenwood, 1991; Abbott et al., 1992).

In summary, humoral and cellular immune mediators accumulate in the vicinity of the initiating T lymphocyte–microglia interaction; cytokine-mediated up-regulation of MHC expression (Navikas and Link, 1996) further increases the potential for local immune reactivity; the full repertoire of immune cells and mediators is therefore brought into the pro-inflammatory lesion, creating the local conditions necessary for myelin and oligodendrocyte injury. Which of these directly damages oligodendrocytes and myelin can now be discussed.

The consequences of brain inflammation
(i) *Oligodendrocyte–myelin damage: reversible injury.* As mentioned above, several lines of evidence indicate that anatomical demyelination with or without oligodendrocyte death may not be obligate requirements for the disruption of saltatory conduction; local inflammation alone appears sufficient temporarily to disturb myelin function and induce conduction block. The compressive effect of oedema represents one possible mechanism of temporary myelin sheath dysfunction in these circumstances, but the exposure of oligodendrocytes and myelin to immune and inflammatory mediators might also account for reversible injury.

In vitro studies have shown that injury of the oligodendrocyte–myelin unit is not necessarily an 'all or nothing' process, of lethal or no effect. Reversible damage, with transient injury of oligodendrocytes followed by complete recovery, may be induced by a number of agents. At appropriate concentrations, *complement* or T cell-derived *perforin*, for example, can each induce a rapid and substantial rise in intracellular calcium and a fall in cellular ATP content (Scolding et al., 1989b; Jones et al., 1991). During complement injury, the initial calcium transient may be followed by a series of calcium oscillations (Wood et al., 1993), while ATP levels return towards normal over 30–40 min of monophasic attack. The calcium changes are directly associated with changes in the morphological appearance of the cell surface which reflect a protection or recovery mechanism. Damaging membrane pores formed by either of these injurious agents are removed by concentration in vesicles which are shed from the cell surface (Figure 2.6).

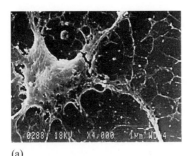
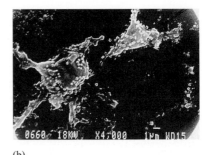

(a)   (b)

Figure 2.6 Reversible oligodendrocyte injury by complement. Cultured rat oligodendrocytes are shown in scanning electron micrographs. Normally, the surface is smooth (a); within minutes of attack by sublethal concentrations of complement, vesicles appear on the cell surface (b). These are rapidly shed from the cell surface; they are rich in complement membrane attack complexes and represent the means by which oligodendrocytes are able to protect themselves against complement injury.

In the peripheral nervous system, calcium flux in myelinated fibres causes conduction block without Schwann cell death (Smith and Hall, 1988); calcium ionophores also cause demyelination in the CNS (Smith and Hall, 1994). Oligodendrocytes possess a number of cell-specific calcium-dependent enzymes, including a neutral protease responsible for MBP degradation (Banik *et al.*, 1985; Chakrabarti *et al.*, 1988; Banik, 1992) and a protein kinase (Turner *et al.*, 1982), and calcium changes are likely significantly to disturb normal metabolism and function of the oligodendrocyte–myelin unit. Reversible oligodendrocyte injury by complement membrane attack complexes therefore represents one potential cellular substrate for temporary disruption of myelin function.

Tumour necrosis factor may also induce transient oligodendrocyte injury, with some evidence in cultured oligodendrocytes exposed to TNF-α of depressed metabolic activity without loss of membrane integrity (D'Souza *et al.*, 1996b), and indeed of reversible effects on differentiation (Agresti *et al.*, 1996), although *in vitro* studies show no effect on conduction in myelinated axons (Dugandzija and Shrager, 1995; Smith and Felts, 1997). By contrast, *nitric oxide* has been shown capable of inducing reversible conduction block (Redford *et al.*, 1997) and this too may therefore be involved in transient injury to the oligodendrocyte–myelin unit.

The possibility that inflammatory mediators may reversibly injure oligodendrocytes and temporarily disturb myelin function *in vivo* in multiple sclerosis has therefore to be considered. Of course, this is not to suggest that each is not also capable in higher doses, or different circumstances, of causing irreversible injury and oligodendrocyte cell death. While there is no direct evidence for the involvement of T cell-derived perforin in oligodendrocyte injury in multiple sclerosis, complement (leaking into the CNS across the poorly functioning blood–brain barrier and locally produced (Morgan and Gasque, 1996)), TNF (produced by infiltrating lymphocytes and activated resident microglia (Probert and Selmaj, 1997)) and nitric oxide have all been implicated (Zajicek *et al.*, 1992; Butt and Jenkins, 1994; Scolding *et al.*, 1994; Redford *et al.*, 1995).

(ii) *Antibody, complement and oligodendrocytes*. Conventionally, complement involvement in pathological events requires local activation of the normally quiescent (or rather, closely controlled) complement cascade, often by fixed, target cell-specific antibodies. In parallel with studies of T cell specificities, data concerning myelin–oligodendrocyte specific antibodies in multiple sclerosis are by no means lacking. Circulating PLP-, MAG- and MOG-reactive B cells are commoner in multiple sclerosis than healthy controls (Baig *et al.*, 1991; Sun, 1993). There is little evidence of altered circulating antibody reactivities in multiple sclerosis, but in CSF, antibodies or B cell reactivities to MOG (Xiao *et al.*, 1991), MAG (Moller *et al.*, 1989), MBP (Cruz *et al.*, 1987; Link *et al.*, 1990; Olsson *et al.*, 1990) and PLP (Warren and Catz, 1994) are identifiable. MOG- and MAG-specific antibodies can cause complement-dependent oligodendrocyte injury and demyelination *in vitro* and in animal models (Linington *et al.*, 1988, 1989b; Scolding, unpublished observations).

Cerebrospinal fluid oligoclonal IgG shows very little reactivity overall to CNS antigens (Cruz *et al.*, 1987) and the specificity of the greater proportion remains undetermined (Olsson, 1992; Sun, 1993). Nevertheless, the remarkably consistent and indeed constant presence of oligoclonal immunoglobulin bands in multiple sclerosis further implicates B cell processes.

An additional and apparently disease-specific mechanism of complement involvement in multiple sclerosis has been suggested, largely based on *in vitro* studies. Rat oligodendrocytes activate complement in the absence of antibody and are thereafter susceptible to complement-mediated damage on exposure to normal syngeneic serum (Scolding *et al.*, 1989a). The same has not been shown with human (cultured) oligodendrocytes (Ruijs *et al.*, 1990; Zajicek *et al.*, 1995). Nevertheless, human oligodendrocytes do not constitutively express many of the important and otherwise widely distributed membrane regulatory proteins which protect against homologous complement attack (Scolding *et al.*, 1998). Furthermore, it has been reported that complement activation occurs within the human CNS in areas of non-inflammatory blood–brain barrier breakdown (Lindsberg *et al.*, 1996). The burden of evidence at present suggests, however, that while complement is likely to be involved in the development of tissue damage in multiple sclerosis, activation is more likely to occur via conventional antibody-dependent classical pathway.

Intrathecal complement activation occurs in patients with isolated or recurrent episodes of demyelination, resulting in the appearance of the short-lived activation products C3a and C4a in CSF (Jans *et al.*, 1984), and a reduction in spinal fluid levels of native complement components consumed by activation (Morgan *et al.*, 1984; Sanders *et al.*, 1986). The concentration of C9 increases with improved clinical status resulting from treatment with methylprednisolone (Compston *et al.*, 1986), the efficacy of which is related to a reduction in tissue oedema (Kesselring *et al.*, 1989) and a restoration of blood–brain barrier function (Miller *et al.*, 1992). Immunocytochemical studies show deposits of C9 and complement membrane attack complexes in a perivascular distribution in association with demyelinated lesions (Compston *et al.*, 1989); more recent investigations demonstrate C9 neoantigen in areas of active demyelination and within macrophages actively phagocytosing myelin (Storch *et al.*, 1998). Complement deposits are demonstrable in EAE (Linington *et al.*, 1989a), where the role of complement in myelin injury has been defined by complement-depletion studies (Linington *et al.*, 1989b; Piddlesden *et al.*, 1991, 1994). Finally, studies of CSF from patients with inflammatory demyelination reveal the presence of oligodendrocyte-derived, complement-rich vesicles, implying reversible complement attack of these cells *in vivo* (Scolding *et al.*, 1989b).

(iii) *Tumor necrosis factor-α*. Evidence that TNF-α and the related cytokine lymphotoxin (TNF-β) cause selective oligodendrocyte death *in vitro* (Selmaj and Raine, 1988; Selmaj *et al.*, 1991c) has been disputed (Satoh *et al.*, 1991; Zajicek *et al.*, 1992; Wood *et al.*, 1993; Dugandzija and Shrager, 1995; Vartanian *et al.*, 1995). However, deleterious changes affecting oligoden-drocyte metabolic processes, nuclear morphology and myelin extensions are repeatedly described (Jenkins and Ikeda, 1992; Butt and Jenkins, 1994; D'Souza *et al.*, 1996). Tumour necrosis factor and lymphotoxin are also present in lesions from patients with multiple sclerosis (Hofman *et al.*, 1989; Selmaj *et al.*, 1991a; Merrill and Benveniste, 1996), and CSF concentrations of TNF have been correlated with disease progression and severity (Beck *et al.*, 1988; Sharief and Hentges, 1991). Finally, anti-TNF antibody treatment of experimental animals prevents the development of EAE (Beck *et al.*, 1988; Ruddle *et al.*, 1990; Selmaj *et al.*, 1991b). TNF-α has a multitude of other activities (Vassalli, 1992; Probert and Selmaj, 1997), including activation of endothelial cells (Brett *et al.*, 1989), up-regulation of ICAM-1 and blood–brain barrier disruption (Brett *et al.*, 1989; Redford *et al.*, 1995; Navikas and Link, 1996; Selmaj, 1996), suggesting other possible roles for this key cytokine. Interestingly, TNF knockout models suggest a potent anti-inflammatory role for this cytokine (Liu *et al.*, 1998).

(iv) *Nitric oxide and other mediators of oligodendrocyte injury*. Other soluble inflammatory mediators might also contribute to myelin and oligodendrocyte injury and death. Phagocyte-associated factors, such as free oxygen radicals and proteolytic enzymes have also been implicated in oligodendrocyte–myelin damage (Kim and Kim, 1991), as have excitotoxins such as glutamate (Oka *et al.*, 1993; Gallo *et al.*, 1996).

More specifically, there is an increasing emphasis on the possible role of nitric oxide (Parkinson *et al.*, 1997); again this is toxic to oligodendrocytes *in vitro* (Mitrovic *et al.*, 1994, 1995) and microglial toxicity to oligodendrocytes is at least in part mediated through nitric oxide (Merrill *et al.*, 1993). Nitric oxide is capable of inducing reversible conduction block in demyelinated axons and may also damage axons (Redford, *et al.*, 1997)

As described in a little more detail above (p . 40), lymphocytes may also contribute directly to oligodendrocyte and myelin injury. Infiltrating γδ T lymphocytes may lyse HSP-expressing oligodendrocytes (Selmaj *et al.*, 1992; Freedman *et al.*, 1997). Similarly, *fas* ligand-expressing lymphocytes may be capable of killing *fas*-positive oligodendrocytes in multiple sclerosis lesions (D'Souza *et al.*, 1996b). Microglia in lesions also express *fas* ligand. *fas*-mediated oligodendrocyte death (*in vitro*) shows no features of apoptosis (D'Souza *et al.*, 1996b) (unlike *fas* killing of other cell types); dying oligodendrocytes *in situ* in multiple sclerosis do not show evidence of apoptosis (Bonetti and Raine, 1997).

(v) *The consequences of inflammation: a summary*. It is therefore tempting to suggest that, in the early stages of inflammatory demyelination, a T cell/microglial interaction causes local cytokine release, in turn precipitating disturbed blood–brain barrier function and the accumulation of soluble and cellular inflammatory mediators. Injury and impaired function of the oligodendrocyte–myelin unit follows exposure to the latter, and this may account for conduction block in myelinated axons.

Two factors may contribute towards the selectivity of cell damage. The first, not dependent on immunological specificity and commonly termed the 'bystander effect', is the apparent vulnerability of oligodendrocytes – or relative robustness of other cell types. Selective damage to cultured oligodendrocytes is reported with complement, TNF, proteases, glutamate, nitric oxide and other free oxygen radicals. Rather than suggesting multiple defects in the normal cellular mechanisms protecting against each of these agents, this may rather reflect the extreme metabolic stress imposed on the oligodendrocyte by its unique specialized function, myelination: thus, minor additional insults during active myelin synthesis may induce irreversible damage. The second is dependent on the immune system. It is overwhelmingly likely that the T cell reactivity responsible for initially generating local inflammation is (i) directed against oligodendrocyte or myelin antigens and (ii) accompanied by B cell reactions against the same targets. Gaining access to their target(s) through the leaky blood–brain barrier, antibodies binding to their target then activate complement, generating damaging membrane attack complexes and also opsonizing oligodendrocytes and myelin for macrophages and activated microglia.

Microglia, demyelination and oligodendrocyte injury
Whilst inflammatory mediators and, perhaps, oedema may account for potentially reversible myelin and oligodendrocyte injury, it is likely that phagocytosis of myelin by macrophages, together with oligodendrocyte death from a variety of insults, accounts for irreversible demyelination and its clinical sequelae. Classical histopathological accounts of multiple sclerosis described 'gitter cells' (Dawson, 1916), foamy, lipid-laden cells cytoplasm in close proximity to degenerating myelin sheaths. Repeated histopathological studies have left little doubt that these phagocytes are responsible for stripping away myelin lamellae from the sheath, ultimately denuding the axon (Lampert, 1967; Prineas, 1985) – as indeed illustrated by Babinski in some of the earliest accounts of the pathology of disseminated sclerosis. In the absence of immunohistological markers distinguishing macrophages from activated microglia, the relative contributions of resident microglia and infiltrating macrophages to myelin phagocytosis remain unresolved; both are probably involved.

In vitro studies indicate that resting microglia or macrophages may be induced to adhere to oligodendrocytes, and to phagocytose and ingest myelin, by the addition of oligodendrocyte specific antibodies. Activated macrophages and microglia will behave similarly in the presence of complement alone (Scolding and Compston, 1991; Zajicek *et al.*, 1992). A role in cell death is also possible: TNF-α expressed on the microglial cell surface may be considerably more toxic to oligodendrocytes than soluble TNF (Zajicek *et al.*, 1992).

Neuropathological studies provide some corroboration of the role for antibody and complement in myelin opsonization suggested by these *in vitro* findings. Prineas and Connell (1978) described coated pits on phagocytes within plaques, implying receptor mediated endocytosis; the presence of immunoglobulins coating the macrophage surface suggested a role for specific antibody. Gay and Esiri (1991) identified complement components and immunoglobulin within phagocytic cells in active lesions.

Axon loss in multiple sclerosis
The mechanisms of axon damage remain largely unexplored (Scolding and Franklin, 1998). Although the recent pathological studies suggest damage by inflammatory processes in the acute phase (Ferguson *et al.*, 1997; Trapp *et al.*, 1998), functionally relevant loss seems unlikely to explain the pathophysiology of relapsing–remitting multiple sclerosis. An attractive possibility is that axons which have become demyelinated are no longer robust. In lesions with persistent, demyelination-induced, conduction block, axons may degenerate as a direct consequence of their enforced and prolonged electrical silence – as is known to happen throughout the CNS, including electrically inactive retinal ganglion cells (Lipton, 1986). Oligodendrocytes secrete trophic factors important for neuronal survival (Meyer-Franke *et al.*, 1995), and their loss might also contribute directly to secondary axonal atrophy (Raine and Cross, 1989). Thus it is possible that axon degeneration in multiple sclerosis is at least in part a consequence of persistent functional impairment caused by long-standing demyelination, rather than its pathophysiological cause (Figure 2.3). This possibility adds to the rationale for pursuing therapeutic remyelination strategies (see below) (Scolding, 1997; Scolding and Franklin, 1999). Attempting to reconstruct normal CNS cellular environments by glial cell transplantation may, by re-populating lesions with oligodendrocytes and by encouraging remyelination, be the most appropriate way to ensure axon preservation in multiple sclerosis.

Immune reactivity in multiple sclerosis

Can the variability of T and B cell immune specificities also be explained by and incorporated into this model? At the time of the initial bout of CNS inflammation and oligodendrocyte–myelin injury, oligodendrocyte and myelin antigens are released into an area containing large numbers of activated T lymphocytes and microglial cells with antigen-presenting capacity. Secondary cellular and humoral immune reactions directed against antigens from and on myelinating cells would thereby be generated. Epitope spread is now a well-described and accepted phenomenon (Lehmann *et al.*, 1992, 1993; Ransohoff *et al.*, 1994; Vanderlugt and Miller, 1996), clearly demonstrated in EAE (Yu *et al.*, 1996a, b), where a variety of cellular and humoral immune reactions against PLP, MOG and other CNS antigens all occur in rats initially inoculated only with purified MBP (Linington and Lassmann, 1987; McCarron *et al.*, 1990). It is proposed that this secondary immunization plays a crucial role in sustaining persistent inflammatory demyelination, and direct evidence that this occurs during the development of multiple sclerosis is beginning to emerge (Tuohy *et al.*, 1997).

Episodes of blood–brain barrier disturbance would consistently amplify the inflammatory process once the lymphocyte repertoire includes populations of T and B cells specific for myelin antigens. Imaging studies reveal that 20 or more episodes of barrier leakage may occur annually in the individual patient, and transient leakage may recur repeatedly at the same site leading to more chronic and persistent barrier compromise (Miller *et al.*, 1988; Koopmans *et al.*, 1989a; Thompson *et al.*, 1990).

The low levels of specific cellular and humoral immune responses directed against a number of oligodendrocyte–myelin antigens, including MBP, PLP-galactocerebroside and MOG, found variably in patients with multiple sclerosis (see above), can therefore be explained as a secondary but nevertheless crucial phenomenon. Combinations of antibodies and T lymphocytes directed against different oligodendrocyte–myelin antigens might assume pathogenetic significance in different patients at different times or stages of disease; those patients with a particular MHC and TCR genetic background may be more likely to mount secondary responses to particular encephalitogenic peptides and so to develop recurrent episodes of inflammatory demyelination.

A summary: the pathogenesis of multiple sclerosis

The following sequence of events – some probable rather than definite – therefore emerges (Figure 2.3). At the onset, T lymphocytes are activated in the periphery. The commonest suggestion is that this crucial immunological episode centres upon an antigen carried by contagion, probably viral and probably common, the (later) idiosyncratic cascade depending on the host gene complement rather than the organism. The responsible antigen may mimic an oligodendrocyte–myelin epitope (Wucherpfennig and Strominger, 1995).

At a later stage – probably much later and perhaps as a consequence of non-specific reactivation of this immune response following viral infection or other events – a small number of these activated T cells, in common with other circulating activated T cells, traverse the blood–brain barrier. Within the perivascular brain parenchyma, they encounter the unknown target self-antigen presented to the TCR by perivascular macrophages and microglia. This interaction represents the initiating nidus of focal CNS inflammation, promoting local maintenance and propagation of the originally systemic immune response. Cytokine production up-regulates expression of adhesion molecules on circulating lymphocytes and blood–brain barrier endothelia, and directly increases the permeability of the barrier, causing increased binding and migration of inflammatory cells into brain parenchyma, together with an influx of humoral immune mediators, culminating in the formation of a perivascular hypercellular inflammatory infiltrate.

Oligodendrocyte and myelin damage is contingent upon this T cell-dependent event and probably involves several mechanisms. This, among the repertoire of humoral and cellular immune mediators accumulating in the vicinity of the initiating T lymphocyte : microglia interaction, is responsible for damaging oligodendrocytes and myelin may prove impossible to resolve. In this early phase, myelin function might be disturbed simply by the compressive effect of oedema. The restoration of blood–brain integrity might subsequently allow oligodendrocyte recovery and restitution of saltatory conduction through myelinated fibres. Animal models suggest that antibodies directed against oligodendrocyte–myelin surface components are important for targeting damage, activating complement and opsonizing for macrophage/microglial attack. Others have proposed non-specific bystander damage by cytotoxic cytokines, enzymes and oxygen radicals secreted by activated T cells and microglia, including TNF-α, lymphotoxin, nitric oxide and myelin-degrading proteases. Ultimately, the damaged myelin sheath is engulfed and removed by microglia; astrocytes invade, hypertrophy and proliferate, and the classical gliotic oligodendrocytopenic demyelinated plaque is formed.

Future approaches to treating multiple sclerosis: immunomodulation and repair

As mentioned above, the details of emerging and future immunotherapeutic approaches, and indeed the strategies underlying their development, demand their own chapter; it is nevertheless valid at this point to ask a simple question: has an improved understanding of the background to tissue damage in multiple sclerosis (see Figure 2.3) led to the development of useful and novel immunotherapeutic approaches in multiple sclerosis? The short and sad answer is obvious to the practising clinician. Experimental allergic encephalomyelitis is one of the very few animal models of pensionable age (Rivers et al., 1933), and yet not a single treatment, among the innumerable agents ameliorating, curing or preventing EAE, has successfully travelled from laboratory to clinic.

This said, the pathogenetic model described above has only recently emerged, and requires (and receives) further refinement. It is nevertheless worth briefly mentioning how a number of putative new treatments now being assessed have been directly based upon it. T cell:endothelial interactions represent an obvious target for therapeutic intervention. Agents interfering with this relationship might inhibit T lymphocyte entry into the CNS, abrogating the subsequent inflammatory cascade, while the unique profile of cell adhesion molecules carried by cerebral endothelia could allow tissue specificity for this approach. Studies of EAE in rodents have illustrated the potential of therapeutic antibodies directed against the adhesion molecule $\alpha_4\beta_1$ integrin – inflammation is blocked and clinical disease prevented – and phase 1 trials adopting this strategy are now underway.

Treatment of experimental animals with TCR-derived antigens, aimed at generating immune responses directed against encephalitogenic T lymphocytes of defined TCR specificity, or with antibodies against MBP-peptide specific TCRs, have produced encouraging results, although a similar approach cannot be advocated in multiple sclerosis until those peptides important in the initial T cell:microglial interactions which precipitate blood–brain barrier impairment have been elucidated – and the important phenomenon of epitope spread may indicate a poor future for strategies ultimately based on the grail-like 'multiple sclerosis antigen'. This said, copolymer-1 or glatirimer acetate, a random polymer which suppresses EAE induction in a number of species, has been reported to have a statistically significant impact upon both relapse frequency (approximately one-third reduction) and disability in a controlled trial (Johnson *et al.*, 1998), and further investigations are underway. At the time of writing, it does not have a product licence in Europe.

Less specific depletion of lymphocytes or their subpopulations, using cytotoxic monoclonal antibodies which have been 'humanized' (to help prevent host responses against the therapeutic antibody), are currently under investigation (Moreau *et al.*, 1994). Although these studies are at an early stage, the initial results – assessing disease activity both clinically (number of relapses) and radiologically (using MRI) – are promising. However, other lymphocyte-specific monoclonal antibodies, directed against the surface markers CD4 (which targets lymphocytes) and CD3 (all T cells), assessed in larger studies, showed no benefit (van Oosten *et al.*, 1997).

The repair of demyelinated lesions

The historical concept of the brain as a tissue almost uniquely incapable of repair is commonly attributed to Cajal. In fact, the opposite is closer to the truth. Cajal summarized others' assertions of the irreparability of brain damage: "everything may die, nothing may regenerate", but went on to suggest, on the basis of his own extensive experimental work, that "this defective capacity for regeneration does not depend on essential, fatal and unchangeable conditions ... the central neurones (do) possess *ab initio* the capacity of rebuilding their structure" (Cajal, 1913). His sanguine view has been revisited, intensely scrutinized and substantially confirmed in recent years. This is true writ large and, more specifically, in multiple sclerosis; there is increasing evidence for significant but ill-sustained remyelination in a minority of early lesions (Prineas *et al.*, 1993; Raine and Wu, 1993). Taken in conjunction with a substantial body of work over the last two decades showing clearly that experimentally demyelinated lesions in animals can be successfully repaired by the transplantation of glial cells (Duncan, 1996; Rosenbluth, 1996; Franklin and Blakemore, 1997), these findings have led to increasing optimism that strategies to supplement myelin repair may in the future prove valuable in patients with multiple sclerosis (Scolding, 1997).

Successful remyelination in the rodent can be established by the transplantation of expanded populations of neonatal oligodendrocyte progenitor cells (Groves *et al.*, 1993). These progenitors, originally isolated from and characterized in cultures derived from neonatal rat optic nerve, have been intensively studied (Figure 2.7); they possess a unique morphology and immunostaining phenotype, are proliferative and, at least *in vitro*, exhibit a bipotential capacity for differentiation into either oligodendrocytes or a type of astrocyte originally named the 'type 2' astrocyte (Raff *et al.*, 1983).

Controversy persisted for many years after the (*in vitro*) description of the oligodendrocyte-type 2 astrocyte (O-2A) progenitor, on the question of its relevance *in vivo*, but recent evidence suggests a counterpart does exist *in vivo*, although the astrocyte differentiation pathway may rarely be engaged

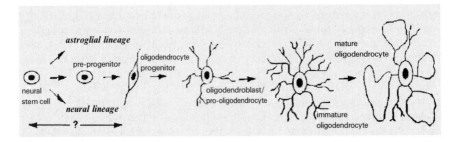

Figure 2.7 The lineage of oligodendrocytes. Mature oligodendrocytes, with a number of branching processes, each of which may elaborate myelin membranes, develop in a number of defined stages. The earliest clearly characterized precursor is the proliferative, bipolar (so-called) O-2A progenitor (see Figure 2.2a); more primitive cells than this are currently the subject of intense research.

(Levison and Goldman, 1993) – perhaps particularly or even exclusively during injury, rather than in health or normal development (Franklin and Blakemore, 1995; Skoff, 1996).

A very similar progenitor is present in cultures derived from the adult rodent CNS (FfrenchConstant and Raff, 1986), and while attempts to extrapolate these observations to human glial cell biology have proved more difficult, a similar proliferative oligodendrocyte progenitor has now been described *in vitro* and *in situ*, in the adult human brain (Scolding *et al.*, 1995). Although this observation has obvious relevance for human demyelinating disease, it has yet to be shown that this cell is capable of myelination *in vitro* or *in vivo* in experimental animals, or whether it is responsible for partial remyelination described in multiple sclerosis – although the progenitor has now been identified in acute multiple sclerosis lesions, increasing the likelihood of its involvement with myelin repair (Figure 2.8).

Schwann cells represent a potential alternative source of myelinating cells for transplantation. Despite their origin and home in the peripheral nervous system, they have been shown to contribute to spontaneous (central) remyelination in multiple sclerosis (Feigin and Popoff, 1966) and, in transplantation studies in the rodent, have been shown to be capable not only of forming compact myelin around axons, but also of restoring saltatory conduction (Blakemore *et al.*, 1987; Baronvan Evercooren *et al.*, 1992; Felts and Smith, 1992; Honmou *et al.*, 1996). Human Schwann cells may readily be prepared and expanded from peripheral nerve biopsy (Rutkowski *et al.*, 1995; Van den Berg *et al.*, 1995).

Clearly, repairing numerous, disseminated lesions in patients with multiple sclerosis is unrealistic. However, certain specifically-sited lesions cause disproportionately severe functional disturbance and disability. The optic nerve is one example; others include the spinal cord and the superior cerebellar peduncle. Targeting such lesions singly for interventions, using direct injection of remyelinating cells or, conceivably, pro-myelination growth factors (Woodruff and Franklin, 1997) might present the optimum prospect of allowing detectable and useful benefit following limited and defined intervention. Another alternative is non-targeted systemic treatment: Rodriguez and his group have shown clearly a striking effect of systemic

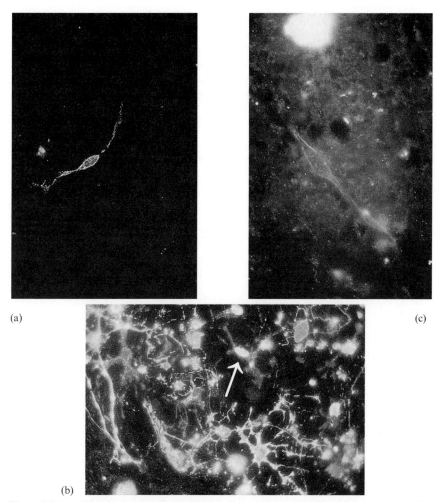

(a)

(c)

(b)

Figure 2.8 A proliferative human oligodendrocyte progenitor can be cultured from normal adult tissue and is present in multiple sclerosis lesions. In cell cultures prepared from normal adult human white matter, small numbers of bipolar cells with the morphological, immunocyto-chemical and behavioural characteristics of immature oligodendrocyte progenitors are found (a); such cells proliferate when grown on human astrocyte monolayers (b). Shown using a different staining technique (identifying the platelet-derived growth factor receptor), similar progenitors are also present in acute inflammatory lesions of multiple sclerosis (c).

immunoglobulins in enhancing experimental myelin repair (Rodriguez and Lennon, 1990; Rodriguez and Miller, 1994).

Hazards and uncertainties remain. The importance of axon loss is increasingly recognized and must be yet further defined before the potential value of remyelinating therapies can be elucidated. The inflammatory process must also be, if not completely halted, at least seriously impeded. Nevertheless, anticipated therapeutic advances may present a new opportunity to exploit an immunologically quiescent environment, and to examine the possibility that the limited endogenous capacity for remyelination might be enhanced using appropriate soluble factors, and/or by implanting human oligodendrocyte progenitors or Schwann cells maintained and expanded in tissue culture. In this way, the realistic prospect is presented that experimental strategies already under assessment might yield treatments that prevent progressive deterioration and permanent disability by the combined approach of protecting oligodendrocytes and myelin, and promoting myelin repair.

References

Abbott, N. J., Revest, P. A. and Romero, I. A. (1992) Astrocyte–endothelial interaction: physiology and pathology. *Neuropathol. Appl. Neurobiol.*, **18**, 424–433.

Acha, O. H., Steinman, L. and McDevitt, H. O. (1989) T cell receptors in murine autoimmune diseases. *Annu. Rev. Immunol.*, **7**, 371–405.

Adams, C. W. (1975) The onset and progression of the lesion in multiple sclerosis. *J. Neurol. Sci.*, **25**, 165–182.

Agresti, C., Durso, D. and Levi, G. (1996) Reversible inhibitory effects of interferon-gamma and tumour necrosis factor-alpha on oligodendroglial lineage cell proliferation and differentiation *in vitro*. *Eur. J. Neurosci.*, **8**, 1106–1116.

Allen, I. V. (1991) Pathology of multiple sclerosis. In *McAlpine's Multiple Sclerosis* (Matthews, W. B., ed.). London: Churchill Livingstone.

Antel, J. P., Arnason, B. G. and Medof, M. E. (1979) Suppressor cell function in multiple sclerosis: correlation with clinical disease activity. *Ann. Neurol.*, **5**, 338–342.

Antel, J. P., Freedman, M. S., Brodovsky, S., Francis, G. S. and Duquette, P. (1989) Activated suppressor cell function in severely disabled patients with multiple sclerosis. *Ann. Neurol.*, **25**, 204–207.

Asselman, P., Chadwick, D. W. and Marsden, D. C. (1975) Visual evoked responses in the diagnosis and management of patients suspected of multiple sclerosis. *Brain*, **98**, 261–282.

Baig, S., Olsson, T., Yu, P. J., Hojeberg, B., Cruz, M. and Link, H. (1991) Multiple sclerosis: cells secreting antibodies against myelin-associated glycoprotein are present in cerebrospinal fluid. *Scand. J. Immunol.*, **33**, 73–79.

Bakker, D. A. and Ludwin, S. K. (1987) Blood–brain barrier permeability during Cuprizone-induced demyelination. Implications for the pathogenesis of immune-mediated demyelinating diseases. *J. Neurol. Sci.*, **78**, 125–137.

Banik, N. L. (1992) Pathogenesis of myelin breakdown in demyelinating diseases: role of proteolytic enzymes. *Crit. Rev. Neurobiol.*, **6**, 257–271.

Banik, N. L., McAlhaney, W .W. and Hogan, E. L. (1985) Calcium-stimulated proteolysis in myelin: evidence for a Ca^{2+}-activated neutral proteinase associated with purified myelin of rat CNS. *J. Neurochem.*, **45**, 581–588.

Barker, C. F. and Billingham, R. E. (1977) Immunologically privileged sites. *Adv. Immunol.*, **25**, 1–54.

Barnes, D., Hughes, R. C., Morris, R. W., Wadejones, O., Brown, P., Britton, T. *et al.* (1997) Randomised trial of oral and intravenous methylprednisolone in acute relapses of multiple sclerosis. *Lancet*, **349**, 902–906.

Barnes, D., Munro, P. M., Youl, B. D., Prineas, J. W. and McDonald, W. I. (1991) The longstanding MS lesion. A quantitative MRI and electron microscopic study. *Brain*, **114**, 1271–1280.

Baronvan Evercooren, A., Gansmuller, A., Duhamel, E., Pascal, F. and Gumpel, M. (1992) Repair of a myelin lesion by Schwann cells transplanted in the adult mouse spinal cord. *J. Neuroimmunol.*, **40**, 235–242.

Beall, S. S., Biddison, W. E., McFarlin, D. E., McFarland, H. F. and Hood, L. E. (1993) Susceptibility for multiple sclerosis is determined, in part, by inheritance of a 175-kb region of the TcR V beta chain locus and HLA class II genes. *J. Neuroimmunol.*, **45**, 53–60.

Beck, J., Rondot, P., Catinot, L., Falcoff, E., Kirchner, H. and Wietzerbin, J. (1988) Increased production of interferon gamma and tumor necrosis factor precedes clinical manifestation in multiple sclerosis: do cytokines trigger off exacerbations? *Acta Neurol. Scand.*, **78**, 318–323.

Beck, R. W., Cleary, P. A., Anderson, M. M. J., Keltner, J. L., Shults, W. T., Kaufman, D. I., *et al.* (1992) A randomized, controlled trial of corticosteroids in the treatment of acute optic neuritis. The Optic Neuritis Study Group (see comments). *N. Engl. J. Med.*, **326**, 581–588.

Beck, R. W., Cleary, P. A., Trobe, J. D., Kaufman, D. I., Kupersmith, M. J., Paty, D. W. *et al.* (1993) The effect of corticosteroids for acute optic neuritis on the subsequent development of multiple sclerosis. The Optic Neuritis Study Group (see comments). *N. Engl. J. Med.*, **329**, 1764–1769.

Beck, R. W. (1995) The optic neuritis treatment trial: three-year follow-up results (letter). *Arch. Ophthalmol.*, **113**, 136–137.

Bell, R. B., Lindsey, J. W., Sobel, R. A., Hodgkinson, S. and Steinman, L. (1993) Diverse T cell receptor V beta gene usage in the central nervous system in experimental allergic encephalomyelitis. *J. Immunol.*, **150**, 4085–4092.

Bellamy, A. S., Calder, V. L., Feldmann, M. and Davison, A. N. (1985) The distribution of interleukin-2 receptor bearing lymphocytes in multiple sclerosis: evidence for a key role of activated lymphocytes. *Clin. Exp. Immunol.*, **61**, 248–256.

Ben, N. A., Wekerle, H., Cohen, I. R. (1981) The rapid isolation of clonable antigen-specific T lymphocyte lines capable of mediating autoimmune encephalomyelitis. *Eur. J. Immunol.*, **11**, 195–199.

Benedikz, J., Magnusson, H. and Guthmundsson, G. (1994) Multiple sclerosis in Iceland, with observations on the alleged epidemic in the Faroe Islands. *Ann. Neurol.*, **36 (Suppl 2)**, S175–S179

Blakemore, W. F., Crang, A. J. and Patterson, R. C. (1987) Schwann cell remyelination of CNS axons following injection of cultures of CNS cells into areas of persistent demyelination. *Neurosci. Lett.*, **77**, 20–24.

Bonetti, B. and Raine, C. S. (1997) Multiple sclerosis: oligodendrocytes display cell death-related molecules *in situ* but do not undergo apoptosis. *Ann. Neurol.*, **42**, 74–84.

Boolell, M., Gepi-Attee, S., Gingell, J. C. and Allen, M. J. (1996) Sildenafil, a novel effective oral therapy for male erectile dysfunction. *Br. J. Urol.*, **78**, 257–261.

Booss, J., Esiri, M. M., Tourtellotte, W. W. and Mason, D. Y. (1983) Immunohistological analysis of T lymphocyte subsets in the central nervous system in chronic progressive multiple sclerosis. *J. Neurol. Sci.*, **62**, 219–232.

Bradbury, M. W. (1993) The blood–brain barrier. *Exp. Physiol.*, **78**, 453–472.

Bradbury, M. W., Cserr, H. F. and Westrop, R. J. (1981) Drainage of cerebral interstitial fluid into deep cervical lymph of the rabbit. *Am. J. Physiol.*, **240**, F329–F336

Brett, J., Gerlach, H., Nawroth, P., Steinberg, S., Godman, G. and Stern, D. (1989) Tumor necrosis factor/cachectin increases permeability of endothelial cell monolayers by a mechanism involving regulatory G proteins. *J. Exp. Med.*, **169**, 1977–1991.

Brock, S., Veromaa, T., Weissman, I. L., Gijbels, K. and Steinman, L. (1994) Infection and multiple sclerosis: a possible role for superantigens? *Trends Microbiol.*, **2**, 250–254.

Brown, W. J. (1978) The capillaries in acute and subacute multiple sclerosis plaques: a morphometric analysis. *Neurology*, **28**, 84–92.

Butt, A. M. and Jenkins, H. G. (1994) Morphological changes in oligodendrocytes in the intact mouse optic nerve following intravitreal injection of tumour necrosis factor. *J. Neuroimmunol.*, **51**, 27–33.

Cajal, S. R (1913) *Degeneration and Regeneration of the Nervous System*. 1928 Edn (Milford, H., ed.), pp. 734–760. London: OUP.

Calder, V., Owen, S., Watson, C., Feldmann, M. and Davison, A. (1989) MS: a localized immune disease of the central nervous system. *Immunol. Today*, **10**, 99–103.

Cannella, B., Cross, A. H. and Raine, C. S. (1990) Upregulation and coexpression of adhesion molecules correlate with relapsing autoimmune demyelination in the central nervous system. *J. Exp. Med.*, **172**, 1521–1524.

Cannella, B., Cross, A. H. and Raine, C. S. (1991) Adhesion-related molecules in the central nervous system. Upregulation correlates with inflammatory cell influx during relapsing experimental autoimmune encephalomyelitis. *Lab. Invest.*, **65**, 23–31.

Cannella, B. and Raine, C. S. (1995) The adhesion molecule and cytokine profile of multiple sclerosis lesions (see comments). *Ann. Neurol.*, **37**, 424–435.

Capello, E., Voskuhl, R. R., McFarland, H. F. and Raine, C. S. (1997) Multiple sclerosis: Re-expression of a developmental gene in chronic lesions correlates with remyelination. *Ann. Neurol.*, **41**, 797–805.

Chakrabarti, A. K., Yoshida, Y., Powers, J. M., Singh, I., Hogan, E. L. and Banik, N. L. (1988) Calcium-activated neutral proteinase in rat brain myelin and subcellular fractions. *J. Neurosci. Res.*, **20**, 351–358.

Charcot, M. (1868) Histologie de la sclérose en plaques. *Gaz. Hôsp.*, **141**, 554–555, 557–558.

Chofflon, M., Weiner, H. L., Morimoto, C. and Hafler, D. A. (1989) Decrease of suppressor inducer (CD4$^+$2H4$^+$) T cells in multiple sclerosis cerebrospinal fluid (see comments). *Ann. Neurol.*, **25**, 494–499.

Chou, Y. K., Bourdette, D. N., Offner, H., Whitham, R., Wang, R. Y., Hashim, G. A., *et al.* (1992) Frequency of T cells specific for myelin basic protein and myelin proteolipid protein in blood and cerebrospinal fluid in multiple sclerosis. *J. Neuroimmunol.*, **38**, 105–113.

Claudio, L., Kress, Y., Factor, J. and Brosnan, C. F. (1990) Mechanisms of edema formation in experimental autoimmune encephalomyelitis. The contribution of inflammatory cells. *Am. J. Pathol.*, **137**, 1033–1045.

Claudio, L., Kress, Y., Norton, W. T. and Brosnan, C. F. (1989) Increased vesicular transport and decreased mitochondrial content in blood–brain barrier endothelial cells during experimental autoimmune encephalomyelitis. *Am. J. Pathol.*, **135**, 1157–1168.

Compston, A. (1997) Genetic epidemiology of multiple sclerosis. *J. Neurol. Neurosurg. Psychiat.*, **62**, 553–561.

Compston, D. A. and Hughes, P. J. (1984) Peripheral blood lymphocyte sub-populations and multiple sclerosis. *J. Neuroimmunol.*, **6**, 105–114.

Compston, D. A., Morgan, B. P., Oleesky, D., Fifield, R. and Campbell, A. K. (1986) Cerebrospinal fluid C9 in demyelinating disease. *Neurology*, **36**, 1503–1506.

Compston, D. A. S., Morgan, B. P., Campbell, A. K., Wilkins, P., Cole, G., Thomas, N. D., *et al.* (1989) Immunocytochemical localization of the terminal complement complex in multiple sclerosis. *Neuropathol. Appl. Neurobiol.*, **15**, 307–316.

Compston, D. (1997) Genetic epidemiology of multiple sclerosis. *J. Neurol. Neurosurg. Psychiat.*, **62**, 553–561.

Confavereux C., Aimard, G. and Devic, M. (1980) Course and prognosis of multiple sclerosis assessed by the computerized data processing of 349 patients. *Brain*, **103**, 281–300.

Crockard, A. D., McNeill, T. A., McKirgan, J. and Hawkins, S. A. (1988) Determination of activated lymphocytes in peripheral blood of patients with multiple sclerosis. *J. Neurol. Neurosurg. Psychiat.*, **51**, 139–141.

Cross, A. H. and Raine, C. S. (1991) Central nervous system endothelial cell-polymorphonuclear cell interactions during autoimmune demyelination. *Am. J. Pathol.*, **139**, 1401–1409.

Cross, A. H., Cannella, B., Brosnan, C. F. and Raine, C. S. (1990) Homing to central nervous system vasculature by antigen-specific lymphocytes. I. Localization of ^{14}C-labeled cells during acute, chronic, and relapsing experimental allergic encephalomyelitis. *Lab. Invest.*, **63**, 162–170.

Cross, A. H., Cannella, B., Brosnan, C. F. and Raine, C. S. (1991) Hypothesis: antigen-specific T cells prime central nervous system endothelium for recruitment of nonspecific inflammatory cells to effect autoimmune demyelination. *J. Neuroimmunol.*, **33**, 237–244.

Cruz, M., Olsson, T., Ernerudh, J., Hojeberg, B. and Link, H. (1987) Immunoblot detection of oligoclonal anti-myelin basic protein IgG antibodies in cerebrospinal fluid in multiple sclerosis. *Neurology*, **37**, 1515–1519.

Cserr, H. F. and Knopf, P. M. (1992) Cervical lymphatics, the blood–brain barrier and the immunoreactivity of the brain: a new view. *Immunol. Today*, **13**, 507–512.

D'Souza, S. D., Alinauskas, K. A. and Antel, J. P. (1996a) Ciliary neurotrophic factor selectively protects human oligodendrocytes from tumor necrosis factor-mediated injury. *J. Neurosci.*

Res., **43**, 289–298.

D'Souza, S. D., Bonetti, B., Balasingam, V., Cashman, N. R., Barker, P. A., Troutt, A. B., *et al.* (1996b) Multiple sclerosis: Fas signaling in oligodendrocyte cell death. *J. Exp. Med.*, **184**, 2361–2370.

Daniel, P. M., Lam, D. K. and Pratt, O. E. (1983) Relation between the increase in the diffusional permeability of the blood–central nervous system barrier and other changes during the development of experimental allergic encephalomyelitis in the Lewis rat. *J. Neurol. Sci.*, **60**, 367–376.

Davie, C. A., Hawkins, C. P., Barker, G. J., Brennan, A., Tofts, P. S., Miller, D. H., *et al.* (1994) Serial proton magnetic resonance spectroscopy in acute multiple sclerosis lesions. *Brain*, **117**, 49–58.

Davie, C. A., Barker, G. J., Webb, S., Tofts, P. S., Thompson, A. J., Harding, A. E., *et al.* (1995) Persistent functional deficit in multiple sclerosis and autosomal dominant cerebellar ataxia is associated with axon loss. *Brain*, **118**, 1583–1592.

Davis, F. A., Srefoski, D. and Quandt, F. N. (1995) Mechanism of action of 4–aminopyridine in the symptomatic treatment of multiple sclerosis. *Ann. Neurol.*, **37**, 684.

Dawson, J. W. (1916) The histology of disseminated sclerosis. *Edinburgh Med. J.*, **17**, 229–410.

De Stefano, N., Matthews, P. M. and Arnold, D. L. (1995) Reversible decreases in N-acetylaspartate after acute brain injury. *Magn. Reson. Med.*, **34**, 721–727.

De Stefano, N., Matthews, P. M., Antel, J. P., Preul, M., Francis, G. and Arnold, D. L. (1995) Chemical pathology of acute demyelinating lesions and its correlation with disability. *Ann. Neurol.*, **38**, 901–909.

Dean, G. (1967) Annual incidence, prevalence, and mortality of multiple sclerosis in white South-African-born and in white immigrants to South Africa. *Br. Med. J.*, **2**, 724–730.

Delasnerie, L. N. and Alperovitch, A. (1992) Migration and age at onset of multiple sclerosis: some pitfalls of migrant studies. *Acta Neurol. Scand.*, **85**, 408–411.

Dhib, J. S., Lewis, K., Bradburn, E., McFarlin, D. E. and McFarland, H. F. (1990) Measles virus polypeptide-specific antibody profile in multiple sclerosis. *Neurology*, **40**, 430–435.

Dugandzija, N. S., Shrager, P. (1995) Survival, development, and electrical activity of central nervous system myelinated axons exposed to tumor necrosis factor *in vitro*. *J. Neurosci. Res.*, **40**, 117–126.

Duncan, I. D. (1996) Glial cell transplantation and remyelination of the central nervous system. *Neuropathol. Appl. Neurobiol.*, **22**, 87–100.

Durelli, L., Cocito, D., Riccio, A., Barile, C., Bergamasco, B., Baggio, G. F., *et al.* (1986) High-dose intravenous methylprednisolone in the treatment of multiple sclerosis: clinical–immunologic correlations. *Neurology*, **36**, 238–243.

Ebers, G. C. and Sadovnick, A. D. (1994) The role of genetic factors in multiple sclerosis susceptibility. *J. Neuroimmunol.*, **54**, 1–17.

Ebers, G. C., Sadovnick, A. D. and Risch, N. J. (1995) A genetic basis for familial aggregation in multiple sclerosis. Canadian Collaborative Study Group (see comments). *Nature*, **377**, 150–151.

Ehrlich, P. (1885) *Das Sauerstaff-Bedurfniss des Organesmus.* Berlin: Hiorschwald.

Elian, M., Nightingale, S. and Dean, G. (1990) Multiple sclerosis among United Kingdom-born children of immigrants from the Indian subcontinent, Africa and the West Indies (see comments). *J. Neurol. Neurosurg. Psychiat.*, **53**, 906–911.

Ellison, M. D., Krieg, R. J. and Povlishock, J. T. (1990) Differential central nervous system responses following single and multiple recombinant interleukin-2 infusions. *J. Neuroimmunol.*, **28**, 249–260.

Fazekas, F., Offenbacher, H., Fuchs, S., Schmidt, R., Niederkorn, K., Horner, S., *et al.* (1988) Criteria for an increased specificity of MRI interpretation in elderly subjects with suspected multiple sclerosis. *Neurology*, **38**, 1822–1825.

Feigin, I. and Popoff, H. (1966) Regeneration of myelin in multiple sclerosis: the role of mesenchymal cells in such regeneration and in myelin formation in the peripheral nervous system. *Neurology*, **16**, 364–372.

Felts, P. A. and Smith, K. J. (1992) Conduction properties of central nerve fibers remyelinated by Schwann cells. *Brain Res.*, **574**, 178–192.

Felts, P. A. and Smith, K. J. (1994) The use of potassium channel blocking agents in the therapy of demyelinating diseases. *Ann. Neurol.* **36**, 454.

Felts, P. A., Kapoor, R. and Smith, K. J. (1995) A mechanism for ectopic firing in central demyelinated axons. *Brain*, **118**, 1225–1231.

Ferguson, B., Matyszak, M. K., Esiri, M. M. and Perry, V. H. (1997) Axonal damage in acute multiple sclerosis lesions. *Brain*, **120**, 393–399.

FfrenchConstant, C. and Raff, M. C. (1986) Proliferating bipotential glial progenitor cells in adult rat optic nerve. *Nature*, **319**, 499–502.

Filippini, G., Comi, G. C., Cosi, V., Bevilacqua, L., Ferrarini, M., Martinelli, V., *et al.* (1994) Sensitivities and predictive values of paraclinical tests for diagnosing multiple sclerosis. *J. Neurol.*, **241**, 132–137.

Fog, T. (1965) The topography of plaques in multiple sclerosis with special reference to cerebral plaques. *Acta Neurol. Scand. Suppl.*, **15**, 1–161.

Ford, A. L., Foulcher, E., Lemckert, F. A., Sedgwick, J. D. (1996) Microglia induce CD4 T lymphocyte final effector function and death. *J. Exp. Med.*, **184**, 1737–1745.

Fowler, C. J. and Henry, M. M. (1996) Gastrointestinal dysfunction in multiple sclerosis. *Semin. Neurol.*, **16**, 277–279.

Francis, D. A., Compston, D. A., Batchelor, J. R. and McDonald, W. I. (1987) A reassessment of the risk of multiple sclerosis developing in patients with optic neuritis after extended follow-up. *J. Neurol. Neurosurg. Psychiat.*, **50**, 758–765.

Franklin, R. J. M. and Blakemore, W. F. (1995) Glial-cell transplantation and plasticity in the O-2A lineage – implications for CNS repair. *Trends Neurosci.*, **18**, 151–156.

Franklin, R. J. M. and Blakemore, W. F. (1997) Transplanting oligodendrocyte progenitors into the adult CNS. *J. Anat.*, **190**, 23–33.

Freedman, M. S., Bitar, R. and Antel, J. P. (1997) Gammadelta T-cell–human glial cell interactions. II. Relationship between heat shock protein expression and susceptibility to cytolysis. *J. Neuroimmunol.*, **74**, 143–148.

Frisen, L. and Hoyt, W. F. (1974) Insidious atrophy of retinal nerve fibers in multiple sclerosis. Funduscopic identification in patients with and without visual complaints. *Arch. Ophthalmol.*, **92**, 91–97.

Fugger, L., Sandberg, W. M., Morling, N., Ryder, L. P. and Svejgaard, A. (1990) The germline repertoire of T-cell receptor beta chain genes in patients with relapsing/remitting multiple sclerosis or optic neuritis. *Immunogenetics*, **31**, 278–280.

Gallo, P., Piccinno, M. G., Tavolato, B. and Siden, A. (1991) A longitudinal study on IL-2, sIL-2R, IL-4 and IFN-gamma in multiple sclerosis CSF and serum. *J. Neurol. Sci.*, **101**, 227–232.

Gallo, V., Zhou, J. M., McBain, C. J., Wright, P., Knutson, P. L. and Armstrong, R. C. (1996) Oligodendrocyte progenitor cell proliferation and lineage progression are regulated by glutamate receptor-mediated K^+ channel block. *J. Neurosci.*, **16**, 2659–2670.

Gay, D. and Esiri, M. (1991) Blood–brain barrier damage in acute multiple sclerosis plaques. An immunocytological study. *Brain*, **114**, 557–572.

Giovannoni, G., Lai, M., Thorpe, J., Kidd, D., Chamoun, V., Thompson, A. J., *et al.* (1997) Longitudinal study of soluble adhesion molecules in multiple sclerosis: correlation with gadolinium enhanced magnetic resonance imaging. *Neurology*, **48**, 1557–1565.

Goldmuntz, E. A., Brosnan, C. F. and Norton, W. T. (1986) Prazosin treatment suppresses increased vascular permeability in both acute and passively transferred experimental autoimmune encephalomyelitis in the Lewis rat. *J. Immunol.*, **137**, 3444–3450.

Goldstein, J. L., Anderson, R. G. and Brown, M. S. (1979) Coated pits, coated vesicles, and receptor-mediated endocytosis. *Nature*, **279**, 679–685.

Goswami, K. K., Randall, R. E., Lange, L. S. and Russell, W. C. (1987) Antibodies against the paramyxovirus SV5 in the cerebrospinal fluids of some multiple sclerosis patients. *Nature*, **327**, 244–247.

Graham, E. M., Francis, D. A., Sanders, M. D. and Rudge, P. (1989) Ocular inflammatory changes in established multiple sclerosis. *J. Neurol. Neurosurg. Psychiat.*, **52**, 1360–1363.

Greenfield, J. G. and King, L. S. (1936) Observations on the histopathology of the cerebral lesions in disseminated sclerosis. *Brain*, **59**, 445–459.

Greenwood, J. (1991) Mechanisms of blood–brain barrier breakdown. *Neuroradiology*, **33**, 95–100.

Groves, A. K., Barnett, S. C., Franklin, R. J. M., Crang, A. J., Mayer, M., Blakemore, W. F., *et al.* (1993) Repair of demyelinated lesions by transplantation of purified O-2A progenitor cells. *Nature*, **362**, 453–455.

Hafler, D. A., Benjamin, D. S., Burks, J. and Weiner, H. L. (1987) Myelin basic protein and proteolipid protein reactivity of brain- and cerebrospinal fluid-derived T cell clones in multiple sclerosis and postinfectious encephalomyelitis. *J. Immunol.*, **139**, 68–72.

Harris, J. O., Frank, J. A., Patronas, N., McFarlin, D. E. and McFarland, H. F. (1991) Serial gadolinium-enhanced magnetic resonance imaging scans in patients with early, relapsing–remitting multiple sclerosis: implications for clinical trials and natural history. *Ann. Neurol.*, **29**, 548–555.

Hartung, H. P., Archelos, J. J., Zielasek, J., Gold, R., Koltzenburg, M., Reiners, K. H., *et al.* (1995) Circulating adhesion molecules and inflammatory mediators in demyelination: a review. *Neurology*, **45**, S22—S32.

Hawkins, C. P., Mackenzie, F., Tofts, P., Du, B. E. and McDonald, W. I. (1991) Patterns of blood–brain barrier breakdown in inflammatory demyelination. *Brain*, **114**, 801–810.

Hawkins, C. P., Munro, P. M., Mackenzie, F., Kesselring, J., Tofts, P. S., Du, B. E., *et al.* (1990) Duration and selectivity of blood–brain barrier breakdown in chronic relapsing experimental allergic encephalomyelitis studied by gadolinium–DTPA and protein markers. *Brain*, **113**, 365–378.

Hayashi, T., Burks, J. S. and Hauser, S. L. (1988) Expression and cellular localization of major histocompatibility complex antigens in active multiple sclerosis lesions. *Ann. N. Y. Acad. Sci.*, **540**, 301–305.

Hayes, G. M., Woodroofe, M. N. and Cuzner, M. L. (1987) Microglia are the major cell type expressing MHC class II in human white matter. *J. Neurol. Sci.*, **80**, 25–37.

Hedlund, G., Sandberg, W. M. and Sjogren, H. O. (1989) Increased proportion of $CD4^+CDw29^+CD45RUCHL-1^+$ lymphocytes in the cerebrospinal fluid of both multiple sclerosis patients and healthy individuals. *Cell Immunol.*, **118**, 406–412.

Hickey, W. F., Hsu, B. L. and Kimura, H. (1991) T-lymphocyte entry into the central nervous system. *J. Neurosci. Res.*, **28**, 254–260.

Hillert, J., Leng, C. and Olerup, O. (1991) No association with germline T cell receptor beta-chain gene alleles or haplotypes in Swedish patients with multiple sclerosis. *J. Neuroimmunol.*, **32**, 141–147.

Hillert, J., Leng, C. and Olerup, O. (1992) T-cell receptor alpha chain germline gene polymorphisms in multiple sclerosis (see comments). *Neurology*, **42**, 80–84.

Hilton, P., Hertogs, K. and Stanton, S. L. (1983) The use of desmopressin (DDAVP) for nocturia in women with multiple sclerosis. *J. Neurol. Neurosurg. Psychiat.*, **46**, 854–855.

Hirano, A., Dembitzer, H. M., Becker, N. H., Levine, S. and Zimmerman, H. M. (1970) Fine structural alterations of the blood–brain barrier in experimental allergic encephalomyelitis. *J. Neuropathol. Exp. Neurol.*, **29**, 432–440.

Hofman, F. M., Hinton, D. R., Johnson, K. and Merrill, J. E. (1989) Tumor necrosis factor identified in multiple sclerosis brain. *J. Exp. Med.*, **170**, 607–612.

Honmou, O., Felts, P. A., Waxman, S. G. and Kocsis, J. D. (1996) Restoration of normal conduction properties in demyelinated spinal cord axons in the adult rat by transplantation of exogenous Schwann cells. *J. Neurosci.*, **16**, 3199–3208.

Hoverd, P. A. and Fowler, C. J. (1998) Desmopressin in the treatment of daytime urinary frequency in patients with multiple sclerosis. *J. Neurol. Neurosurg. Psych.*, **65**, 778–780.

Hughes, R. A. (1994) Immunotherapy for multiple sclerosis (editorial). *J. Neurol. Neurosurg. Psychiat.*, **57**, 3–6.

Jans, H., Heltberg. A., Zeeberg, I., Kristensen. J. H., Fog, T. and Raun, N. E. (1984) Immune complexes and the complement factors C4 and C3 in cerebrospinal fluid and serum from patients with chronic progressive multiple sclerosis. *Acta Neurol. Scand.*, **69**, 34–38.

Janzer, R. C. and Raff, M. C. (1987) Astrocytes induce blood–brain barrier properties in endothelial cells. *Nature*, **325**, 253–257.

Jenkins, H. G. and Ikeda, H. (1992) Tumour necrosis factor causes an increase in axonal transport of protein and demyelination in the mouse optic nerve. *J. Neurol. Sci.*, **108**, 99–104.

Johnson, K. P., Brooks, B. R., Cohen, J. A., Ford, C. C., Goldstein, J., Lisak, R. P., *et al.* (1998) Extended use of glatiramer acetate (Copaxone) is well tolerated and maintains its clinical effect on multiple sclerosis relapse rate and degree of disability. *Neurology*, **50**, 701–708.

Johnson, R. T. (1994) The virology of demyelinating diseases. *Ann. Neurol.*, **36 (Suppl)**, S54—S60

Jones, J., Frith, S., Piddlesden, S., Morgan, B. P., Compston, D. A., Campbell, A. K., *et al.* (1991) Imaging Ca2$^+$ changes in individual oligodendrocytes attacked by T-cell perforin. *Immunology*, **74**, 572–577.

Joshi, N., Usuku, K. and Hauser, S. L. (1993) The T-cell response to myelin basic protein in familial multiple sclerosis: diversity of fine specificity, restricting elements, and T-cell receptor usage. *Ann. Neurol.*, **34**, 385–393.

Kermode, A. G., Thompson, A. J., Tofts, P., MacManus, D. G., Kendall, B. E., Kingsley, D. P., *et al.* (1990) Breakdown of the blood–brain barrier precedes symptoms and other MRI signs of new lesions in multiple sclerosis. Pathogenetic and clinical implications. *Brain*, **113**, 1477–1489.

Kesselring, J., Miller, D. H., MacManus, D. G., Johnson, G., Milligan, N. M., Scolding, N., *et al.* (1989) Quantitative magnetic resonance imaging in multiple sclerosis: the effect of high dose intravenous methylprednisolone. *J. Neurol. Neurosurg. Psychiat.*, **52**, 14–17.

Kidd, D. and Thompson, A. J. (1997) Prospective study of neurorehabilitation in multiple sclerosis. *J. Neurol. Neurosurg. Psychiat.*, **62**, 423–424.

Kim, Y. S. and Kim, S. U. (1991) Oligodendroglial cell death induced by oxygen radicals and its protection by catalase. *J. Neurosci. Res.*, **29**, 100–106.

Koopmans, R. A., Li, D. K., Oger, J. J., Kastrukoff, L. F., Jardine, C., Costley, L., *et al.* (1989a) Chronic progressive multiple sclerosis: serial magnetic resonance brain imaging over six months. *Ann. Neurol.*, **26**, 248–256.

Koopmans, R. A., Li, D. K., Oger, J. J., Mayo, J., Paty, D. W. (1989b) The lesion of multiple sclerosis: imaging of acute and chronic stages. *Neurology*, **39**, 959–963.

Koprowski, H., Defreitas, E. C., Harper, M. E., Sandberg, W. M., Sheremata, W. A., Robert, G. M., *et al.* (1985) Multiple sclerosis and human T-cell lymphotropic retroviruses. *Nature*, **318**, 154–160.

Kujala, P., Portin, R. and Ruutiainen, J. (1997) The progress of cognitive decline in multiple sclerosis – A controlled 3–year follow-up. *Brain*, **120**, 289–297.

Kuroda, Y., Shibasaki, H. (1987) CSF mononuclear cell subsets in active MS: lack of disease-specific alteration. *Neurology*, **37**, 497–499.

Kurtzke, J. F. (1977) Geography in multiple sclerosis. *J. Neurol.*, **215**, 1–26.

Kurtzke, J. F. (1993) Epidemiologic evidence for multiple sclerosis as an infection (published erratum appears in *Clin. Microbiol. Rev.*, **7**(1), 141). *Clin. Microbiol. Rev.*, **6**, 382–427.

Lampert, P. (1967) Electron microscopic studies on ordinary and hyperacute experimental allergic encephalomyelitis. *Acta Neuropathol. Berl.*, **9**, 99–126.

Lassmann, H. (1983) *The Comparative Pathology of Chronic Relapsing Experimental Allergic Encephalomyelitis and Multiple Sclerosis*, pp. 37–72. New York: Springer-Verlag.

Lassmann, H., Zimprich, F., Vass, K. and Hickey, W. F. (1991a) Microglial cells are a component of the perivascular glia limitans. *J. Neurosci. Res.*, **28**, 236–243.

Lassmann, H., Rossler, K., Zimprich, F. and Vass, K. (1991b) Expression of adhesion molecules and histocompatibility antigens at the blood–brain barrier. *Brain Pathol.*, **1**, 115–123.

Lassmann, H., Suchanek, G. and Ozawa, K. (1994) Histopathology and the blood-cerebrospinal fluid barrier in multiple sclerosis. *Ann. Neurol.*, **36**, S42—S46.

Lee, K. H., Hashimoto, H., Hooge, J. P., Kastrukoff, L. F., Oger, J. J., Li, D. K., *et al.* (1991) Magnetic resonance imaging of the head in the diagnosis of multiple sclerosis: a prospective 2-year follow-up with comparison of clinical evaluation, evoked potentials, oligoclonal banding, and CT. *Neurology*, **41**, 657–660.

Lehmann, P. V., Forsthuber, T., Miller, A. and Sercarz, E. E. (1992) Spreading of T-cell autoimmunity to cryptic determinants of an autoantigen. *Nature*, **358**, 155–157.

Lehmann, P. V., Sercarz, E. E., Forsthuber, T., Dayan, C. M. and Gammon, G. (1993) Determinant spreading and the dynamics of the autoimmune T-cell repertoire (see comments). *Immunol. Today*, **14**, 203–208.

Levison, S. W. and Goldman, J. E. (1993) Both oligodendrocytes and astrocytes develop from progenitors in the sub-ventricular zone of postnatal rat forebrain. *Neuron*, **10**, 201–212.

Lightman, S., McDonald, W. I., Bird, A. C., Francis, D. A., Hoskins, A., Batchelor, J. R., *et al.* (1987) Retinal venous sheathing in optic neuritis. Its significance for the pathogenesis of multiple sclerosis. *Brain*, **110**, 405–414.

Lindsberg, P. J., Ohman, J., Lehto, T., Karjalainenlindsberg, M. L., Pactau, A., Wuorimaa, T., *et al.* (1996) Complement activation in the central nervous system following blood–brain barrier damage in man. *Ann. Neurol.*, **40**, 587–596.

Linington, C., Lassmann, H. (1987) Antibody responses in chronic relapsing experimental allergic encephalomyelitis: correlation of serum demyelinating activity with antibody titre to the myelin/oligodendrocyte glycoprotein (MOG). *J. Neuroimmunol.*, **17**, 61–69.

Linington, C., Bradl, M., Lassmann, H., Brunner, C. and Vass, K. (1988) Augmentation of demyelination in rat acute allergic encephalomyelitis by circulating mouse monoclonal antibodies directed against a myelin/oligodendrocyte glycoprotein. *Am. J. Pathol.*, **130**, 443–454.

Linington, C., Lassmann, H., Morgan, B. P. and Compston, D. A. (1989a) Immunohistochemical localization of terminal complement component C9 in experimental allergic encephalomyelitis. *Acta Neuropathol. Berl.*, **79**, 78–85.

Linington, C., Morgan, B. P., Scolding, N. J., Wilkins, P., Piddlesden, S. and Compston, D. A. S. (1989b) The role of complement in the pathogenesis of experimental allergic encephalomyelitis. *Brain*, **112**, 895–911.

Link, H., Baig, S., Olsson, O., Jiang, Y. P., Hojeberg, B. and Olsson, T. (1990) Persistent anti-myelin basic protein IgG antibody response in multiple sclerosis cerebrospinal fluid. *J. Neuroimmunol.*, **28**, 237–248.

Lipton, S. A. (1986) Blockade of electrical-activity promotes the death of mammalian retinal ganglion-cells in culture. *Proc. Natl Acad. Sci. USA*, **83**, 9774–9778.

Liu, J., Marino, M. W., Grail, G., Dunn, A., Bettadapnra, J. *et al.* (1998) TNF is a potent anti-inflammatory cytokine in autoimmune mediated demyelination. *Nature Medicine*, **4**, 78–83.

Losseff, N. A., Wang, L., Lai, H. M., Yoo, D. S., Gawne, C. M., McDonald, W. I., *et al.* (1996a) Progressive cerebral atrophy in multiple sclerosis. A serial MRI study. *Brain*, **119**, 2009–2019.

Losseff, N. A., Webb, S. L., O'Riordan, J. I., Page, R., Wang, L., Barker, G. J., *et al.* (1996b) Spinal cord atrophy and disability in multiple sclerosis. A new reproducible and sensitive MRI method with potential to monitor disease progression. *Brain*, **119**, 701–708.

Lucchinetti, C. F., Bruck, W., Rodriguez, M., Lassmann, H. (1996) Distinct patterns of multiple sclerosis pathology indicates heterogeneity on pathogenesis. *Brain Pathol.*, **6**, 259–274.

Lumsden, C. E. (1951) Fundamental problems in the pathology of multiple sclerosis and allied demyelinating diseases. *Br. Med. J.*, 1035–1043.

Lumsden, C. E. (1955) Pathology. In *Multiple Sclerosis* (McAlpine, D., Compston, N. D. and Lumsden, C. E., eds), pp. 208–239. London: Livingstone.

McAlpine, D., Compston, N. D. and Lumsden, C. E. (1955) Early symptomatology. In *Multiple Sclerosis* (McAlpine, D., Compston, N. D. and Lumsden, C. E., eds), pp. 64–89. London: Livingstone.

McCarron, R. M., Fallis, R. J. and McFarlin, D. E. (1990) Alterations in T cell antigen specificity and class II restriction during the course of chronic relapsing experimental allergic encephalomyelitis. *J. Neuroimmunol.*, **29**, 73–79.

McDonald, W. I. (1994) Rachelle Fishman–Matthew Moore Lecture. The pathological and clinical dynamics of multiple sclerosis. *J. Neuropathol. Exp. Neurol.*, **53**, 338–343.

McDonald, W. I. (1996) Mechanisms of relapse and remission in multiple sclerosis. In *The Neurobiology of Disease* (Bostock, H., Kirkwood, P. A. and Pullen, A. H., eds), pp. 118–123. Cambridge: Cambridge University Press.

McDonald, W. I. and Sears, T. A. (1970) The effects of experimental demyelination on conduction in the central nervous system. *Brain*, **93**, 583–598.

McLean, B. N. and Thompson, E. J. (1989) Antibodies against the paramyxovirus SV5 are not specific for cerebrospinal fluid from multiple sclerosis patients. *J. Neurol. Sci.*, **92**, 261–266.

Martin, S., Maruta, K., Burkart, V., Gillis, S. and Kolb, H. (1988) IL-1 and IFN-gamma increase vascular permeability. *Immunology*, **64**, 301–305.

Matsui, M., Mori, K. J., Saida, T. (1990) Cellular immunoregulatory mechanisms in the central nervous system: characterization of noninflammatory and inflammatory cerebrospinal fluid lymphocytes. *Ann. Neurol.*, **27**, 647–651.

Matthews, W. B. (1991a) Symptoms and signs. Initial symptoms. In *McAlpine's Multiple Sclerosis* (Matthews, W. B., ed.), pp. 43–46. London: Churchill Livingstone.

Matthews, W. B. (1991b) Symptoms and signs. Paroxysmal. In *McAlpine's Multiple Sclerosis* (Matthews, W. B., ed.), pp. 64–69. London: Churchill Livingstone.

Matthews, W. B. and Small, D. G. (1979) Serial recording of visual and somatosensory evoked potentials in multiple sclerosis. *J. Neurol. Sci.*, **40**, 11–21.

Mayne, M., Krishnan, J., Metz, L., Natu, A., Auty, A., Satai, B. M. and Power, C. (1998) Infrequent detection of human herpes virus 6 DNA in peripherial blood mononuclear cells from multiple sclerosis patients. *Ann. Neurol.*, **44**, 391–394.

Merrill, J. E. and Benveniste, E. N. (1996) Cytokines in inflammatory brain lesions: helpful and harmful. *Trends. Neurosci.*, **19**, 331–338.

Merrill, J. E., Ignarro, L. J., Sherman, M. P., Melinek, J. and Lane, T. E. (1993) Microglial cell cytotoxicity of oligodendrocytes is mediated through nitric oxide. *J. Immunol.*, **151**, 2132–2141.

Meyerfranke, A., Kaplan, M. R., Pfrieger, F. W., Barres, B. A. (1995) Characterization of the signaling interactions that promote the survival and growth of developing retinal ganglion cells in culture. *Neuron*, **15**, 805–819.

Miller, D. H., Grossman, R. I., Reingold, S. C., McFarland, H. F. (1998) The role of magnetic resonance techniques in understanding and managing multiple sclerosis. *Brain*, **121**, 3–24.

Miller, D. H., Rudge, P., Johnson, G., Kendall, B. E., MacManus, D. G., Moseley, I. F., *et al.* (1988) Serial gadolinium enhanced magnetic resonance imaging in multiple sclerosis. *Brain*, **111**, 927–939.

Miller, D. H., Thompson, A. J., Morrissey, S. P., MacManus, D. G., Moore, S. G., Kendall, B. E., *et al.* (1992) High dose steroids in acute relapses of multiple sclerosis: MRI evidence for a possible mechanism of therapeutic effect. *J. Neurol. Neurosurg. Psychiat.*, **55**, 450–453.

Miller, H. G., Gibbons, J. L. (1953) Acute disseminated encephalomyelitis and acute disseminated sclerosis: results of treatment with ACTH. *Lancet*, **ii**, 1345–1349.

Milligan, N. M., Newcombe, R. and Compston, D. A. (1987) A double-blind controlled trial of high dose methylprednisolone in patients with multiple sclerosis: 1. Clinical effects. *J. Neurol. Neurosurg. Psychiat.*, **50**, 511–516.

Mitrovic, B., Ignarro, L. J., Montestruque, S., Smoll, A. and Merrill, J. E. (1994) Nitric oxide as a potential pathological mechanism in demyelination: its differential effects on primary glial cells *in vitro*. *Neuroscience*, **61**, 575–585.

Mitrovic, B., Ignarro, L. J., Vinters, H. V., Akers, M. A., Schmid, I., Uittenbogaart, C., *et al.* (1995) Nitric oxide induces necrotic but not apoptotic cell death in oligodendrocytes. *Neuroscience*, **65**, 531–539.

Moller, J. R., Johnson, D., Brady, R. O., Tourtellotte, W. W. and Quarles, R. H. (1989) Antibodies to myelin-associated glycoprotein (MAG) in the cerebrospinal fluid of multiple sclerosis patients. *J. Neuroimmunol.*, **22**, 55–61.

Moreau, T., Coles, A., Wing M., Isaacs, J., Hale, G., Waldmann, H., *et al.* (1996) Transient increase in symptoms associated with cytokine release in patients with multiple sclerosis. *Brain*, **119**, 225–237.

Moreau, T., Thorpe, J., Miller, D., Moseley, I., Hale, G., Waldmann, H., *et al.* (1994) Preliminary evidence from magnetic resonance imaging for reduction in disease activity after lymphocyte depletion in multiple sclerosis. *Lancet*, **344**, 298–301.

Morgan, B. P. and Gasque, P. (1996) Expression of complement in the brain: Role in health and disease. *Immunol. Today*, **17**, 461–466.

Morgan, B. P., Campbell, A. K. and Compston, D. A. (1984) Terminal component of complement (C9) in cerebrospinal fluid of patients with multiple sclerosis. *Lancet*, **ii**, 251–254.

Morimoto, C., Hafler, D. A., Weiner, H. L., Letvin, N. L., Hagan, M., Daley, J., *et al.* (1987) Selective loss of the suppressor-inducer T-cell subset in progressive multiple sclerosis. Analysis with anti-2H4 monoclonal antibody. *N. Engl. J. Med.*, **316**, 67–72.

Morrissey, S. P., Miller, D. H., Kendall, B. E., Kingsley, D. P., Kelly, M. A., Francis, D. A., *et al.* (1993) The significance of brain magnetic resonance imaging abnormalities at presentation with clinically isolated syndromes suggestive of multiple sclerosis. A 5-year follow-up study. *Brain*, **116**, 135–146.

Murphy, J. B. and Sturm, E. (1923) Conditions determining the transplantation of tissues in the brain. *J. Exp. Med.*, **39**, 183–197.

Naparstek, Y., Cohen, I. R., Fuks, Z. and Vlodavsky, I. (1984) Activated T lymphocytes produce a matrix-degrading heparan sulphate endoglycosidase. *Nature*, **310**, 241–244.

Navikas, V. and Link, H. (1996) Review: cytokines and the pathogenesis of multiple sclerosis. *J. Neurosci. Res.*, **45**, 322–333.

Nielsen, L., Larsen, A. M., Munk, M. and Vestergaard, B. F. (1997) Human herpesvirus-6 immunoglobulin G antibodies in patients with multiple sclerosis. *Acta Neurolog. Scand.*, **95 (Suppl)**, 76–78.

Nishimura, M., Adachi, A., Maeda, M., Akiguchi, I., Ishimoto, A. and Kimura, J. (1990) Human T lymphotrophic virus type I may not be associated with multiple sclerosis in Japan. *J. Immunol.*, **144**, 1684–1688.

Norrby, E. (1978) Viral antibodies in multiple sclerosis. *Prog. Med. Virol.*, **24**, 1–39.

Oka, A., Belliveau, M. J., Rosenberg, P. A. and Volpe, J. J. (1993) Vulnerability of oligodendroglia to glutamate: Pharmacology, mechanisms, and prevention. *J. Neuroscience*, **13**, 1441–1453.

Oldendorf, W. H. and Towner, H. F. (1974) Blood–brain barrier and DNA changes during the evolution of experimental allergic encephalomyelitis. *J. Neuropathol. Exp. Neurol.*, **33**, 616–631.

Olsson, T. (1992) Immunology of multiple sclerosis. *Curr. Opin. Neurol. Neurosurg.*, **5**, 195–202.

Olsson, T., Baog, S., Hojeberg, B. and Link, H. (1990) Antimyelin basic protein and antimyelin antibody-producing cells in multiple sclerosis. *Ann. Neurol.*, **27**, 132–136.

Olsson, T., Sun, J., Hillert, J., Hojeberg, B., Ekre, H. P., Andersson, G., *et al.* (1992) Increased numbers of T cells recognizing multiple myelin basic protein epitopes in multiple sclerosis. *Eur. J. Immunol.*, **22**, 1083–1087.

Olsson, T., Zhi, W. W., Hojeberg, B., Kostulas, V., Jiang, Y. P., Anderson, G., *et al.* (1990) Autoreactive T lymphocytes in multiple sclerosis determined by antigen-induced secretion of interferon-gamma. *J. Clin. Invest.*, **86**, 981–985.

Omlin, F. X., Webster, H. D., Palkovits, C. G., Cohen, S. R. (1982) Immunocytochemical localization of basic protein in major dense line regions of central and peripheral myelin. *J. Cell Biol.*, **95**, 242–248.

Ozawa, K., Suchanek, G., Breitschopf, H., Bruck, W., Budka, H., Jellinger, K., *et al.* (1994) Patterns of oligodendroglia pathology in multiple sclerosis. *Brain*, **117**, 1311–1322.

Palace, J. and Rothwell, P. (1997) New treatments and azathioprine in multiple sclerosis. *Lancet*, **350**, 261.

Parkinson, J. F., Mitrovic, B. and Merrill, J. E. (1997) The role of nitric oxide in multiple sclerosis (see comments). *J. Mol. Med.*, **75**, 174–186.

Paterson, P. Y. and Day, E. D. (1981) Current perspectives of neuroimmunologic disease: multiple sclerosis and experimental allergic encephalomyelitis (1,2). *Clin. Immunol. Rev.*, **1**, 581–697.

Perier, O. and Gregoire, A. (1965) Electron microscopic features of multiple sclerosis lesions. *Brain*, **88**, 937–952.

Perron, H., Garson, J. A., Bedin, F., Beseme, F., Paranhosbaccala, G., Komurianpradel, F., *et al.* (1997) Molecular identification of a novel retrovirus repeatedly isolated from patients with multiple sclerosis. *Proc. Natl Acad. Sci. USA*, **94**, 7583–7588.

Peters, G. (1968) Multiple sclerosis. In *Pathology of the Nervous System* (Minckler, J., ed.), pp.

821–843. New York: McGraw-Hill.

Piddlesden, S., Lassmann, H., Laffafian, I., Morgan, B. P. and Linington, C. (1991) Antibody-mediated demyelination in experimental allergic encephalomyelitis is independent of complement membrane attack complex formation. *Clin. Exp. Immunol.*, **83**, 245–250.

Piddlesden, S. J., Storch, M. K., Hibbs, M., Freeman, A. M., Lassmann, H. and Morgan, B. P. (1994) Soluble recombinant complement receptor 1 inhibits inflammation and demyelination in antibody-mediated demyelinating experimental allergic encephalomyelitis. *J. Immunol.*, **152**, 5477–5484.

Poduslo, J. F. and Braun, P. E. (1975) Topographical arrangement of membrane proteins in the intact myelin sheath. Lactoperoxidase incorporation of iodine into myelin surface proteins. *J. Biol. Chem.*, **250**, 1099–1105.

Poser, C. M., Paty, D. W., Scheinberg, L., McDonald, W. I., Davis, F. A., Ebers, G. C., *et al.* (1983) New diagnostic criteria for multiple sclerosis: guidelines for research protocols. *Ann. Neurol.*, **13**, 227–231.

Poser, S. (1978) *Multiple Sclerosis: An Analysis of 812 Cases by Means of Electronic Data Processing*. Berlin: Springer-Verlag.

Prineas, J. W. (1975) Pathology of the early lesion in multiple sclerosis. *Human Pathol.*, **6**, 531–554.

Prineas, J. W. (1985) The neuropathology of multiple sclerosis. In *Demyelinating Diseases* (Vincken, P.J., Bruyn, G. W. and Klawans, H. L., eds), pp. 213–257. Amsterdam: Elsevier Science.

Prineas, J. W. and Connell, F. (1978) The fine structure of chronically active multiple sclerosis plaques. *Neurology*, **28**, 68–75.

Prineas, J. W. and Connell, F. (1979) Remyelination in multiple sclerosis. *Ann. Neurol.*, **5**, 22–31.

Prineas, J. W., Kwon, E. E., Cho, E. S. and Sharer, L. R. (1984) Continual breakdown and regeneration of myelin in progressive multiple sclerosis plaques. *Ann. N. Y. Acad. Sci.*, **436**, 11–32.

Prineas, J. W., Kwon, E. E. and Goldenberg, P. Z. (1989) Multiple sclerosis: oligodendrocyte proliferation and differentiation in fresh lesions. *Lab. Invest.*, **61**, 489–503.

Prineas, J. W., Barnard, R. O., Kwon, E. E., Sharer, L. R. and Cho, E. S. (1993) Multiple sclerosis: remyelination of nascent lesions. *Ann. Neurol.*, **33**, 137–151.

Probert, L. and Selmaj, K. (1997) TNF and related molecules: trends in neuroscience and clinical applications. *J. Neuroimmunol.*, **72**, 113–117.

Raff, M. C., Miller, R. H. and Noble, M. (1983) A glial progenitor cell that develops *in vitro* into an astrocyte or an oligodendrocyte depending on culture medium. *Nature*, **303**, 390–396.

Raine, C. S. (1983) Multiple sclerosis and chronic EAE: comparative ultrastructural neuropathology. In *Multiple Sclerosis* (Hallpike, J. F., Adams, C. W. and Tourtellotte, W. W., eds), p. 413. London: Chapman & Hall.

Raine, C. S. (1991) Multiple sclerosis: a pivotal role for the T cell in lesion development. *Neuropathol. Appl. Neurobiol.*, **17**, 265–274.

Raine, C. S. (1994a) Multiple sclerosis: immune system molecule expression in the central nervous system. *J. Neuropathol. Exp. Neurol.*, **53**, 328–337.

Raine, C. S. (1994b) The Dale E. McFarlin Memorial Lecture: the immunology of the multiple sclerosis lesion. *Ann. Neurol.*, **36 (Suppl)**, S61—S72.

Raine, C. S. (1997) The Norton Lecture: A review of the oligodendrocyte in the multiple sclerosis lesion. *J. Neuroimmunol.*, **77**, 135–152.

Raine, C. S. and Cross, A. H. (1989) Axonal dystrophy as a consequence of long-term demyelination. *Lab. Invest.*, **60**, 714–725.

Raine, C. S. and Wu, E. (1993) Multiple sclerosis: remyelination in acute lesions. *J. Neuropathol. Exp. Neurol.*, **52**, 199–204.

Raine, C. S., Scheinberg, L. and Waltz, J. M. (1981) Multiple sclerosis. Oligodendrocyte survival and proliferation in an active established lesion. *Lab. Invest.*, **45**, 534–546.

Raine, C. S., Cannella, B., Duijvestijn, A. M. and Cross, A. H. (1990) Homing to central nervous system vasculature by antigen-specific lymphocytes. II. Lymphocyte/endothelial cell adhesion during the initial stages of autoimmune demyelination. *Lab. Invest.*, **63**, 476–489.

Ransohoff, R. M., Tuohy, V. and Lehmann, P. (1994) The immunology of multiple sclerosis: new intricacies and new insights. *Curr. Opin. Neurol.*, **7**, 242–249.

Rasminsky, M. (1973) The effects of temperature on conduction in demyelinated single nerve fibers. *Arch. Neurol.*, **28**, 287–292.

Rasminsky, M. (1980) Ephaptic transmission between single nerve fibres in the spinal nerve roots of dystrophic mice. *J. Physiol. Lond.*, **305**, 151–169.

Redford, E. J., Hall, S. M. and Smith, K. J. (1995) Vascular changes and demyelination induced by the intraneural injection of tumour necrosis factor. *Brain*, **118**, 869–878.

Redford, E. J., Kapoor, R. and Smith, K. J. (1997) Nitric oxide donors reversibly block axonal conduction: demyelinated axons are especially susceptible. *Brain*, **120**, 2149–2157.

Rio Hortega, P. (1921) Estudios sobre la neuroglia. La glia de escasas radiciones (oligodendroglia). *Biol. Real. Soc. Esp. d. Hist. Nat.*, **January**.

RiveraQuinones, C., McGavern, D., Schmelzer, J. D., Hunter, S. F., Low, P. A. and Rodriguez, M. (1998) Absence of neurological deficits following extensive demyelination in a class I-deficient murine model of multiple sclerosis. *Nat. Med.*, **4**, 187–193.

Rivers, T. M., Sprunt, D. M. and Berry, G. P. (1933) Observations on attempts to produce acute disseminated encephalomyelitis in monkeys. *J. Exp. Med.*, **58**, 39–53.

Robertson, N. P., O'Riordan, J. I., Chataway, J., Kingsley, D. P., Miller, D. H., Clayton, D., *et al.* (1997) Offspring recurrence rates and clinical characteristics of conjugal multiple sclerosis. *Lancet*, **349**, 1587–1590.

Rodriguez, M. and Lennon, V. A. (1990) Immunoglobulins promote remyelination in the central nervous system. *Ann. Neurol.*, **27**, 12–17.

Rodriguez, M. and Miller, D. J. (1994) Immune promotion of CNS remyelination. *Prog. in Brain Res.*, **103**, 343–355.

Rose, A. S., Kuzma, J. W., Kurtzke, J. F., Namerow, N. S., Sibley, W. A. and Tourtellotte, W. W. (1970) Cooperative study in the evaluation of therapy in multiple sclerosis. ACTH vs. placebo – final report. *Neurology*, **20**, 1–59.

Rose, J., Gerken, S., Lynch, S., Pisani, P., Varvil, T., Otterud, B., *et al.* (1993) Genetic susceptibility in familial multiple sclerosis not linked to the myelin basic protein gene (see comments). *Lancet*, **341**, 1179–1181.

Rosenbluth, J. (1996) Glial transplantation in the treatment of myelin loss or deficiency. In *The Neurobiology of Disease: Contributions from Neuroscience to Clinical Neurology* (Bostock, H., Kirkwood, P. A. and Pullen, A. H., eds), pp. 124–148. Cambridge: Cambridge University Press.

Roth, M. P., Dolbois, L., Borot, N., Pontarotti, P., Clanet, M. and Coppin, H. (1995) Myelin oligodendrocyte glycoprotein (MOG) gene polymorphisms and multiple sclerosis: no evidence of disease association with MOG. *J. Neuroimmunol.*, **61**, 117–122.

Ruddle, N. H., Bergman, C. M., McGrath, K. M., Lingenheld, E. G., Grunnet, M. L., Padula, S. J., *et al.* (1990) An antibody to lymphotoxin and tumor necrosis factor prevents transfer of experimental allergic encephalomyelitis. *J. Exp. Med.*, **172**, 1193–1200.

Ruijs, T. C. G., Olivier, A. and Antel, J. P. (1990) Serum cytotoxicity to human and rat oligodendrocytes in culture. *Brain Res.*, **517**, 99–104.

Rutkowski, J. L., Kirk, C. J., Lerner, M. A. and Tennekoon, G. I. (1995) Purification and expansion of human schwann cells *in vitro*. *Nat. Med.*, **1**, 80–83.

Sabel, B. A. (1997) Unrecognized potential of surviving neurons: Within-systems plasticity, recovery of function, and the hypothesis of minimal residual structure. *Neuroscientist*, **3**, 366–370.

Sabin, F. R. (1916) The origin and development of the lymphatic system. *Johns Hopkins Hosp. Rep.*, **17**, 347–440.

Salmi, A., Reunanen, M., Ilonen, J. and Panelius, M. (1983) Intrathecal antibody synthesis to virus antigens in multiple sclerosis. *Clin. Exp. Immunol.*, **52**, 241–249.

Sanders, M. E., Koski, C. L., Robbins, D., Shin, M. L., Frank, M. M. and Joiner, K. A. (1986) Activated terminal complement in cerebrospinal fluid in Guillain–Barré syndrome and multiple sclerosis. *J. Immunol.*, **136**, 4456–4459.

Satoh, J., Kastrukoff, L. F. and Kim, S. U. (1991) Cytokine-induced expression of intercellular adhesion molecule-1 (ICAM-1) in cultured human oligodendrocytes and astrocytes. *J. Neuropathol. Exp. Neurol.*, **50**, 215–226.

Sawcer, S., Goodfellow, P. N. and Compston, A. (1997) The genetic analysis of multiple sclerosis. *Trends Genet.*, **13**, 234–239.

Scolding, N., Linington, C. and Compston, A. (1989) Immune mechanisms in the pathogenesis of demyelinating diseases. *Autoimmunity*, **4**, 131–142.

Scolding, N. J. (1997) Strategies for repair and remyelination in demyelinating diseases. *Curr. Opin. Neurol.*, **10**, 193–200.

Scolding, N. J. and Compston, D. A. S. (1991) Oligodendrocyte-macrophage interactions *in vitro* triggered by specific antibodies. *Immunology*, **72**, 127–132.

Scolding, N. J. and Franklin, R. (1998) Axon loss in multiple sclerosis. *Lancet*, **352**, 340–341.

Scolding, N. J. and Franklin, R. J. M. (1999) Remyelination in demyelinating disease. In *Multiple Sclerosis* (Miller, D. H., ed.). London: Baillière Tindall. In press.

Scolding, N. J., Morgan, B. P., Houston, A., Campbell, A. K., Linington, C. and Compston, D. A. S. (1989a) Normal rat serum cytotoxicity against syngeneic oligodendrocytes. Complement activation and attack in the absence of anti-myelin antibodies. *J. Neurolog. Sci.*, **89**, 289–300.

Scolding, N. J., Morgan, B. P., Houston, W. A. J, Linington, C., Campbell, A. K. and Compston, D. A. S. (1989b) Vesicular removal by oligodendrocytes of membrane attack complexes formed by activated complement. *Nature*, **339**, 620–622.

Scolding, N. J., Rayner, P. J., Sussman, J., Shaw, C. and Compston, D. A. S. (1995) A proliferative adult human oligodendrocyte progenitor. *NeuroReport*, **6**, 441–445.

Scolding, N. J., Zajicek, J. P., Wood, N. and Compston, D. A. S. (1994) The pathogenesis of demyelinating disease. *Prog. Neurobiol.*, **43**, 143–173.

Sedgwick, J. D. (1997) T-lymphocyte activation and regulation in the central nervous system. *Biochem. Soc. Trans.*, **25**, 673–679.

Selmaj, K. (1996) Pathophysiology of the blood–brain barrier. *Springer Semin. Immunopathol.*, **18**, 57–73.

Selmaj, K. W. and Raine, C. S. (1988) Tumor necrosis factor mediates myelin and oligodendrocyte damage *in vitro*. *Ann. Neurol.*, **23**, 339–346.

Selmaj, K., Raine, C. S., Cannella, B. and Brosnan, C. F. (1991a) Identification of lymphotoxin and tumor necrosis factor in multiple sclerosis lesions. *J. Clin. Invest.*, **87**, 949–954.

Selmaj, K., Raine, C. S. and Cross, A. H. (1991b) Anti-tumor necrosis factor therapy abrogates autoimmune demyelination. *Ann. Neurol.*, **30**, 694–700.

Selmaj, K., Raine, C. S., Farooq, M., Norton, W. T. and Brosnan, C. F. (1991c) Cytokine cytotoxicity against oligodendrocytes: Apoptosis induced by lymphotoxin. *J. Immunology*, **147**, 1522–1529.

Selmaj, K., Brosnan, C. F. and Raine, C. S. (1992) Expression of heat shock protein-65 by oligodendrocytes *in vivo* and *in vitro*: implications for multiple sclerosis. *Neurology*, **42**, 795–800.

Sharief, M. K. and Hentges, R. (1991) Association between tumor necrosis factor-alpha and disease progression in patients with multiple sclerosis (see comments). *N. Engl. J. Med.*, **325**, 467–472.

Sharief, M. K. and Thompson, E. J. (1993) Correlation of interleukin-2 and soluble interleukin-2 receptor with clinical activity of multiple sclerosis. *J. Neurol. Neurosurg. Psychiat.*, **56**, 169–174.

Sheremata, W. A., Poskanzer, D. C., Withum, D. G., Macleod, C. L. and Whiteside, M. E. (1985) Unusual occurrence on a tropical island of multiple sclerosis (letter). *Lancet*, **ii**, 618.

Simmons, R. D., Buzbee, T. M., Linthicum, D. S., Mandy, W. J., Chen, G. and Wang, C. (1987) Simultaneous visualization of vascular permeability change and leukocyte egress in the central nervous system during autoimmune encephalomyelitis. *Acta Neuropathol. Berl.*, **74**, 191–193.

Simmons, R. D. and Willenborg, D. O. (1990) Direct injection of cytokines into the spinal cord causes autoimmune encephalomyelitis-like inflammation (see comments). *J. Neurol. Sci.*, **100**, 37–42.

Skoff, R. P. (1996) The lineages of neuroglial cells. *Neuroscientist*, **2**, 335–344.

Sloan, D. J., Wood, M. J. and Charlton, H. M. (1991) The immune response to intracerebral neural grafts. *Trends. Neurosci.*, **14**, 341–346.

Smith, K. J. (1996) Conduction properties of central demyelinated axons: the generation of symptoms in demyelinating disease. In *The Neurobiology of Disease* (Bostock, H., Kirkwood, P. A. and Pullen, A. H., eds), pp. 95–117. Cambridge: Cambridge University Press.

Smith, K. J. and Hall, S. M. (1988) Peripheral demyelination and remyelination initiated by the calcium-selective ionophore ionomycin: *in vivo* observations. *J. Neurol. Sci.*, **83**, 37–53.

Smith, K. J. and Hall, S. M. (1994) Central demyelination induced *in vivo* by the calcium ionophore ionomycin. *Brain*, **117**, 1351–1356.

Smith, K. J. and McDonald, W. I. (1982) Spontaneous and evoked electrical discharges from a central demyelinating lesion. *J. Neurol. Sci.*, **55**, 39–47.

Smith, K. J., Blakemore, W. F. and McDonald, W. I. (1979) Central remyelination restores secure conduction. *Nature*, **280**, 395–396.

Smith, K. J., Bostock, H. and Hall, S. M. (1982) Saltatory conduction precedes remyelination in axons demyelinated with lysophosphatidyl choline. *J. Neurol. Sci.*, **54**, 13–31.

Sobel, R. A. (1989) T-lymphocyte subsets in the multiple sclerosis lesion. *Res. Immunol.*, **140**, 208–211.

Sobel, R. A. (1995) The pathology of multiple sclerosis. *Neurolog. Clin.*, **13**, 1–21.

Sobel, R. A., Mitchell, M. E. and Fondren, G. (1990) Intercellular adhesion molecule-1 (ICAM-1) in cellular immune reactions in the human central nervous system. *Am. J. Pathol.*, **136**, 1309–1316.

Soderstrom, M., Link, H., Sun, J. B., Fredrikson, S., Kostulas, V., Hojeberg, B., *et al.* (1993) T cells recognizing multiple peptides of myelin basic protein are found in blood and enriched in cerebrospinal fluid in optic neuritis and multiple sclerosis. *Scand. J. Immunol.*, **37**, 355–368.

Soderstrom, M., Link, H., Sun, J. B., Fredrikson, S., Wang, Z. Y. and Huang, W. X. (1994) Autoimmune T cell repertoire in optic neuritis and multiple sclerosis: T cells recognizing multiple myelin proteins are accumulated in cerebrospinal fluid. *J. Neurol. Neurosurg. Psychiat.*, **57**, 544–551.

Sola, P., Merelli, E., Marasca, R., Poggi, M., Luppi, M., Montorsi, M., *et al.* (1993) Human herpesvirus 6 and multiple sclerosis: survey of anti-HHV–6 antibodies by immunofluorescence analysis and of viral sequences by polymerase chain reaction. *J. Neurol. Neurosurg. Psychiat.*, **56**, 917–919.

Soldan, S. S., Berti, R., Salem, N., Secchiero, P., Flamand, L., Calabresi, P. A., *et al.* (1997) Association of human herpes virus 6 (HHV-6) with multiple sclerosis: Increased IgM response to HHV-6 early antigen and detection of serum HHV-6 DNA. *Nature Medicine*, **3**, 1394–1397.

Stinissen, P., Raus, J. and Zhang, J. (1997) Autoimmune pathogenesis of multiple sclerosis: role of autoreactive T lymphocytes and new immunotherapeutic strategies. *Crit. Rev. Immunol.*, **17**, 33–75.

Storch, M. K., Piddlesden, S., Haltia, M., Iivanainen, M., Morgan, P. and Lassmann, H. (1998) Multiple sclerosis: In situ evidence for antibody and complement-mediated demyelination. *Ann. Neurol.*, **43**, 465–471.

Sun, J., Link, H., Olsson, T., Xiao, B. G., Andersson, G., Ekre. H. P., *et al.* (1991a) T and B cell responses to myelin–oligodendrocyte glycoprotein in multiple sclerosis. *J. Immunol.*, **146**, 1490–1495.

Sun, J. B. (1993) Autoreactive T and B cells in nervous system diseases. *Acta Neurol. Scand. Suppl.*, **142**, 1–56.

Sun, J. B., Olsson, T., Wang, W. Z., Xiao, B. G., Kostulas, V., Fredrikson, S., *et al.* (1991b) Autoreactive T and B cells responding to myelin proteolipid protein in multiple sclerosis and controls. *Eur. J. Immunol.*, **21**, 1461–1468.

Suzuki, K., Andrews, J. M., Walty, J. M. and Terry, R. D. (1969) Ultrastructural studies of multiple sclerosis. *Lab. Invest.*, **20**, 444–454.

Thompson, A. J. (1996) Multiple sclerosis: symptomatic treatment. *J. Neurol.*, **243**, 559–565.

Thompson, A. J., Miller, D. H., MacManus, D. G. and McDonald, W. I. (1990) Patterns of disease activity in multiple sclerosis (letter; comment). *Br. Med. J.*, **301**, 44–45.

Thompson, A. J., Polman, C. H., Miller, D. H., McDonald, W. I., Brochet, B., Filippi, M., *et al.* (1997) Primary progressive multiple sclerosis. *Brain*, **120**, 1085–1096.

Tienari, P. J., Wikstrom, J., Sajantila, A., Palo, J. and Peltonen, L. (1992) Genetic susceptibility to multiple sclerosis linked to myelin basic protein gene (see comments). *Lancet*, **340**, 987–991.

Trapp, B. D., Peterson, J., Ransohoff, R. M., Rudick, R. A., Mork, S. and Bo, L. (1998) Axon transection in the lesions of multiple sclerosis. *N. Engl. J. Med.*, **338**, 278–285.

Tuohy, V. K., Yu, M., Weinstock Guttman, B. and Kinkel, R. P. (1997) Diversity and plasticity of self-recognition during the development of multiple sclerosis. *J. Clin. Invest.*, **99**, 1682–1690.

Turner, R. S., Chou, C. H., Kibler, R. F. and Kuo, J. F. (1982) Basic protein in brain myelin is phosphorylated by endogenous phospholipid-sensitive Ca^{2+}-dependent protein kinase. *J. Neurochem.*, **39**, 1397–1404.

Van den Berg, L. H., Bar, P. R., Sodaar, P., Mollee, I., Wokke, J. J. H. and Logtenberg, T. (1995) Selective expansion and long-term culture of human Schwann cells from sural nerve biopsies. *Ann. Neurol.*, **38**, 674–678.

Van Oosten, B. W., Lai, M., Hodgkinson, S., Barkhof, F., Miller, D. H., Moseley, I. F., *et al.* (1997) Treatment of multiple sclerosis with the monoclonal anti-CD4 antibody cM-T412: results of a randomized, double-blind, placebo-controlled, MR-monitored phase II trial. *Neurology*, **49**, 351–357.

Vanderlugt, C. J. and Miller, S. D. (1996) Epitope spreading. *Curr. Opin. Immunol.*, **8**, 831–836.

Vartanian, T., Li, Y., Zhao, M. and Stefansson, K. (1995) Interferon-gamma-induced oligodendrocyte cell death: implications for the pathogenesis of multiple sclerosis. *Mol. Med.*, **1**, 732–743.

Vass, K., Lassmann, H., Wekerle, H. and Wisniewski, H. M. (1986) The distribution of Ia antigen in the lesions of rat acute experimental allergic encephalomyelitis. *Acta Neuropathol. Berl.*, **70**, 149–160.

Vassalli, P. (1992) The pathophysiology of tumor necrosis factors. *Annu. Rev. Immunol.*, **10**, 411–452.

Vidovic, M., Sparacio, S. M., Elovitz, M. and Benveniste, E. N. (1990) Induction and regulation of class II major histocompatibility complex mRNA expression in astrocytes by interferon-gamma and tumor necrosis factor-alpha. *J. Neuroimmunol.*, **30**, 189–200.

Waksman, B. H. and Reynolds, W. E. (1984) Multiple sclerosis as a disease of immune regulation. *Proc. Soc. Exp. Biol. Med.*, **175**, 282–294.

Walter, M. A., Gibson, W. T., Ebers, G. C. and Cox, D. W. (1991) Susceptibility to multiple sclerosis is associated with the proximal immunoglobulin heavy chain variable region. *J. Clin. Invest.*, **87**, 1266–1273.

Warren, K. G. and Catz, I. (1994) Relative frequency of autoantibodies to myelin basic protein and proteolipid protein in optic neuritis and multiple sclerosis cerebrospinal fluid. *J. Neurol. Sci.*, **121**, 66–73.

Waxman, S. G. (1997) Molecular remodeling of neurons in multiple sclerosis: what we know, and what we must ask about brain plasticity in demyelinating diseases. *Adv. Neurol.*, **73**, 109–120.

Weinshenker, B. G. and Ebers, G. C. (1987) The natural history of multiple sclerosis. *Can. J. Neurol. Sci.*, **14**, 255–261.

Weinshenker, B. G., Bass, B., Rice, G. P., Noseworthy, J., Carriere, W., Baskerville, J., *et al.* (1989) The natural history of multiple sclerosis: a geographically based study. I. Clinical course and disability. *Brain*, **112**, 133–146.

Whittle, I. R., Hooper, J. and Pentland, B. (1998) Thalamic deep-brain stimulation for movement disorders due to multiple sclerosis. *Lancet*, **351**, 109–110.

Wood, A., Wing, M. G., Benham, C. D. and Compston, D. A. (1993) Specific induction of intracellular calcium oscillations by complement membrane attack on oligodendroglia. *J. Neurosci.*, **13**, 3319–3332.

Wood, N. W., Holmans, P., Clayton, D., Robertson, N. and Compston, D. A. (1994) No linkage or association between multiple sclerosis and the myelin basic protein gene in affected sibling pairs. *J. Neurol. Neurosurg. Psychiat.*, **57**, 1191–1194.

Wood, N. W., Sawcer, S. J., Kellar, W. H., Holmans, P., Clayton, D., Robertson, N., *et al.* (1995a) Susceptibility to multiple sclerosis and the immunoglobulin heavy chain variable region. *J. Neurol.*, **242**, 677–682.

Wood, N. W., Sawcer, S. J., Kellar, W. H., Holmans, P., Clayton, D., Robertson, N., *et al.* (1995b) The T-cell receptor beta locus and susceptibility to multiple sclerosis. *Neurology*, **45**, 1859–1863.

Woodruff, R. H. and Franklin, R. J. M. (1997) Growth factors and remyelination in the CNS. *Histol. Histopathol.*, **12**. In press

Wucherpfennig, K. W. (1994) Autoimmunity in the central nervous system: mechanisms of antigen presentation and recognition. *Clin. Immunol. Immunopathol.*, **72**, 293–306.

Wucherpfennig, K. W. and Strominger, J. L. (1995) Molecular mimicry in T cell-mediated autoimmunity: viral peptides activate human T cell clones specific for myelin basic protein. *Cell*, **80**, 695–705.

Wucherpfennig, K. W., Weiner, H. L. and Hafler, D. A. (1991) T-cell recognition of myelin basic protein (see comments). *Immunol. Today*, **12**, 277–282.

Xiao, B. G., Linington, C. and Link, H. (1991) Antibodies to myelin–oligodendrocyte glycoprotein in cerebrospinal fluid from patients with multiple sclerosis and controls. *J. Neuroimmunol.*, **31**, 91–96.

Yednock, T. A., Cannon, C., Fritz, L. C., Sanchez-Madrid, F., Steinman, L. and Karin, N. (1992) Prevention of experimental autoimmune encephalomyelitis by antibodies against alpha-4–beta-1 integrin. *Nature*, **356**, 63–66.

Youl, B. D., Turano, G., Miller, D. H., Towell, A. D., Macmanus, D. G., Moore, S. G., *et al.* (1991) The pathophysiology of acute optic neuritis. An association of gadolinium leakage with clinical and electrophysiological deficits. *Brain*, **114**, 2437–2450.

Yu, M., Johnson, J. M., Tuohy, V. K. (1996a) A predictable sequential determinant spreading cascade invariably accompanies progression of experimental autoimmune encephalomyelitis: a basis for peptide-specific therapy after onset of clinical disease. *J. Exp. Med.*, **183**, 1777–1788.

Yu, M., Johnson, J. M. and Tuohy, V. K. (1996b) Generation of autonomously pathogenic neo-autoreactive Th1 cells during the development of the determinant spreading cascade in murine autoimmune encephalomyelitis. *J. Neurosci. Res.*, **45**, 463–470.

Zajicek, J., Wing, M., Skepper, J. and Compston, A. (1995) Human oligodendrocytes are not sensitive to complement: A study of CD59 expression in the human central nervous system. *Lab. Invest.*, **73**, 128–138.

Zajocek, J. P., Wing, M., Scolding, N. J. and Compston, D. A. S. (1992) Interactions between oligodendrocytes and microglia. A major role for complement and tumour necrosis factor in oligodendrocyte adherence and killing. *Brain*, **115**, 1611–1631.

Zamvil, S. S. and Steinman, L. (1990) The T lymphocyte in experimental allergic encephalomyelitis. *Annu. Rev. Immunol.*, **8**, 579–621.

Zhang, Y., Burger, D., Saruhan, G., Jeannet, M. and Steck, A. J. (1993) The T-lymphocyte response against myelin-associated glycoprotein and myelin basic protein in patients with multiple sclerosis. *Neurology*, **43**, 403–407

Inflammatory demyelinating disease (II): syndromes and disorders related to multiple sclerosis

Neil Scolding

Introduction	74
Syndromes of isolated demyelination	74
Diffuse or disseminated syndromes	82
Apparent variants of multiple sclerosis	86
References	88

Introduction

A number of disorders are characterized by clinical pictures which exhibit a clear relationship with that of multiple sclerosis, whilst nevertheless remaining distinct. Biochemical, radiological and pathological features may also be shared to variable degrees. The most obvious difference is in clinical course; a relapsing and remitting pattern is exclusive to multiple sclerosis, while some of the related disorders have a more aggressive or even fulminating course. Other differences are historical and partly reflect the nosological evolution of the demyelinating diseases. Some early clinical and pathological descriptions are difficult to accommodate within current pigeon holes, but an attempt may be made to include these disorders whose often eponymous epithets occasionally survive.

Syndromes of isolated demyelination

Optic neuritis

The term optic neuritis refers to a clinical syndrome comprising subacute monocular visual loss, often accompanied by pain on eye movement (68% of cases (Bradley and Whitty, 1967)), and almost invariably associated with spontaneous and near complete recovery over a course of weeks to months. Use of the term implies an unknown aetiology. Approximately 70% of patients with multiple sclerosis experience optic neuritis at some stage during the course of their disease (Shibasaki *et al.*, 1981) and in 18–20% it is the first manifestation of the disease (Mathews, 1991). Optic neuritis is not invariably followed by the development of multiple sclerosis, but there are no useful clinical clues indicating whether or not optic neuritis in any one individual heralds multiple sclerosis.

Clinical features
The predominant symptoms have been mentioned. Objectively, a central scotoma is usually found, although other monocular field defects are well-

described (Bradley and Whitty, 1967). Colour vision is usually impaired and light intolerance may be mentioned. A sluggish and incomplete direct pupillary response to light, contrasting (if the other eye is normal) with a normal consensual response – moving a torch beam from contralateral to affected pupil results in dilation of the latter – constitutes the Marcus Gunn pupil or afferent pupillary defect. The optic disc appears normal in around 60% of cases and swollen to a variable degree in the remainder. Persistent visual symptoms following recovery are unusual, 50% having normal vision at 1 month, 75% at 6 months (Bradley and Whitty, 1967), although objective or electrophysiological abnormalities may be permanent.

Measuring visual evoked potentials provides a quantifiable record of impaired optic nerve function, but in practice rarely aids the diagnosis, lacking specificity. A normal result in a patient with suspected disease should encourage further searching for alternative causes of visual impairment, including ocular disease, but may also raise the possibility of hysteria. An abnormal result in the symptomatically unaffected nerve is prognostically useful, suggesting bilateral disease with an increased risk of later development of multiple sclerosis (Compston et al., 1978; Sandberg et al., 1990). Magnetic resonance imaging (MRI) can also reveal changes in optic neuritis; its principal role is in excluding alternative diagnoses, though there is evidence that prognostication is also possible – long lesions and those occupying the intracanalicular portion of the optic nerve are associated with poorer recovery (Youl et al., 1991).

Bilateral simultaneous optic neuritis is unusual (approximately 7% of cases (Bradley and Whitty, 1967)) and warrants a more assiduous search for an identifiable cause. Clinically unsuspected Leber's hereditary optic neuropathy may account for approximately 20% of such cases (Morrissey et al., 1995) and may be excluded by careful fundoscopy (preferably using a slit lamp), which shows tortuous vessels with capillary dilatation and telangiectasia, with no increase in vascular permeability apparent on fluorescein angiography, contrasting with optic neuritis. Mitochondrial DNA analysis is now an important component of investigation, occasionally revealing Leber's associated mutations in the absence of obvious fundal abnormalities (Morrissey et al., 1995). (More usually, Leber's disease is suspected by the occurrence of a severe and sequential optic neuropathy typically in a young man with a family history indicating matrilineal inheritance.)

The differential diagnosis also includes toxins, B_{12} deficiency, other inflammatory disorders (particularly sarcoidosis, vasculitis and lupus, see p. 163), ischaemia, infections, mitochondrial disease (Leber's hereditary optic neuropathy) and optic nerve, chiasmal or other local tumours. The latter may be intrinsic (classically gliomata or optic nerve sheath meningiomata, which may be suggested by the presence of opto-ciliary shunt vessels) or extrinsic (pituitary and craniopharyngiomata).

In conventional or idiopathic inflammatory demyelinating optic neuritis, recurrence in one or other eye will occur in between 15 and 35% of cases (Francis et al., 1987; Sandberg et al., 1990), while progression to multiple sclerosis ultimately occurs in 50–85% of cases (Bradley and Whitty, 1968; Francis et al., 1987). There are no reliable clinical features which influence the risk of progression to multiple sclerosis, but on investigation the presence of multifocal white matter lesions at the time of presentation of optic neuritis, seen in 50–70% of cases overall (Ormerod *et al.*, 1986) increases the risk to 82% in 5 years, while a normal brain MRI carries a predictive risk of between 6 and 24% at 5 years (Morrissey *et al.*, 1993), 16% in the largest study (the Optic Neuritis Treatment Trial; Brodsky *et al.*, 1997). Although rarely sought, the occurrence of oligoclonal bands in the spinal fluid also increases the likelihood of developing disseminated disease, nine of 13 patients with a positive result developing multiple sclerosis in one series (Sandberg *et al.*, 1990). The Optic Neuritis Treatment Trial (see below) yielded further information: 11 of 13 patients with oligoclonal bands developed multiple sclerosis within 2 years, but it was clear that spinal fluid analysis added little or nothing to the prognostic information yielded by MRI (Rolak *et al.*, 1996). Other studies, however, report precisely the opposite – that cerebrospinal fluid (CSF) immunoglobulin studies have a better predictive value than MRI (Jacobs *et al.*, 1997).

As mentioned in Chapter 2, a carefully executed large randomized trial of intravenous methylprednisolone (1 g daily for 3 days) in the treatment of acute optic neuritis (Beck *et al.*, 1992) showed treatment to increase the speed, but not the overall extent, of recovery. Additional retrospective analysis suggested a further and unexpected beneficial effect of decreasing the risk of developing multiple sclerosis in the following 2 years (Beck *et al.*, 1993), although the difference between control and methylprednisolone-treated patients had vanished by 3 years (Beck, 1995). Although clearly of interest, this observation – not a primary aim of the trial – awaits confirmation.

Pathological processes in optic neuritis
Pathological observations in acute optic neuritis are understandably lacking, but studies of chronic lesions in patients dying with multiple sclerosis provides no evidence of any differences between the pathological processes in optic nerve lesions and those elsewhere. Patches of demyelinated axons, deficient in oligodendrocytes but containing numerous and hypertrophied astrocytes, are apparent, commonly centred upon venules. Similarly, immunological investigations, including haplotype analysis, spinal fluid immunoglobulin and complement changes, and studies of peripheral lymphocyte phenotype and function, all reveal abnormalities in optic neuritis broadly comparable with those in multiple sclerosis (Compston, 1986).

Notwithstanding the lack of histological data, studies of patients with optic neuritis have, because of the clinical eloquence of lesions within the optic nerve, the unique opportunity (with ophthalmoscopy) to visualize directly neurones, axons and blood vessels at the origin of the optic nerve, and because of the accessibility of lesions to electrophysiological and imaging investigation, allowed substantial contributions to be made to our understanding of the pathological processes underlying inflammatory demyelination. These have been discussed in more detail in the preceding chapter, but three key observations may briefly be mentioned.

First is the finding of retinal vascular leakage, either on direct fundoscopy or fluorescein angiography, which correlates pathologically with perivenous inflammatory infiltration with lymphocytes and plasma cells (Fog, 1965;

Arnold *et al.*, 1984). This provides powerful support for a primary pathological process centred upon the blood–retinal – and, by implication, the blood–brain barrier – in multiple sclerosis, there being in the retina (of course) no myelin to provide an alternative immunological or inflammatory stimulus.

Secondly, correlative analysis of the temporal sequence of changes in the clinical features, electrophysiological abnormalities and (gadolinium-enhanced) MRI findings in acute optic neuritis has yielded important insights into the relative roles of oedema, inflammation and demyelination in the pathological development of lesions (see Chapter 2). Thus, loss of normal myelin function (which of course does not necessarily equate with anatomical demyelination) occurred very early in the course of disease (within 48 h); a direct effect of local inflammation on saltatory conduction was suggested. Symptomatic remission correlated with the resolution of inflammation, while evidence of demyelination was persistent (Youl *et al.*, 1991; McDonald, 1996).

Third, fundoscopic observations in 1974 provided direct evidence of neuronal loss in the retinal nerve fibre layer of patients with previous optic neuritis and multiple sclerosis (Frisen and Hoyt 1974), an important observation whose implications are more fully discussed in Chapter 2.

Transverse myelitis

Despite a number of immediate and obvious similarities – a syndromic disorder of monophasic course, affecting a single focus within the CNS, presumed often to have an inflammatory basis, usually a diagnosis of exclusion, and occurring in isolation or in the context of multiple sclerosis – transverse myelitis and optic neuritis are only distantly related. 'Idiopathic' transverse myelitis has in fact a rather different clinical phenotype to the spinal cord involvement more commonly seen in multiple sclerosis, their pathological relationship is less certain and entirely unrelated alternative underlying diagnoses more commonly emerge in patients with this syndrome compared to those with suspected optic neuritis.

Transverse myelitis most commonly affects the thoracic cord (approximately 80% of cases (Berman *et al.*, 1981; Jeffery *et al.*, 1993), and the usual clinical picture suggests involvement of the whole spinal cord at the affected level. This contrasts with myelitis occurring in the context of established multiple sclerosis, where a partial cord lesion is more typical (Scott *et al.*, 1998). Thus, while episodes of deafferentation of one upper limb caused by inflammation in or near the dorsal root entry zone, or of pure sensory disturbance in both legs due to a partial thoracic lesion, would be common in multiple sclerosis, the more usual picture in acute myelitis is one of paralysis, sensory loss and incontinence progressing over perhaps 24–48 h, sometimes more (Ropper and Poskanzer, 1978). Back pain is often prominent, and a fever and meningism may be present. Also in contrast with multiple sclerosis, men and women are equally affected. A history of preceding infection is found in approximately one-third of cases, in the majority (80%), of the upper respiratory tract (Berman *et al.*, 1981). Objectively, the flaccid paraparetic or paraplegic picture of spinal shock with useless bladder and/or bowel sphincter function is found, often with a sensory level accompanied by a band of hyperaesthesia, allodynia or hyperpathia. (This syndrome can, of course, occur in or herald multiple sclerosis, but only rarely.)

The differential diagnosis is wide and includes any compressive cord disorder, so that urgent imaging of the spinal cord, formerly by contrast myelography, now commonly by MRI, is mandatory: this often reveals that the process is far more extensive longitudinally than the clinical picture – or indeed the name – implies (Figure 3.1). Structural compression having been excluded, spinal fluid examination is important to exclude direct infectious causes, such as herpes viruses (Klastersky et al., 1972). Dermatological manifestations of zoster infection precede spinal involvement by up to a fortnight – or may be altogether absent; the myelopathy may spare the dorsal columns and produce a largely motor picture (Devinsky et al., 1991). Retroviruses, both HIV and HTLV-1, can cause a transverse myelopathy, and serological testing should be instigated, although in both cases presentation is usually rather less acute. Systemic lupus erythematosus (SLE) can cause a severe and acute myelopathy (Mok et al., 1998). In idiopathic transverse myelitis, an increased mononuclear cell count and protein level is usual and oligoclonal bands may be detected; the spinal fluid is, however, normal in up to 40% of patients (Berman et al., 1981). A more recent study reported raised protein and/or cell counts in 94% of (31) patients, none of whom had oligoclonal bands (Al Deeb et al., 1997).

The third main cause of this picture – neither compressive nor inflammatory/infective – is spinal cord ischaemia. This, like idiopathic transverse myelitis, is usually a diagnosis of exclusion. Occasionally the context renders an infarct the inevitable diagnosis – an expanding, dissecting or surgically challenged aortic aneurysm, for example. Evidence of occlusive vascular disease elsewhere, or of embolizing heart disease (including endocarditis), might also suggest an ischaemic cord lesion, while the often sought and rarely heard dorsal bruit indicates a local vascular malformation. More commonly, spinal cord infarction is inferred, but not proven, largely on the basis of the abruptness of onset of cord symptoms. Meningovascular syphilis is now rather a rare cause of spinal cord infarction.

There are no controlled trials of treatment of acute myelitis. High-dose intravenous corticosteroids are commonly administered and the established value of this treatment in traumatic cord lesions, where similar secondary mechanisms of oedema and ischaemia are implicated, provide some rationale for this approach.

The prognosis for patients with transverse myelitis is at best middling. In the Israel series of 62 patients (Berman et al., 1981) – one of the largest reported – approximately one-third had a good recovery, one-third fair and one-third poor. Five percent (three patients) died in the acute stage from respiratory failure or sepsis. No patient who had not improved by 3 months recovered thereafter. Back pain and spinal shock are poor prognostic indicators (Ropper and Poskanzer, 1978). In the Israel study, only one patient went on to develop multiple sclerosis, while of a UK group of 34 cases, seven (studied 5–42 years later) developed multiple sclerosis (Lipton and Teasdall, 1973). Relapsing transverse myelitis, with neither clinical nor radiological evidence of disease elsewhere in the nervous system (and with negative testing for oligoclonal bands), occurs in a very small proportion of patients (Tippett et al., 1991).

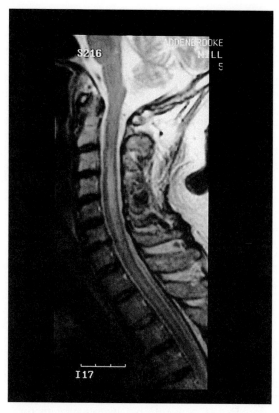

Figure 3.1 Magnetic resonance imaging (MRI) in transverse myelitis. In a patient with classical features of transverse myelitis, the MRI scan often reveals disease extending over many levels. Here, expansion of the cervical cord is apparent, with high signal visible from C_3 to at least T_3.

Although other studies have addressed the likelihood of multiple sclerosis being diagnosed in patients presenting with myelopathies, most have either investigated all (suspected) inflammatory cord lesions (Miller *et al.*, 1987, 1989) or concentrated on partial cord syndromes of the type more commonly seen in multiple sclerosis (Ford *et al.*, 1992; Jeffery *et al.*, 1993). In such patients, the risk of developing multiple sclerosis is 60–90% in those who are found on brain MRI examination to have white matter lesions and only 6–10% in those who do not – a figure close to that for patients with complete cord syndromes (Miller *et al.*, 1987, 1989; Ford *et al.*, 1992; Morrissey *et al.*, 1993). As with optic neuritis, the presence of oligoclonal bands also increases the risk; Morrisey *et al.* found no patients who developed multiple sclerosis having had neither MRI lesions nor oligoclonal bands. It should be re-emphasized, however, that patients in these studies did not, on the whole, have typical transverse myelitis.

The pathological process in transverse myelitis
A history of preceding infection in a third or more of patients diagnosed clinically as having transverse myelitis suggests a post-infectious inflamma-

tory process which may be more akin to acute disseminated encephalomyelitis (ADEM; see below) in the CNS, and the Guillain–Barré syndrome (GBS) peripherally, than multiple sclerosis. The clinical and pathological similarities between transverse myelitis, ADEM and experimental allergic encephalomyelitis (EAE) have drawn comment in the literature: histologically, an inflammatory necrotic process, with perivascular lymphocytic infiltration and microglial proliferation, is apparent. There is axonal loss as well as secondary demyelination, grey matter being involved but usually to a lesser extent than white (Greenfield and Turner, 1939; Ropper and Poskanzer, 1978). In one study, peripheral blood lymphocyte reactivity to myelin basic protein (MBP) – an efficient inducer of EAE – was found in seven out of 10 patients with transverse myelitis (Abramsky and Teitelbaum, 1977).

Devic's disease or neuromyelitis optica

F. Clifford Albutt (1870) first drew attention to a disorder characterized by a subacutely progressive optic nerve (uni- or bilateral) and spinal cord syndrome – the two sites often affected simultaneously, occasionally in close succession (Albutt, 1870). The more lasting eponymous association, however, followed Devic's report in 1894, though *neuromyelitis optica* has also become a commonly used descriptive epithet (Devic, 1895).

Devic's *syndrome* represents the phenotype common to at least three underlying disease processes. Thus it is often part of the spectrum of multiple sclerosis, where the burden of disease happens to have fallen asymmetrically upon the spinal cord and optic nerves – pathologically, or with MRI, disseminated lesions are apparent elsewhere in the central nervous system (CNS). In these cases, a conventional histological picture of perivascular inflammation and primary demyelination is found (Lumsden, 1951). Secondly, other inflammatory disorders may cause a similar clinical picture, notoriously SLE (April and Vansonnenberg, 1976), but also vasculitic syndromes, sarcoidosis and Behçet's disease. Usually, but not invariably, systemic manifestations are apparent.

Whilst these descriptions may be encompassed within the rubric Devic's *syndrome*, both groups of patients should be excluded from the diagnostic label of Devic's *disease*, a term which should be reserved for those patients with no clinical or paraclinical evidence of disease elsewhere in the CNS and in whom other systemic or vasculitic disorders have been excluded.

In an important studying of eight patients with such a picture, Mandler *et al.* confirmed a unique clinical and pathological phenotype clearly separable from multiple sclerosis (Mandler *et al.*, 1993). Perhaps unexpectedly, in five cases the course was relapsing, monophasic in the remainder, while (also of interest) optic neuritis was unilateral in every case. Within a 4 year period, five patients had died and two were severely disabled; one improved but was reported to be dependent on lymphocytoplasmaphoresis. Spinal fluid examination typically failed to show oligoclonal bands (six of seven cases); the cell count was significantly elevated, however, with a mean of 59 leukocytes. Cranial MRI was normal. These observations have been broadly confirmed (O'Riordan *et al.*, 1996). Recent studies suggest azothioprine with steroids may hold some therapeutic promise (Mandle *et al.*, 1998).

The pathological processes in neuromyelitis optica appear intermediate between those of multiple sclerosis and transverse myelitis or ADEM. The spinal cord picture is one of necrosis and axonal loss with demyelination, often accompanied by cavitation, while the optic nerve lesion more closely resembles primary demyelination, though here too cavitation is occasionally seen. In Mandler's study, no pathological changes were found elsewhere in the brain, reflecting the imaging observations and helping to confirm the disorder as a separate entity.

A very low incidence of conversion to clinical multiple sclerosis appears to occur in 'true' Devic's syndrome (Stansbury, 1949).

Foix–Alajuanine Syndrome and acute necrotising myelitis

In 1926, Foix and Alajouanine described a syndrome they called *subacute necrotic myelitis* (Foix and Alajouanine, 1926). Adult males were predominantly affected by an illness characterized clinically by a spastic paralysis progressing over a course of 2–3 months, with sensory loss followed by incontinence; a flaccid, areflexic and amyotrophic phase ensued. Signs of systemic illness, with a fever, meningism and often severe local pain were common. Spinal fluid changes (cyto-albuminic dissociation with markedly elevated protein levels) – and in later cases, imaging – revealed evidence of a spinal block, from a markedly swollen cord. In fact, cellular reaction in the spinal fluid, often substantial, can occur in either disorder.

In the same decade, a disorder of similar nature but substantially more rapid in onset – with complete paralysis within 1–2 days of onset – was described, termed *acute necrotising myelitis* (reviewed in Hoffman, 1955). Hoffman drew attention to the occurrence of a preceding infection in approximately one-third of cases.

Pathological examination in both disorders revealed broadly similar findings, with a profoundly severe necrotic process affecting grey and white matter, accompanied by an inflammatory infiltrate and a brisk astrocytic reaction. Characteristically in Foix–Alajuanine syndrome, the lumbo-sacral cord was most affected, the thoracic cord less so. Subsequent attention was directed towards a possible underlying veno-occlusive process: thrombin deposition, thickening the walls of vessels, was common and often prominent, though venous infarction less so and not present in the cases originally described. Hoffman also pointed out that many cases have no vascular changes at all.

As with transverse myelitis – with which the syndrome clearly may merge, although classically the later phase of flaccidity, wasting and areflexia is stressed as unique to necrotising myelitis (Hoffman, 1955) – high doses of intravenous methylprednisolone may substantially improve the outcome. Surgical intervention not uncommonly is considered unavoidable, usually to exclude compression and/or local pyogenic infection, and it is possible (though entirely conjectural) that decompression may critically improve perfusion, preventing infarction secondary to the swelling.

A similar syndrome is described in conjunction with lymphomatous or leukaemic cancers or with adenocarcinoma, and with infections, including herpes and AIDS (Ojeda, 1984; Britton *et al.*, 1985; Wiley *et al.*, 1987).

Diffuse or disseminated syndromes

Acute disseminated encephalomyelitis

The syndrome known as ADEM (Lisak, 1994) essentially includes post-infectious encephalomyelitis and post-vaccinal encephalomyelitis, and a proportion of cases in which no antecedent infectious or inflammatory event is identifiable historically, microbiologically or serologically. (Originally the term *post-vaccinal encephalomyelitis* was naturally used specifically for cases following smallpox inoculation. While *post-vaccination encephalomyelitis* is now the more commonly used general term, *post-vaccinal encephalomyelitis* is still occasionally seen but in most instances has lost its Jennerian specificity.) It is part of the spectrum of acute inflammatory demyelinating diseases affecting the CNS, monophasic (usually) and with a more severe and aggressive phenotype than acute events or relapses in multiple sclerosis; it is, however, less severe than the often fatal acute haemorrhagic encephalomyelitis (see below).

The historically described disorders which occurred following rabies vaccination and after measles virus infection essentially represent prototypic ADEM. 'Neuroparalytic accidents' in patients receiving Jenner's smallpox (actually cowpox) vaccine were noted after its more widespread introduction in 1853 and in patients receiving Pasteur's rabies vaccine, introduced in 1885. It was not until the 1920s, however, that the disorder appeared to gain more formal and widespread recognition (Ford, 1928; Bassoe and Grinker, 1930; Turnbull and McIntosh, 1997). Pasteur's inoculum was prepared from rabbit spinal cord (injected with fixed rabies virus); the origin and cause of post-smallpox inoculation encephalomyelitis is less clear as vaccine preparation does not involve neural tissues.

Post-vaccination encephalomyelitis continues to be seen after rabies vaccine containing neural tissue (Swamy et al., 1984), such as the Semple preparation (extracted from rabbit brain and used particularly in developing countries) and duck embryo vaccine, which also contains minimal amounts of neural tissue. Occasional reports associating ADEM (and transverse myelitis) with other non-neural vaccines, including hepatitis B, influenza, measles, pertussis and diphtheria continue to appear (Fenichel, 1982) and to evoke controversy. Post-infectious encephalomyelitis is reduced in incidence following the introduction of widespread measles vaccination, but still occurs (Johnson et al., 1984; Johnson, 1994). Other infectious (or para-infectious) precipitants include in particular mycoplasma (and other atypical pneumonic infections), Herpesviruses, rubella, leptospira and Borrelia (Johnson et al., 1985; Johnson, 1996). Non-specific or unidentified viral illnesses can also antecede ADEM.

Clinical features
Acute disseminated encephalomyelitis occurs predominantly, though by no means exclusively, in childhood. The timing of the first symptoms varies slightly with the precipitant: typically 1–14 days after non-neural vaccines, 1 week or less after the appearance of a rash in exanthematous illnesses and 13 weeks (or more) after rabies inoculation (Fenichel, 1982; Swamy et al., 1984; Lisak, 1994; Johnson, 1996).

A prodromal illness of fever, myalgia and general malaise, lasting a few days, appears more common in post-vaccination disease than after infections. Subsequently, widely varying neurological features occur (Lisak, 1994); their onset is rapid, with progression over hours to a peak in days. An encephalopathy, with or without meningismus, is usual (and almost invariable in measles-associated disease (Swamy *et al.*, 1984)) and this may progress to coma. Seizures are more often seen in post-infectious disease than after vaccines, but focal signs, including those indicating brainstem or hemisphere disorder, and cranial neuropathies occur in both varieties. Cerebellar ataxia is notoriously associated with varicella (and carries an excellent prognosis, although whether this represents an infectious or a para-infectious process remains unresolved). Transverse myelitis (see above) may occur in isolation or in conjunction with cerebral manifestations.

The peripheral nervous system may be involved particularly in post-rabies disease, where a predilection for radicular complications is found (Swamy *et al.*, 1984). Of course, conventional GBS can follow inoculations or infectious processes, and combined GBS and ADEM after infections is also well-described.

Spontaneous recovery is the rule, usually over a course of weeks to months. Fatal disease is not rare, however (approximately 10–20%), while recovery is often incomplete. In Swamy's series, one-third of those who survived had a partial recovery at approximately 18 months, though the deficit was often not severe; two-thirds had made a complete recovery (Swamy *et al.*, 1984). Relapsing disease is rare and raises the alternative diagnostic possibility of multiple sclerosis.

The diagnosis is commonly made from the typical clinical picture. No tests are pathognomic, but a lymphocytic pleocytosis with raised protein levels are common CSF findings. A polymorphonucleocytosis may also be found, as may oligoclonal immunoglobulin bands in some patients (Kesselring *et al.*, 1990), although others suggest the spinal fluid is more often normal and oligoclonal bands not present. Multifocal MRI lesions similar to those seen in multiple sclerosis are observed, but diagnostically useful differences in their distribution have been described (Kesselring *et al.*, 1990) – a particular tendency for lesions to be found extensively and symmetrically in the cerebral and cerebellar white matter, and occasionally in the basal ganglia, was noted, while additional assessment of gadolinium enhancement might also be expected to help delineate the disorders when there is diagnostic uncertainty: only acute lesions are thought to enhance and since ADEM is conventionally a monophasic disorder, all identifiable lesions should be of the same age. A mixture of enhancing and non-enhancing lesions might therefore suggest the temporal dissemination of multiple sclerosis. Serial MRI studies can serve the same purpose.

High-dose corticosteroids, usually given as intravenous methylprednisolone, are generally advised in ADEM, though there remains no formal documentary evidence of efficacy. Swamy *et al.* (1984) described a response to intravenous cyclophosphamide in some patients not responding to steroids. The roles of plasmapheresis and intravenous immunoglobulin have also yet to be formally assessed, although the latter has been recommended in the unusual instance of recurrent disease (Hahn *et al.*, 1996).

Disease processes in ADEM

Whatever the precipitant, the histopathological appearances in ADEM subtypes do not differ. There is marked perivascular inflammation comprising lymphocytes, plasma cells and macrophages, with lesions widely disseminated throughout the CNS: a preponderance in white matter is seen, but the grey is not spared, by contrast with multiple sclerosis. In other respects, the degree of similarity with multiple sclerosis varies a little according to different authors. Myelin is lost, but whether this mainly represents primary rather than secondary demyelination is not wholly clear. Areas of necrosis may be found (though some authors would suggest such change indicates a diagnosis of acute haemorrhagic encephalomyelitis rather than ADEM), and the presence of meningeal inflammation may also provide some distinction from multiple sclerosis. An astrocytic response is common to both disorders.

The clinical recognition and pathological descriptions of post-vaccination encephalomyelitis in the 1920s and 1930s triggered the first experiments in which animal models of inflammatory demyelination were described. Rivers' group inoculated monkeys with brain extracts and found them to develop ataxia and weakness. Pathologically, perivascular inflammation and demyelination were found, and similarities between what became known as experimental allergic encephalomyelitis and post-vaccination encephalomyelitis, the disorder upon which it was directly modelled, were immediately apparent (Rivers *et al.*, 1933; Rivers and Schwentker, 1935).

Ferraro and Jervis (1940) extended the parallels, suggesting similarities at the histopathological level with multiple sclerosis. Although subsequent studies of the pathology of EAE maintained and emphasized a greater resemblance with ADEM than multiple sclerosis (Ferraro and Roizin, 1954) – not surprisingly, considering the mode of induction – and have continued (notwithstanding changes in species of experimental animal and method of inducing disease) so to do, it has remained the case that EAE is most commonly perceived and studied as a model of multiple sclerosis rather than of ADEM.

(This said, models with greater clinical similarities with multiple sclerosis than acute EAE have emerged. Chronic relapsing EAE (CR-EAE) may be induced in certain immature strains of guinea pigs and in the SJL/J mouse, while acute EAE in the Lewis rat, a disorder in which there is much inflammation but little primary demyelination, may be converted into a model with pronounced demyelination by the additional injection (following induction with, for example, sensitized MBP-specific T cells) of a monoclonal antibody directed against a surface component of oligodendrocytes and myelin, myelin–oligodendrocyte glycoprotein (Lassmann, 1983; Linington *et al.*, 1988).)

The close parallels between ADEM and EAE, and the common use in rodent models of MBP as the encephalitogenic inoculum, stimulated investigations seeking MBP-reactivity in ADEM patients. In general terms, a more compelling case implicating anti-MBP responses can be assembled in ADEM than in multiple sclerosis, as might be predicted by the pathological relationships. Thus, in an important study, Haffler's group isolated and analysed 57 T cell clones from plaques and several hundred from cerebrospinal fluid samples from patients with inflammatory demyelination

(Hafler *et al.*, 1987). In those from patients with multiple sclerosis, none was identified that was specific for either of the major myelin proteins MBP or proteolipid protein (PLP); in contrast, clones with reactivity against MBP were found in five of nine CSF samples from patients with ADEM. Similarly, peripheral blood reactivity to MBP is more striking and consistent in patients with post-infectious ADEM than those with multiple sclerosis, and disappears with clinical recovery (Lisak *et al.*, 1974; Lisak and Zweiman, 1977).

A possible contribution from humoral mechanisms is suggested by the finding of serum antibodies directed against MBP and galactocerebroside in patients with post-rabies inoculation ADEM (Hemachudha *et al.*, 1987, 1988); intrathecal synthesis of these antibodies was also convincingly demonstrated. In studies of post-infectious ADEM, however, no serum antibodies against MBP were found (Lisak *et al.*, 1974).

In summary, it appears likely that parallel B and T cell-mediated reactions are responsible for generating CNS inflammatory damage in ADEM (Johnson, 1987; Lisak, 1994). Establishing the relative primacy of humoral and cellular immune responses may be as difficult as it is inconsequential.

In the case of post-infectious ADEM, it is likely that molecular mimicry between virus and myelin antigens is responsible for initiating disease – as suggested with the more hypothetical viral connection in multiple sclerosis. Sequences of myelin proteins which have significant homologies with incriminated viruses are described (Jahnke *et al.*, 1985). For many years after the original descriptions of post-infectious encephalomyelitis, the question of whether this was an 'allergic' reaction or a direct (but delayed) CNS invasion by the infecting pathogen remained contentious (and studies apparently but not surprisingly demonstrating 'infectivity' of affected CNS material naturally did little to resolve the issue). A more complicated residual question of whether CNS invasion at some time in the course of infection was a necessary precipitant of ADEM has only more recently been answered, careful studies confirming the absence of viral invasion of the CNS in post-measles ADEM (Gendelman *et al.*, 1984). Thus, simple systemic infection in susceptible individuals appears sufficient for the development of ADEM. In the case of post-vaccinal ADEM involving CNS-derived tissue, the causes of myelin-directed immune reactivity are rather more transparent.

Acute haemorrhagic leukoencephalomyelitis

Acute haemorrhagic leukoencephalomyelitis (AHLE) or Weston–Hurst disease (Hurst, 1941), is an altogether more severe disorder, bearing a relationship with ADEM parallel to that of necrotising myelitis with transverse myelitis (Lisak, 1994). It is rare, and may represent essentially a hyperacute form of ADEM: there is frequently a history of antecedent upper respiratory tract infection, though often rather non-specific.

The clinical course is more rapid in onset and more severe, with pronounced systemic features; seizures are frequent and coma was present in all of the first 10 cases reported (Crawford, 1954). Cerebrospinal fluid analysis often reveals a raised intracranial pressure, and a pleomorphic cellular reaction with lymphocytes and also neutrophils and significant numbers of red cells, reflecting the haemorrhagic process.

High doses of steroids are conventionally used: their value is unproven and likely to remain so given the rarity of this disorder.

Pathologically, a severe and widespread inflammatory demyelinating process is supplemented by perivascular necrosis and microhaemorrhages. Macroscopically, the haemorrhagic element is conspicuous, areas varying from point size to a few millimetres, occasionally becoming confluent. They are found exclusively in the white matter, and most strikingly in the centrum semi-ovale and deeper cerebral areas. Changes reminiscent of fibrinoid necrosis within the walls of small blood vessels, mainly venules, are described (Crawford, 1954).

An unusually severe form of experimental disease, hyperacute EAE, strongly resembles AHLE pathologically. Although the mode of disease induction varies from that of other forms of EAE, the reason for the more devastating phenotypic and histopathological changes is no clearer in hyperacute EAE than it is in AHLE.

Apparent variants of multiple sclerosis

During the early part of this century, a number of disorders were described which are now thought to represent clinical and/or pathological variants of multiple sclerosis. The first to be recognized was Marburg's disease.

Marburg disease; acute multiple sclerosis

Marburg (1906) described three patients studied at autopsy after monophasic short acute or subacute illnesses (Marburg, 1906). Myelin destruction was extensive, but still in discrete lesions, and axonal loss often marked. Multiple sclerosis with a strikingly aggressive or malignant course, often rapidly fatal, continues to be recognized, occasionally occurring after one or two isolated demyelinating events (by way of clinical contrast with ADEM). Although pathogenetic differences accounting for the idiosyncratic course have not been explored, the distinction is justified on clinical grounds, patients with the Marburg variant more often receiving intense immunotherapy – though (again) no definitive information concerning efficacy is available.

Lassmann's group (Ozawa et al., 1994), in a recent careful study of the histopathology of multiple sclerosis concentrating particularly on the fate of the oligodendrocyte, drew attention to significant differences between cases with a conventional course, and those with aggressive disease of the Marburg type. Defining the latter as patients with acute multiple sclerosis, using Marburg's own criteria of "a very severe progressive or relapsing neurological disease that led to extensive neurological deficits and death within 1 year after onset", these authors confirmed Marburg's pathological observations, finding widespread changes quite different from those seen in conventional multiple sclerosis – a substantial inflammatory infiltrate with extensive destruction of not only of oligodendrocytes, but astrocytes, axons, lymphocytes and macrophages. The authors were able reasonably to conclude that quite different disease processes were occurring, justifying preservation of the distinct Marburg epithet (Ozawa et al., 1994; Lucchinetti *et al.*, 1996). More recently an association of Marburg's disease with developmentally immature forms of MBP has been suggested (Wood *et al.*, 1996).

Schilder's diffuse sclerosis

The nosology of Schilder's disease is more complex, but again, retention of the eponym in recognition of a distinct clinical phenotype within the syndrome of multiple sclerosis is probably worthwhile. Schilder's original description concerned a single child who died after a short, monophasic demyelinating illness not unlike Marburg's disease clinically (Schilder, 1912). The pathology was distinct, however, with widespread confluent or diffuse demyelination involving the cerebrum, cerebellum and brainstem, and Schilder used the term encephalitis periaxalis diffusa to emphasize the pathological distinction from Marburg's disorder, encephalitis periaxalis scleroticans. Other pathological features included significant axonal damage (raising the possibility that demyelination might in many areas be secondary or Wallerian, rather than primary), and tendencies for a subcortical rim of white matter to be spared, and for lesions to cavitate.

Confusion concerning the disorder was generated by the two subsequent cases described by Schilder, later analyses suggesting that these were not similar, one probably representing a metabolic leukodystrophy (probably adrenoleukodystrophy; see Poser and van Bogaert (1956), the other subacute sclerosing pan-encephalitis (Lumsden, 1951).

However, Poser (Poser, 1957) reviewed 105 cases of 'diffuse/disseminated' demyelinating disease similar to Schilder's first case and later presented a further analysis of the syndrome (Poser *et al.*, 1986). Pathologically, two-thirds had diffuse sclerosis (as Schilder's original title indicates), but with additional distinct plaques indistinguishable from those of multiple sclerosis, suggesting the existence of a disorder distinct from, but with a clear relationship to, multiple sclerosis. Childhood onset is usual, with a progressive course punctuated by occasional periods of accelerated disease activity. Rarely, spontaneous sustained stabilisation has been observed. The neurological manifestations are similar to those in multiple sclerosis, although dementia and other predominantly cortical features are more prominent, including hemiplegia, cortical blindness and deafness. Adreno-leukodystrophy must be excluded.

Balò's concentric sclerosis

Retention of this term is perhaps less useful than in the foregoing cases. Balò (1928) originally described a disorder which he named encephalitis periaxalis concentrica – closely resembling Schilder's disease (Balò, 1928). The pathological distinction lay in the presence of alternating bands of demyelination and apparently normal and unaffected myelin, forming concentric rings – these can also be strikingly illustrated by MRI (Morioka *et al.*, 1994; Yao *et al.*, 1994; Chen *et al.*, 1996). It was proposed that these findings implied centrifugal diffusion of a myelinoclastic factor, but similar changes are occasionally seen in more conventional multiple sclerosis, and a more recent interpretation is that repeated inflammatory demyelinating episodes at the same site, with intervening periods of myelin repair, could equally explain these lesions. A recent (at least, in this particular context) review is listed (Courville, 1970).

Combined peripheral and central demyelination

A number of contexts are described in which inflammatory demyelination is found in both central and peripheral nerves. Thomas *et al.* described six patients who had clinical, imaging and electrophysiological evidence of multiple sclerosis (clinically definite by Poser criteria) and chronic inflammatory demyelinating neuropathy, the latter confirmed by nerve biopsy (Thomas *et al.*, 1987). Others have reported peripheral electrophysiological evidence of peripheral conduction abnormalities in patients with multiple sclerosis (Weir *et al.*, 1980).

More severe forms of CNS disease may more commonly be associated with peripheral inflammation and demyelination. Lassmann described a patient with multiple sclerosis of the Marburg type, who at post-mortem was found to have central plaques and an inflammatory demyelinating radiculopathy (Lassmann *et al.*, 1981). Best (1985) reported a case in whom the peripheral manifestations were dominant and fatal, and central inflammatory demyelinating lesions found unexpectedly at autopsy (Best, 1985). ADEM is not unusually accompanied by peripheral nerve involvement, whether induced by inoculation (Hemachudha *et al.*, 1987) or infection (Amit *et al.*, 1992).

Extensive peripheral nerve and root demyelination is found in acute EAE (see, e.g. Pender, 1987), and it is surmised that reactivity against antigens common to peripheral and central myelin (e.g. galactocerebroside, MBP), perhaps arising secondarily rather than as part of the initiating immune response, accounts for these instances of combined disease.

References

Abramsky, O. and Teitelbaum, D. (1977) The autoimmune features of acute transverse myelopathy. *Ann. Neurol.*, **2**, 36–40.

Albutt, F. C. (1870) On the ophthalmoscopic signs of spinal cord disease. *Lancet*, **i**, 76–78.

Al Deeb, S. M., Yaqub, B. A., Bruyn, G. W., Biary, N. M. (1997) Acute transverse myelitis – a localized form of postinfectious encephalomyelitis. *Brain* **120**: 1115–1122.

Amit, R., Glick, B., Itzchak, Y., Dgani, Y. and Meyeir, S. (1992) Acute severe combined demyelination. *Childs. Nerv. Syst.*, **8**, 354–356.

April, R. S. and Vansonnenberg, E. (1976) A case of neuromyelitis optica (Devic's syndrome) in systemic lupus erythematosus. Clinicopathologic report and review of the literature. *Neurology*, **26**, 1066–1070.

Arnold, A. C., Pepose, J. S., Hepler, R. S. and Foos, R. Y. (1984) Retinal periphlebitis and retinitis in multiple sclerosis. I. Pathologic characteristics. *Ophthalmology*, **91**, 255–262.

Baló, J. (1928) Encephalitis periaxalis concentrica. *Arch. Neurol. Psychol.*, **19**, 242–264.

Bassoe, P. and Grinker, R. R. (1930) Human rabies and rabies vaccine encephalomyelitis. *Arch. Neurol. Psychol.*, **23**, 1138–1160.

Beck, R. W. (1995) The optic neuritis treatment trial: three-year follow-up results (letter). *Arch. Ophthalmol.*, **113**, 136–137.

Beck, R. W., Cleary, P. A., Anderson, M. M. J., Keltner, J. L., Shults, W. T., Kaufman, D. I., *et al.* (1992) A randomized, controlled trial of corticosteroids in the treatment of acute optic neuritis. The Optic Neuritis Study Group (see comments). *N. Engl. J. Med.*, **326**, 581–588.

Beck, R. W., Cleary, P. A., Trobe, J. D., Kaufman, D. I., Kupersmith, M. J., Paty, D. W., *et al.* (1993) The effect of corticosteroids for acute optic neuritis on the subsequent development of multiple sclerosis. The Optic Neuritis Study Group (see comments). *N. Engl. J. Med.*, **329**, 1764–1769.

Berman, M., Feldman, S., Alter, M., Zilber, N. and Kahana, E. (1981) Acute transverse myelitis: incidence and etiologic considerations. *Neurology*, **31**, 966–971.

Best, P. V. (1985) Acute polyradiculoneuritis associated with demyelinated plaques in the central nervous system: report of a case. *Acta Neuropathol. Berl.*, **67**, 230–234.

Bradley, W. G. and Whitty, C. W. (1967) Acute optic neuritis: its clinical features and their relation to prognosis for recovery of vision. *J. Neurol. Neurosurg. Psychiat.*, **30**, 531–538.

Bradley, W. G. and Whitty, C. W. (1968) Acute optic neuritis: prognosis for development of multiple sclerosis. *J. Neurol. Neurosurg. Psychiat.*, **31**, 10–18.

Britton, C. B., Mesa, T. R., Fenoglio, C. M., Hays, A. P., Garvey, G. G. and Miller, J. R. (1985) A new complication of AIDS: thoracic myelitis caused by herpes simplex virus. *Neurology*, **35**, 1071–1074.

Brodsky, M., Jay, W. and Johnson, P. (1997) The 5-year risk of MS after optic neuritis – Experience of the optic neuritis treatment trial. *Neurology* **49**, 1404–1413.

Chen, C. J., Ro, L. S., Chang, C. N., Ho, Y. S. and Lu, C. S. (1996) Serial MRI studies in pathologically verified Balò's concentric sclerosis. *J. Comput. Assist. Tomogr.*, **20**, 732–735.

Compston, A. (1986) Immunological abnormalities in patients with optic neuritis. In *Optic Neuritis* (Hess, R. F. and Plant, G. T., eds), pp. 86–108. Cambridge: Cambridge University Press.

Compston, D. A., Batchelor, J. R., Earl, C. J. and McDonald, W. I. (1978) Factors influencing the risk of multiple sclerosis developing in patients with optic neuritis. *Brain*, **101**, 495–511.

Courville, C. B. (1970) Concentric sclerosis. In *Handbook of Clinical Neurology* (Vincken, P. J. and Bruyn, G. W., eds), pp. 437–451. Amsterdam: North-Holland.

Crawford, M. H. (1954) Acute haemorrhagic encephalomyelitis. *J. Clin. Pathol.*, **7**, 1–9.

Devic, E. (1895) Myélite aiguë dorso-lombaire avec névrite optique, autopsie. *Congrès Français Med. (Première Session, Lyon)*, **1**, 434–439.

Devinsky, O., Cho, E. S., Petito, C. K. and Price, R. W. (1991) Herpes zoster myelitis. *Brain*, **114**, 1181–1196.

Fenichel, G. M. (1982) Neurological complications of immunization. *Ann. Neurol.*, **12**, 119–128.

Ferraro, A. and Jervis, G. A. (1940) Experimental disseminated encephalopathy in the monkey. *Arch. Neurol. Psychol.*, **43**, 195–209.

Ferraro, A. and Roizin, L. (1954) Neuropathologic variations in experimental allergic encephalomyelitis. *J. Neurol. Neurosurg. Psychiat.*, **13**, 60–89.

Fog, T. (1965) The topography of plaques in multiple sclerosis with special reference to cerebral plaques. *Acta Neurol. Scand. Suppl.*, **15 (Suppl)**, 1–161.

Foix, C. and Alajouanine, T. (1926) La myélite necrotique subaigue. *Rev. Neurol.*, **2**, 1.

Ford, B., Tampieri, D. and Francis, G. (1992) Long-term follow-up of acute partial transverse myelopathy (see comments). *Neurology*, **42**, 250–252.

Ford, F. R. (1928) The nervous complications of measles. With a summary of the literature and publication of 12 additional case reports. *Bull. Johns Hopkins Hosp.*, **43**, 140.

Francis, D. A., Compston, D. A., Batchelor, J. R. and McDonald, W. I. (1987) A reassessment of the risk of multiple sclerosis developing in patients with optic neuritis after extended follow-up. *J. Neurol. Neurosurg. Psychiat.*, **50**, 758–765.

Frisen, L. and Hoyt, W. F. (1974). Insidious atrophy of retinal nerve fibers in multiple sclerosis. Funduscopic identification in patients with and without visual complaints. *Arch. Ophthalmol.* **92**, 91–97.

Gendelman, H. E., Wolinsky, J. S., Johnson, R. T., Pressman, N. J., Pezeshkpour, G. H. and Boisset, G. F. (1984) Measles encephalomyelitis: lack of evidence of viral invasion of the central nervous system and quantitative study of the nature of demyelination. *Ann. Neurol.*, **15**, 353–360.

Greenfield, J. G. and Turner, J. W. A. (1939) Acute and subacute necrotic myelitis. *Brain*, **62**, 227–252.

Hafler, D. A., Benjamin, D. S., Burks, J. and Weiner, H. L. (1987) Myelin basic protein and proteolipid protein reactivity of brain- and cerebrospinal fluid-derived T cell clones in multiple sclerosis and postinfectious encephalomyelitis. *J. Immunol.*, **139**, 68–72.

Hahn, J. S., Siegler, D. J. and Enzmann, D. (1996) Intravenous gammaglobulin therapy in recurrent acute disseminated encephalomyelitis. *Neurology*, **46**, 1173–1174.

Hemachudha, T., Griffin, D. E., Johnson, R. T. and Giffels, J. J. (1988) Immunologic studies of patients with chronic encephalitis induced by post-exposure Semple rabies vaccine. *Neurology*, **38**, 42–44.

Hemachudha, T., Phanuphak, P., Johnson, R. T., Griffin, D. E., Ratanavongsiri, J. and Siriprasomsup, W. (1987) Neurologic complications of Semple-type rabies vaccine: clinical and immunologic studies. *Neurology*, **37**, 550–556.

Hoffman, H. L. (1955) Acute necrotic myelopathy. *Brain*, **78**, 377–393.

Hurst, E. W. (1941) Acute haemorrhagic leucoencephalitis: a previously undefined entity. *Med. J. Aust.*, **28**, 1–6.

Jahnke, U., Fischer, E. H. and Alvord, E. C. J. (1985) Sequence homology between certain viral proteins and proteins related to encephalomyelitis and neuritis. *Science*, **229**, 282–284.

Jeffery, D. R., Mandler, R. N. and Davis, L. E. (1993) Transverse myelitis. Retrospective analysis of 33 cases, with differentiation of cases associated with multiple sclerosis and parainfectious events. *Arch. Neurol.*, **50**, 532–535.

Jacobs, L. D., Kaba, S. E., Miller, C. M., Priore, R. L., Brownscheidle, C. M. (1997) Correlation of clinical, magnetic resonance imaging, and cerebrospinal fluid findings in optic neuritis. *Ann. Neurol.* **41**, 392–398.

Johnson, R. T. (1987) The pathogenesis of acute viral encephalitis and postinfectious encephalomyelitis. *J. Infect. Dis.*, **155**, 359–364.

Johnson, R. T. (1994) The virology of demyelinating diseases. *Ann. Neurol.*, **36 (Suppl)**, S54–S60.

Johnson, R. T. (1996) Acute encephalitis. *Clin. Infect. Dis.*, **23**, 219–224.

Johnson, R. T., Griffin, D. E., Hirsch, R. L., Wolinsky, J. S., Roedenveck, S., Lindo-de-Soriano, I., *et al.* (1984) Measles encephalomyelitis – clinical and immunologic studies. *N. Engl. J. Med.*, **310**, 137–141.

Johnson, R. T., Burke, D. S., Elwell, M., Leake, C. J., Nisalak, A., Hoke, C. H., *et al.* (1985) Japanese encephalitis: immunocytochemical studies of viral antigen and inflammatory cells in fatal cases. *Ann. Neurol.*, **18**, 567–573.

Kesselring, J., Miller, D. H., Robb, S. A., Kendall, B. E., Moseley, I. F., Kingsley, D., *et al.* (1990) Acute disseminated encephalomyelitis. MRI findings and the distinction from multiple sclerosis. *Brain*, **113**, 291–302.

Klastersky, J., Cappel, R., Snoeck, J. M., Flament, J. and Thiry, L. (1972) Ascending myelitis in association with herpes-simplex virus. *N. Engl. J. Med.*, **287**, 182–184.

Lassmann, H. (1983) *The Comparative Pathology of Chronic Relapsing Experimental Allergic Encephalomyelitis and Multiple Sclerosis*, pp. 37–72. New York: Springer-Verlag.

Lassmann, H., Budka, H. and Schnaberth, G. (1981) Inflammatory demyelinating polyradicu-litis in a patient with multiple sclerosis. *Arch. Neurol.*, **38**, 99–102.

Linington, C., Bradl, M., Lassmann, H., Brunner, C. and Vass, K. (1988) Augmentation of demyelination in rat acute allergic encephalomyelitis by circulating mouse monoclonal antibodies directed against a myelin/oligodendrocyte glycoprotein. *Am. J. Pathol.*, **130**, 443–454.

Lipton, H. L. and Teasdall, R. D. (1973) Acute transverse myelopathy in adults. A follow-up study. *Arch. Neurol.*, **28**, 252–257.

Lisak, R. P. (1994) Immune-mediated para-infectious encephalomyelitis. In *Handbook of Neurovirology* (McKendall, R. R. and Stroop, W. G., eds), pp. 173–186. New York: Marcel Dekker.

Lisak, R. P., Behan, P. O., Zweiman, B. and Shetty, T. (1974) Cell-mediated immunity to myelin basic protein in acute disseminated encephalomyelitis. *Neurology*, **24**, 560–564.

Lisak, R. P. and Zweiman, B. (1977) In vitro cell-mediated immunity of cerebrospinal-fluid lymphocytes to myelin basic protein in primary demyelinating diseases. *N. Engl. J. Med.*, **297**, 850–853.

Lucchinetti, C. F., Bruck, W., Rodriguez, M. and Lassmann, H. (1996) Distinct patterns of multiple sclerosis pathology indicates heterogeneity on pathogenesis. *Brain Pathol.*, **6**, 259–274.

Lumsden, C. E. (1951) Fundamental problems in the pathology of multiple sclerosis and allied demyelinating diseases. *Br. Med. J.*, 1035–1043.

McDonald, W. I. (1996) Mechanisms of relapse and remission in multiple sclerosis. In *The Neurobiology of Disease* (Bostock, H., Kirkwood, P. A. and Pullen, A. H., eds), pp. 118–123. Cambridge: Cambridge University Press.

Mandler, R. N., Davis, L. E., Jeffery, D. R. and Kornfeld, M. (1993) Devic's neuromyelitis optica: a clinicopathological study of 8 patients. *Ann. Neurol.*, **34**, 162–168.

Mandler, R. N., Ahmed, W. and Dencoff, J. E. (1998) Devic's neuromyelitis optica: a prospective study of seven patients treated with prednisone and azotrioprine. *Neurology*, **51**, 1219–1220.

Marburg, O. (1906) Die sogenannte 'akute multiple sklerose'. *Jahrbuch für Psychiatrie und Neurologie*, **27**, 211–312.

Mathews, W. B. (1991) Symptoms and signs. Initial symptoms. In *McAlpine's Multiple Sclerosis* (Mathews, W. B., ed.), pp. 43–46. London: Churchill Livingstone.

Miller, D. H., McDonald, W. I., Blumhardt, L. D., Du, B. G., Halliday, A. M., Johnson, G., *et al.* (1987) Magnetic resonance imaging in isolated noncompressive spinal cord syndromes. *Ann. Neurol.*, **22**, 714–723.

Miller, D. H., Ormerod, I. E., Rudge, P., Kendall, B. E., Moseley, I. F. and McDonald, W. I. (1989) The early risk of multiple sclerosis following isolated acute syndromes of the brainstem and spinal cord. *Ann. Neurol.*, **26**, 635–639.

Mok, C. C., Lau, C. S., Chan, E. Y. and Wong, R. W. (1998) Acute transverse myelopathy in systemic erythematosus: clinical presentation, treatment and outcome. *J. Rheumatol.*, **25**, 467–473.

Morioka, C., Komatsu, Y., Tsujio, T., Araki, Y. and Kondo, H. (1994) The evolution of the concentric lesions of atypical multiple sclerosis on MRI. *Radiat. Med.*, **12**, 129–133.

Morrissey, S. P., Miller, D. H., Kendall, B. E., Kingsley, D. P., Kelly, M. A., Francis, D. A., *et al.* (1993) The significance of brain magnetic resonance imaging abnormalities at presentation with clinically isolated syndromes suggestive of multiple sclerosis. A 5-year follow-up study. *Brain*, **116**, 135–146.

Morrissey, S. P., Borruat, F. X., Miller, D. H., Moseley, I. F., Sweeney, M. G., Govan, G. G., *et al.* (1995) Bilateral simultaneous optic neuropathy in adults: clinical, imaging, serological, and genetic studies. *J. Neurol. Neurosurg. Psychiat.*, **58**, 70–74.

O'Riordan, J. I., Gallagher, H. L., Thompson, A. J., Howard, R. S., Kingsley, D. P., Thompson, E. J., *et al.* (1996) Clinical, CSF, and MRI findings in Devic's neuromyelitis optica. *J. Neurol. Neurosurg. Psychiat.*, **60**, 382–387.

O'Riordan, J. I., Thompson, A. J., Kingsley, D. P. E, MacManus, D. G, Kendall, B. E., Rudge, P., McDonald, W. I. and Miller, D. H. (1998). The prognostic value of brain MRI in clinically isolated syndromes of the CNS. A 10-year follow-up study. *Brain*, **121**, 495–503.

Ojeda, V. J. (1984) Necrotizing myelopathy associated with malignancy. A clinicopathologic study of two cases and literature review. *Cancer*, **53**, 1115–1123.

Ormerod, I. E., McDonald, W. I., Du, B. G., Kendall, B. E., Moseley, I. F., Halliday, A. M., *et al.* (1986) Disseminated lesions at presentation in patients with optic neuritis. *J. Neurol. Neurosurg. Psychiat.*, **49**, 124–127.

Ozawa, K., Suchanek, G., Breitschopf, H., Bruck, W., Budka, H., Jellinger, K., *et al.* (1994) Patterns of oligodendroglia pathology in multiple sclerosis. *Brain*, **117**, 1311–1322.

Pender, M. P. (1987) Demyelination and neurological signs in experimental allergic encephalomyelitis. *J. Neuroimmunol.*, **15**, 11–24.

Poser, C. M. (1957) Diffuse-disseminated sclerosis in the adult. *J. Neuropathol. Exp. Neurol.*, **16**, 61–78.

Poser, C. M. and Van Bogaert, L. (1956) Natural history and evolution of the concept of

Schilder's diffuse sclerosis. *Acta Neurol. Scand.*, **31**, 285–331.

Poser, C. M., Goutieres, F., Carpentier, M. A. and Aicardi, J. (1986) Schilder's myelinoclastic diffuse sclerosis (published erratum appears in *Pediatrics* **78**(1), 138). *Pediatrics*, **77**, 107–112.

Rivers, T. M. and Schwentker, F. F. (1935) Encephalomyelitis accompanied by myelin destruction experimentally produced in monkeys. *J. Exp. Med.*, **61**, 689–702.

Rivers, T. M., Sprunt, D. M., Berry, G. P. (1933) Observations on attempts to produce acute disseminated encephalomyelitis in monkeys. *J. Exp. Med.*, **58**, 39–53.

Rolak, L. A., Beck, R. W., Paty, D. W., Tourtellotte, W. W., Whitaker, J. N. and Rudick, R. A. (1996) Cerebrospinal fluid in acute optic neuritis: experience of the optic neuritis treatment trial. *Neurology*, **46**, 368–372.

Ropper, A. H. and Poskanzer, D. C. (1978) The prognosis of acute and subacute transverse myelopathy based on early signs and symptoms. *Ann. Neurol.*, **4**, 51–59.

Sandberg, W. M., Bynke, H., Cronqvist, S., Holtas, S., Platz, P. and Ryder, L. P. (1990) A long-term prospective study of optic neuritis: evaluation of risk factors. *Ann. Neurol.*, **27**, 386–393.

Schilder, P. (1912) Zur Kentniss der sogenannte diffusen sklerosen. *Zeitschrift für die gesammte. Neurologie und Psychiatrie*, **10**, 1–60.

Scott, T. F., Bhagavatula, K., Snyder, P. J. and Chieffe, C. (1998) Transverse myelitis. Comparison with spinal cord presentations of multiple sclerosis. *Neurology*, **50**, 429–433.

Shibasaki, H., McDonald, W. I., Kuroiwa, Y. (1981) Racial modification of clinical picture of multiple sclerosis: comparison between British and Japanese patients. *J. Neurol. Sci.*, **49**, 253–271.

Stansbury, F. C. (1949) Neuromyelitis optica (Devic's disease). Presentation of five cases with pathological study and review of the literature. *Arch. Ophthalmol.*, **42**, 292–335, 465–501.

Swamy, H. S., Shankar, S. K., Chandra, P. S., Aroor, S. R., Krishna, A. S. and Perumal, V. G. (1984) Neurological complications due to beta-propiolactone (BPL)-inactivated antirabies vaccination. Clinical, electrophysiological and therapeutic aspects. *J. Neurol. Sci.*, **63**, 111–128.

Thomas, P. K., Walker, R. W., Rudge, P., Morgan, H. J., King, R. H., Jacobs, J. M., *et al.* (1987) Chronic demyelinating peripheral neuropathy associated with multifocal central nervous system demyelination. *Brain*, **110**, 53–76.

Tippett, D. S., Fishman, P. S. and Panitch, H. S. (1991) Relapsing transverse myelitis (see comments). *Neurology*, **41**, 703–706.

Turnbull, T. M. and McIntosh, B. (1997) Encephalomyelitis following vaccination. *Br. J. Exp. Pat*, **7**, 181–222.

Weir, A. I., Hansen, S. and Ballantyne, J. P. (1980) Motor unit potential abnormalities in multiple sclerosis: further evidence for a peripheral nervous system defect. *J. Neurol. Neurosurg. Psychiat.*, **43**, 999–1004.

Wiley, C. A., Vanpatten, P. D., Carpenter, P. M., Powell, H. C. and Thal, L. J. (1987) Acute ascending necrotizing myelopathy caused by herpes simplex virus type 2. *Neurology*, **37**, 1791–1794.

Wood, D. D., Bilbao, J. M., O'Connors, P. and Moscarello, M. A. (1996) Acute multiple sclerosis (Marburg type) is associated with developmentally immature myelin basic protein. *Ann. Neurol.*, **40**, 18–24.

Yao, D. L., Webster, H. D., Hudson, L. D., Brenner, M., Liu, D. S., Escobar, A. I., *et al.* (1994) Concentric sclerosis (Balò): morphometric and *in situ* hybridization study of lesions in six patients. *Ann. Neurol.*, **35**, 18–30.

Youl, B. D., Turano, G., Miller, D. H., Towell, A. D., MacManus, D. G., Moore, S. G., *et al.* (1991) The pathophysiology of acute optic neuritis. An association of gadolinium leakage with clinical and electrophysiological deficits. *Brain*, **114**, 2437–2450.

Chapter 4

Current and future therapies for multiple sclerosis

David C. Wraith

The pathology of multiple sclerosis	93
T cells and multiple sclerosis	94
Experimental models of multiple sclerosis	95
Current approaches to therapy of multiple sclerosis	96
New drugs in clinical trial for therapy of multiple sclerosis	100
Experimental therapies for multiple sclerosis	104
Towards more specific forms of immunotherapy in multiple sclerosis	107
Conclusions: the specificity pyramid in immunotherapy of multiple sclerosis	111
References	111

The pathology of multiple sclerosis

Multiple sclerosis is a chronic T cell-dependent inflammatory disease of the central nervous system (CNS) characterized by myelin destruction (as described in more detail in Chapter 2). The cause is unknown: the imperfect concordance among identical twins demonstrates, however, that an environmental influence is involved in both the initiation and progression of this disease. Although there is little direct evidence, recent studies suggest the possibility that viral or bacterial antigens could account for the environmental trigger (Wucherpfennig and Strominger, 1995). An involvement of the immune system in multiple sclerosis is implied by the association between human leukocyte antigen (HLA) type and disease (see below). Plasma cells are found within multiple sclerosis plaques and these may account for the presence of oligoclonal immunoglobulin bands in cerebrospinal fluid (CSF). In addition to B cells, T cells and macrophages are found in early lesions (Traugott *et al.*, 1983). Furthermore, involvement of the immune system is supported by the presence of interleukins, interferons (IFNs), tumour necrosis factor (TNF)-α and various T cell subsets in multiple sclerosis plaques. High levels of TNF-α are found in the CSF of patients with chronic progressive multiple sclerosis (Sharief and Hentges, 1991) and some studies correlate increasing production of this cytokine by blood leukocytes with disease progression (Beck *et al.*, 1988).

Up to now, much of our understanding of pathology in multiple sclerosis has come from a combination of post-mortem histology and the close analogy between multiple sclerosis and an experimental model, experimental allergic encephalomyelitis (EAE) (see below). More recently, however, the application of magnetic resonance imaging (MRI) to multiple sclerosis has allowed neurologists to follow disease progression in individual patients (McDonald *et al.*, 1992). The multiple sclerosis plaque can be detected by this technique because it produces an altered image derived from the nuclear magnetic resonance (NMR) signals of mobile protons in the tissue.

Further information is derived from the use of gadolinium-diethylene-triaminepenta-acetic acid. Gadolinium enhances the MRI image and is normally excluded from the CNS by the blood–brain barrier. Regions of breakdown in the blood–brain barrier allow free passage of gadolinium with subsequent enhancement of multiple sclerosis plaques involved in inflammation in that region. This technology therefore allows the differentiation of active (gadolinium enhancing) as opposed to latent (gadolinium non-enhancing) plaques. Developing lesions are associated with breakdown of the blood–brain barrier as revealed by gadolinium enhancement. Importantly, these lesions may disappear quite rapidly and may never contribute to clinical disease. Gadolinium enhancement, however, clearly correlates with the pathological features of disease activity including perivascular infiltration of lymphocytes and macrophages, and associated breakdown of myelin. Newly developing plaques generally display gadolinium enhancement, which emphasizes the pathological significance of immunological activity in the perivascular region. As plaques expand they continue to demonstrate enhancement at their expanding edge. Established lesions lose gadolinium enhancement and may concurrently shrink in size. Pre-existing lesions, however, may also re-activate, as evidenced by renewed gadolinium enhancement.

The extent and severity of pathology in multiple sclerosis, as detected by MRI scanning, is directly related to the severity of disability in patients with benign and secondary progressive multiple sclerosis (Filippi *et al.*, 1995). The overall picture emerging from MRI analysis shows us that multiple sclerosis is a dynamic disease in which breakdown of the blood–brain barrier is a critical event involved in plaque formation. Analysis of post-mortem material has revealed that small plaques; which in active disease, contain inflammatory lymphocytes and monocytes surround a central vein. Larger lesions often have such a rim of inflammatory cells at their outer circumference (Lumsden, 1970). The dramatic co-localization of gadolinium enhancement and perivascular cuffs of inflammatory cells implies that the gadolinium enhancement correlates with inflammation. Such perivascular infiltration is also a central feature of the experimental model of multiple sclerosis, EAE. The power of MRI scanning in conjunction with gadolinium enhancement now allows the neurologist to trace both clinically active and silent disease elements. This obviously provides a crucial marker for efficacy in clinical trials of novel therapeutic agents in multiple sclerosis.

T cells and multiple sclerosis

Multiple sclerosis carries many of the hallmarks of an autoimmune disease. There is a close association between disease and a particular MHC determinant (Oksenberg *et al.*, 1993a), a raised frequency of T cells specific for myelin components (Olsson *et al.*, 1992; Wucherpfennig *et al.*, 1994) and an increased level of autoantibodies to myelin basic protein (MBP) in CSF

(Warren *et al.*, 1995). Between 40 and 70% of multiple sclerosis patients carry the HLA-A3, -B7, -DR2-Dw2 extended haplotype. Molecular analysis has further refined the HLA susceptibility genes to HLA-DRB1*1501-DQA1*0102-DQB1*0602, although there is no clear picture as to which gene is responsible, whether it be a Class II MHC gene or one of the many other HLA-associated genes such as TNF. Finally, multiple sclerosis can be partially controlled but not cured by treatment with immune suppressing agents including antibodies known to deplete $CD4^+$ T cells (see below).

Analysis of T cell specificity and T cell receptor (TCR) usage has been undertaken both *in vivo* and *in vitro*. Studies of T cells from multiple sclerosis patients have highlighted the raised frequency of cells specific for myelin components such as MBP. There is evidence of clonal selection of MBP-specific cells in multiple sclerosis patients and in any one individual it appears that specific clonotypes can persist for a long time (Wucherpfennig *et al.*, 1994). Oksenberg and colleagues have performed an analysis of TCR usage in post-mortem material from patients with multiple sclerosis (Oksenberg *et al.*, 1993b). By studying V region gene rearrangement they have shown a relatively restricted TCR usage correlating with HLA type. Fifty percent of their patients were HLA-DRB1*1501-DQA1*0102-DQB1*0602 positive and these all expressed either V_β5.1 or 5.2 with the majority displaying a particular rearrangement of V_β5.2 in the lesion. The same V_β type was expressed by the majority of MBP-reactive cells isolated by Kotzin *et al.* (1991). While this association is interesting it does not confirm that the TCR isotypes identified by Oksenberg were MBP specific or indeed that they were definitely involved in immune pathology. In a separate study of TCR usage, Wucherpfennig *et al.* found a diverse usage of V_β genes among MBP T cell clones with, if anything, a more restricted V_α representation (Wucherpfennig *et al.*, 1994).

Experimental models of multiple sclerosis

The two best characterized experimental models for multiple sclerosis are EAE and Theiler's virus (TMEV) infection in the mouse. The EAE models have many features in common with the human disease apart from the fact that the disease is induced artificially. There are chronic-relapsing forms of disease induced by injection of whole myelin (Baker *et al.*, 1990), the response to myelin antigens shows linkage to Class II regions of the MHC (Fritz *et al.*, 1985), there is evidence for limited heterogeneity of TCR usage (Acha-Orbea *et al.*, 1988), although this is not always the case (Padula *et al.*, 1991) and histology of the chronic-relapsing form of disease displays striking similarity to multiple sclerosis. As with the acute models of EAE, the Biozzi mouse model displays classical perivascular cuffing involving lymphocytes and monocytes. During relapses, however, there is evidence of parenchymal infiltration reminiscent of secondary-progressive multiple sclerosis (Smith, 1995).

EAE is T cell mediated: it is inhibited by antibodies specific for either CD4 or TCR on the T cell surface (Wraith *et al.*, 1989) and Class II MHC on the antigen-presenting cell surface (Smith *et al.*, 1994). EAE can be transferred to naïve mice by activated T cell clones (Zamvil *et al.*, 1985) and it is readily induced in animals expressing a myelin-specific TCR as a transgene (Goverman *et al.*, 1993; Liu *et al.*, 1995). Theiler's murine encephalitis, on the other hand, shows little evidence of an autoimmune component. The acute phase of the disease is restricted to grey matter but spreads with time to the white matter with associated demyelination. Demyelination can be observed, however, in nude mice indicating that this takes place in the absence of T cells (Roos and Wollmann, 1986). More convincingly, TMEV persistence and demyelination were demonstrated in Class II knockout mice lacking functional $CD4^+$ T cells (Njenga *et al.*, 1996). In the TMEV model $CD4^+$ T cells protect against virus-induced demyelination, whereas in multiple sclerosis these cells contribute to demyelination.

Finally, although epidemiological evidence argues for an environmental agent in the initiation of multiple sclerosis, a single virus has not yet been satisfactorily linked to disease pathogenesis. Recent interest in human herpesvirus-6 (HHV-6) should, however, be noted. This virus causes a subacute leukoencephalitis (SHLE) which in some cases can mimic acute multiple sclerosis (Carrigan *et al.*, 1996). The majority of patients with multiple sclerosis do not, however, display high levels of HHV-6 DNA in their CNS tissue (Challoner *et al.*, 1995). Furthermore, the pathology of SHLE differs from multiple sclerosis in that the lesions are relatively devoid of inflammatory infiltrates. It appears, therefore, that the leukoencephalitis associated with this virus induces a demyelinating disease which produces some symptoms similar to multiple sclerosis but which is most probably a distinct disease.

The evidence to date tells us that multiple sclerosis is similar to the model of inflammatory disease in the CNS (EAE). It is clear that $CD4^+$ T cells play a central role in the EAE model and there is circumstantial evidence in favour of this view in multiple sclerosis. Here we will take the lead from the EAE model in considering possible new therapies for multiple sclerosis and direct our attention towards $CD4^+$ T cells.

Current approaches to therapy of multiple sclerosis

Current approaches are defined as those which have been tested in clinical trials. At this stage, they are largely based on chemical immunosuppression (Table 4.1). The chemical immune suppressive agents can be divided into four categories: alkylating agents, antimetabolites, corticosteroids and antibiotics.

Cyclophosphamide

Alkylating agents transfer alkyl groups to proteins, DNA and RNA. The guanine group of DNA is particularly sensitive and cyclophosphamide is the chosen agent because this drug must be metabolized in the liver to gain activity and can therefore be given either orally or parenterally.

The use of cyclophosphamide has met with varying degrees of success. In one trial, a short high-dose treatment did not produce significant clinical benefit (Likosky *et al.*, 1991). Cyclophosphamide has been tested in combination with other drugs and the degree of success has been somewhat controversial. The Boston study demonstrated some disease stabilization in combination therapy with corticotrophin but the effect was short lived (Carter *et al.*, 1988; Weiner *et al.*, 1993a,b). In a contrasting study, however, combination therapy with oral prednisolone did not reveal any significant benefit from cyclophosphamide (The Canadian Cooperative Multiple Sclerosis Study Group, 1991).

Table 4.1 Current therapeutic strategies in multiple sclerosis

Drug	Mechanism	Comment
Cyclophosphamide	Alkylating agent	Not convincingly successful; Unacceptable side effects
Azathioprine	Purine synthesis inhibitor	Marginal success revealed by meta-analysis; increased risk of cancer
Corticosteroids	Broad range immune suppression	Can delay disease progression? in optic neuritis
Cyclosporin A	Inhibits signal transduction in T cells	Can delay disease progression; unacceptable side effects
Intravenous immunoglobulin	Fc receptor blockade; Cytokine and immune complex modulation; inhibition of complement system	Can delay disease progression but effect short lived

Cyclophosphamide has severe side effects: in addition to bone marrow suppression, the incidence of bladder cancer increases 200-fold after 3 years' treatment. Hair loss occurs; amenorrhoea is common in women. Under such conditions it would be impossible to use the drug in a blinded fashion and this alone could account for the variation in apparent efficacy in clinical trials. The low benefit from use of cyclophosphamide, in combination with its obvious severe side effects argues against the use of this drug for treatment of chronic multiple sclerosis.

Azathioprine

The antimetabolites are designed to interfere with normal cell function and are commonly used in the treatment of cancer. Azathioprine acts by inhibiting purine biosynthesis, and hence decreases the rate of cell replication particularly among B and T lymphocytes.

There have been a number of trials of azathioprine in multiple sclerosis all of which were relatively disappointing. A meta-analysis of the combined data has, however, demonstrated a significant effect on disease progression and relapse rate (Yudkin *et al.*, 1991) of not dissimilar magnitude to that of IFN-β (Palace and Rothwell, 1997). Chronic use of this drug in rheumatoid arthritis and transplantation has revealed an increase in susceptibility to cancer which emphasizes the role of an intact immune system in tumour surveillance; the same risk has not been shown to apply to patients with multiple sclerosis (Confavreux *et al.*, 1996).

Methotrexate

Although little used in the UK or continental Europe, there is some evidence for the efficacy of this dihydrofolate reductase inhibitor in relatively low doses, administered once weekly. Modest benefit in terms of the accumulation of sustained disability was demonstrated in a placebo-controlled trial studying 60 ambulatory patients with chronic progressive multiple sclerosis (Goodkin *et al.*, 1995).

It seems possible that the potential benefits of both methotrexate and azathioprine may warrant reassessment; both have arguably been prematurely rejected.

Corticosteroids

Corticosteroids act by entering cells, binding to intracellular, cytoplasmic receptors and forming complexes. The complexes bind to nuclear acceptor sites and influence the expression of various species of mRNA. Corticosteroids produce multiple effects on the immune system although it is believed that they spare B lymphocytes *in vivo*. High-dose intravenous methylprednisolone allows faster recovery from relapse in multiple sclerosis (Milligan *et al.*, 1987). This may be accounted for in part by the positive effect of methylprednisolone on blood–brain barrier function, as shown by gadolinium-enhanced MRI scanning (Miller *et al.*, 1992). The observation of an unsustained delay in the development of further inflammatory demyelinating episodes following optic neuritis, emerging from the Optic Neuritis Treatment Trial, has been mentioned (Beck *et al.*, 1993, 1995; see Chapters 2 and 3). Corticosteroids provide no benefit in terms of slowing disease progression.

Cyclosporin A

Cyclosporin A is a fungal metabolite originally selected for antibiotic activity. The main site of action of cyclosporin A is within the $CD4^+$ T cell where the drug binds to a cytoplasmic receptor protein, cyclophilin. The complex then interferes with the signal transduction pathway mediated by ligation of the TCR.

Cyclosporin A may have a modest therapeutic effect in multiple sclerosis, but there is broad agreement that it brings with it unacceptable side effects (MS Study Group 1990; Faulds *et al.*, 1993). While there is some evidence that disease progression is slowed by cyclosporin A treatment, there is an increased risk of hypertension and a rise in serum creatinine levels.

The suggested beneficial effect of cyclosporin A in multiple sclerosis, however, provides some indirect support for a role for $CD4^+$ T cells in the disease and emphasizes the need to find less toxic strategies for their immune suppression.

The overall impression from trials with chemical immunosuppressive drugs is that the risk:benefit ratio is poor. Many of these drugs are toxic and, in many cases, they unfortunately provide limited improvement. Corticosteroids cannot slow disease progression but boost recovery from relapses. If anything, steroids are the least toxic of the drugs described above and therefore the most acceptable for routine use.

Intravenous immunoglobulin

Female multiple sclerosis patients often suffer acute exacerbations of disease following childbirth, and in an early study, nine multiple sclerosis patients with a history of post-partum exacerbations were treated with intravenous immunoglobulin immediately after childbirth and again at 6 and 12 weeks (Achiron *et al.*, 1996). None of the treated patients relapsed during the first 6 months following delivery although their disease resumed its normal course with time.

In a European controlled study of intravenous immunoglobulin in multiple sclerosis, a significant reduction in relapse rate, with beneficial effects also on progression, was reported (Fazekas *et al.*, 1997). In a more recent double-blind, placebo-controlled trial, 40 patients (aged 19–60 years) with clinical definite relapsing–remitting multiple sclerosis were studied; those treated with intravenous immunoglobulin exhibited a 38.6% reduction in relapse rate and again a positive effect on progression of disability was suggested (Achiron *et al.*, 1998). Larger placebo-controlled trials are currently in progress, though other studies have suggested that intravenous immunoglobulin does not halt the progression of chronic multiple sclerosis (Francis *et al.*, 1997) and also fails to reverse recently acquired fixed motor deficits (Noseworthy *et al.*, 1997).

The preparations used in these trials consist of intact IgG with a distribution of subclasses similar to normal serum and collected from several thousand healthy blood donors. The immunomodulating effects of intravenous immunoglobulin are wide ranging. Immediate effects include the functional blockade of Fc receptors on splenic macrophages, inhibition of complement-mediated damage, changes in clearance of immune complexes, modulation of the production of pro-inflammatory cytokines and phenotypic changes among circulating leukocytes.

Plasma exchange

Anecdotal evidence for the efficacy of plasma exchange is available, particularly for very severe and aggressive disease (Rodriguez *et al*, 1993). No benefit was apparent, however, in those patients treated with both plasma exchange and cyclophosphamide in the well-controlled Canadian Cooperative Trial (The Canadian Cooperative Multiple Sclerosis Study Group, 1991).

Bone marrow transplantation

Following the tentative success of bone marrow transplantation in some system autoimmune conditions, this approach has now begun to be explored in multiple sclerosis (Burt *et al.*, 1997). Whilst having some enthusiastic proponents, the morbidity of pre-transplant marrow ablative therapy is likely to restrict this technique to all but those with the most aggressive disease.

Total body irradiation appears not to offer promise (Comi *et al.*, 1997; Cook *et al.*, 1997).

New drugs in clinical trial for therapy of multiple sclerosis

Type I interferons

Two new drugs (the type I IFNs and Copolymer-1, renamed glatirimer acetate) have recently undergone clinical trials and both have shown some benefit (Table 4.2). Interferon-α and IFN-β are both anti-viral proteins produced by cells in response to viral infection. Normally they have three functions. First, they inhibit viral replication by interacting with signalling pathways and activating genes that destabilize mRNA and inhibit protein translation. Second, they induce MHC Class I expression thereby making cells more susceptible to lysis by anti-viral CD8$^+$ T cells. Third, they activate NK cells which proceed to kill virus-infected cells.

Table 4.2 New drugs undergoing clinical trial

Drug	Mechanism	Comment
Interferon-β	Inhibits immune cell proliferation; alters cell trafficking; modifies antigen-presenting cell function reduces interferon-γ and tumour necrosis factor-α production	Notable reduction in magnetic resonance imaging activity; efficacy may be reduced by neutralizing antibody
Co-polymer 1	Based on structure of MBP; mechanism in humans unknown	Can delay relapse rate in some patients
Campath-1H	Pan leukocyte cytotoxic antibody; causes long-term depletion of CD4$^+$ cells	Notable reduction in magnetic resonance imaging activity; 're-awakening' of previous lesions can be controlled with methylprednisolone
Anti-CD4	Depletes CD4$^+$ cells	No apparent clinical improvement in small trial

Putative mechanisms in the treatment of multiple sclerosis include inhibition of viral replication and hence the severity of viral infections, a possible trigger for multiple sclerosis relapses. Interferon-β also inhibits IFN-γ-induced up-regulation of Class II MHC (Lu *et al.*, 1995) which could have a profound effect on any T cell-driven inflammatory response. Other anti-inflammatory effects of the type I IFNs include the inhibition of immune cell proliferation; altered cell trafficking into and out of the lymphoid organs and into the CNS; interference with the antigen-presenting capacity of macrophages; reduced synthesis and release of the stimulatory cytokine IFN-γ and of the toxic cytokines lymphotoxin and TNF-α; augmented CD8 suppressor cell function and increased synthesis and release of the suppressive cytokines TGF-β and IL-10 (Faulds and Benfield, 1994).

Interferon-β has received great support in the medical press for some years, partly based on the outcome of the first, large-scale, blinded, randomized, controlled trial (Duquette *et al.*, 1995). This trial involved 372 patients receiving either 1.6 or 8 million international units (MIU) of IFN-β1b (*Betaferon*; Schering) subcutaneously every other day over a 5 year period. Interferon-β was reported to have a persistent beneficial effect on exacerbation rate and on MRI burden, while giving relatively few side effects – flu-like symptoms, local skin reactions, and depression in certain cases. There was a 30% reduction in exacerbation rate in the 8 MIU arm with no significant progression of lesion burden as measured by MRI.

There was, however, no significant effect on the progression of clinical disability, and even in the self-selected cases proceeding to 5 years' treatment (the initial trial design was for 3 years), the reduction in annual relapse rate was statistically significant only for the first 2 years (Duquette *et al.*, 1995). It is also the case that 122 out of 372 randomized patients dropped out before the completion of 3 years and were not included in the analysis. Relapses also were self-reported; 80% of patients correctly guessed they were taking the active drug, raising serious difficulties concerning blinding (Sibley *et al.*, 1994).

A significant titre of neutralizing antibodies developed in the treated group with associated reduction in efficacy. This latter point is disturbing if this dose of IFN-β is to be used for chronic therapy. The dose must be reduced, in a form of combination therapy, in order to avoid the effect of neutralizing antibodies.

A recent trial of IFN-β1b in over 700 patients with secondary progressive multiple sclerosis treated for 2 years reports a significant effect on disability, although it is also true that the mean EDSS, which did not differ between placebo and treated group at baseline, also did not differ significantly at the endpoint (European Study Group, 1998).

Interferon-β1a differs from IFN-β1b in being non-glycosylated and having an amino acid sequence identical to natural human IFN-β; IFN-β1b has a single substitution (at position 17). In a trial of similar size to the above (301 patients), IFN-β1a (*Avonex*, Biogen; given by intramuscular injection once weekly) was shown not only to produce an equivalent (approximately 30%) reduction in relapse rate, but also to delay significantly the accumulation of disability in patients with progressive disease (Jacobs *et al.*, 1996). The study was, however, terminated before the intended 2 years' treatment had been completed for all patients (only 172 of 301 patients completed 2 years); in fact, therefore, the proportion of patients progressing after two years was not significantly different (18 of 85 of the IFN-β1a-treated group, 29 of 87 of those in the placebo group; $p = 0.07$).

Finally, a larger study of 560 patients treated for 2 years with an alternative preparation of IFN-β1a (*Rebif*, Serono; subcutaneously three times a week) revealed again a statistically significant effect on both relapse rate and the accumulation of disability (PRISMS Study Group, 1998).

All three preparations are now licensed. The cost of each is broadly comparable, approximately £10 000 per patient per annum, and this has contributed not insignificantly to the continuing debate concerning the use of this treatment in multiple sclerosis.

High-dose IFN-α may have a similar effect to IFN-β, in reducing MRI signs of disease activity and lymphocyte IFN-γ production in relapsing–remitting multiple sclerosis. In a recent follow-up of a small trial of IFN-α treatment, it was found that disease activity returned to placebo levels immediately after stopping treatment (Durelli *et al.*, 1996). While this shows that the previously observed suppression of disease activity was almost undoubtedly a consequence of drug administration it does emphasize the fact that treatment with type I IFNs treats the disease but does not provide a cure.

Copolymer-1

Copolymer-1 (now known as glatirimer acetate) is a random copolymer of alanine, glutamic acid, lysine and tyrosine in a molar ratio of 6:1.9:4.7:1, which was originally designed to simulate the activity of MBP in inducing EAE (Teitelbaum *et al.*, 1971). Surprisingly, this agent suppressed the induction of EAE, despite cross-reactivity between MBP and copolymer-1 at both the B and T cell level (Arnon and Teitelbaum, 1994). There is evidence, from animal models, that glatirimer acetate induces a form of immune regulation which is capable of moderating disease activity directed against both of the major myelin antigens MBP and proteolipid protein (PLP) (Arnon *et al.*, 1996). If true for multiple sclerosis in humans, this type of approach holds great promise for future improvements in antigen-specific therapy (see below).

Glatirimer acetate has been studied in a multicentre phase II trial of patients with relapsing–remitting multiple sclerosis. In this trial 125 patients received 20 mg glatirimer acetate subcutaneously administered daily over a 2 year period with 126 patients receiving a placebo. There was a 29% reduction in relapse rate and a reported improvement in disability status although the proportion progressing one or more Kurtzke EDSS points did not significantly differ between the two groups (24.6% of the placebo; 21.6 of the treated patients). There was an injection site reaction to glatirimer acetate in 90% of patients and a rare systemic reaction. In a short (less than 6 month) extension of this study, the above clinical benefits were reportedly sustained (Johnson *et al.*, 1998).

Other agents

Recent studies suggest neither pentoxifylline nor sulfasalazine are of significant promise (Noseworthy *et al.*, 1998; Myers *et al.*, 1998).

Campath-1

Increasing specificity for disease has been achieved through the use of antibodies targeting the cells contained in inflammatory infiltrates in multiple sclerosis. Seven patients with multiple sclerosis have been treated with a 10 day course of the humanized monoclonal antibody Campath-1H (Moreau *et al.*, 1994). This antibody is specific for the CDw52 molecule on the surface of lymphocytes and monocytes, and causes rapid lymphopoenia which persists for at least 1 year, no population of circulating T lymphocytes returning to a normal range for at least 6 months. Using MRI analysis as a marker of changes in disease activity, there was a reduction in the incidence of new lesions during the course of treatment compared to a run-up period in this small sample of patients.

Interestingly the use of this antibody is associated with a transient exacerbation of disease resulting from a re-awakening of previously silent MRI lesions. This is probably the result of a transient 'rush' of cytokine production as a result of CDw52 cross-linking at the surface of lymphocytes and monocytes. Peak levels of TNF-α and IFN-γ were noted at 2 h and IL-6 at 4 h after starting antibody treatment (Moreau et al., 1996). The increase in cytokine production and the associated symptoms of multiple sclerosis were inhibited by pre-treatment with methylprednisolone. Campath-1H may stabilize disease for 12 months or more after a single treatment, but its side-effect profile may limits its use to patients with more aggressive disease, perhaps particularly the Marburg variant of multiple sclerosis.

Anti-CD4

Twenty one patients with active multiple sclerosis have been treated with a monoclonal anti-CD4 antibody for 10 days (Racadot et al., 1993). Similarly to Campath-1H treatment, infusion of anti-CD4 led to the production of TNF-α and IL-6. There was no apparent clinical improvement or deterioration resulting from this treatment in the short period of patient monitoring despite significant reduction in CD4 cell count for at least 1 month. The treatment led to the generation of xenogeneic antibodies directed against the infused antibody in half the patient group. In a more recent, larger and potentially definitive study of a group of 72 patients with multiple sclerosis treated in a randomized, double-blind, placebo-controlled, MR-monitored trial with anti-CD4 monoclonal antibody, no MRI effect was apparent in the treated group (van Oosten et al., 1997).

Antibodies for immunotherapy of multiple sclerosis

The choice of monoclonal antibodies over other drugs such as azathioprine and cyclosporin A is based on our wish to climb the specificity ladder in immune suppression. The chemical drugs have serious side effects because of their lack of specificity. With monoclonal antibodies we can begin to target discrete subsets of cells within the body and even within the immune system. The use of Campath-1H in multiple sclerosis shows promising results. In these preliminary trials, the patient group sizes are small because the antibodies are both difficult and expensive to produce.

There are two drawbacks to the use of such antibodies. First, the depletion of CD4$^+$ cells is extremely long lived. This is good for treatment of disease but bad for tumour surveillance and protection from infection in general. Second, antibodies are complex molecules and it will be difficult to avoid the generation of anti-idiotype antibodies with repeated administration. It is perhaps surprising that early results suggest no useful effect of CD4 antibody (using MRI as a surrogate marker), whereas Campath-1H may offer a significant protective effect against new MRI activity – but these results must be regarded as preliminary. There are, however, theoretical advantages in using Campath-1H over CD4-specific antibodies since the former antibody also depletes macrophages which probably play an important role in disease (see above). The cytokine 'rush' after both types of antibody treatment and the long-term depletion of CD4$^+$ cells is similar in both cases although this can be limited by co-administration of methylprednisolone.

Experimental therapies for multiple sclerosis

These are defined as approaches which are at the pre-clinical stage of development following successful application in experimental models of multiple sclerosis such as the EAE model (Table 4.3).

Table 4.3 New drugs awaiting clinical trial

Drug	Mechanism	Comments
Transforming growth factor-β	Potent immunosuppressive agent	Reduces disease severity and relapse rate in experimental allergic encephalomyelitis models
Interleukin-10	Inhibits antigen-presenting cell function of macrophages	Reduces disease severity and relapse rate in experimental allergic encephalomyelitis models
Anti-interleukin-12	Inhibits pro-inflammatory function of interleukin-12	Reduces disease severity and relapse rate in experimental allergic encephalomyelitis models
Anti-tumour necrosis factor-α	Inhibits pro-inflammatory function of tumour necrosis factor-α	Reduces disease severity and relapse rate in experimental allergic encephalomyelitis models
Anti-very large antigen (VLA)-4	Prevents T cell interaction with vascular endothelium at blood–brain barrier	Reduces disease severity and relapse rate in experimental allergic encephalomyelitis models
Rolipram	Type IV phosphodiesterase inhibitor	Reduces disease severity and relapse rate in experimental allergic encephalomyelitis models
Metalloproteinase inhibitors	Block role of metalloproteinases in tumour necrosis factor-α secretion and tissue invasion	Not yet tested in experimental allergic encephalomyelitis models

Cytokines

There is good evidence that multiple sclerosis and EAE are both inflammatory diseases. In general terms, effector arms of the immune system may be divided into two categories. The first arm is pro-inflammatory and anti-humoral: it supports delayed-type hypersensitivity responses and dampens down antibody production. The second arm is pro-humoral and anti-inflammatory. The mediators accounting for this dichotomy in function are cytokines produced by T lymphocytes and monocytes. In the mouse there is a clear distinction between the pro-inflammatory T cell (T_h1) and the pro-humoral T cell in terms of the ILs produced by each cell type. In humans the distinction is less clearcut. Nevertheless, this dichotomy in function raises various possibilities for immune intervention in multiple sclerosis:

1. Administer anti-inflammatory cytokines.
2. Administer antibodies or soluble receptor molecules specific for inflammatory cytokines.
3. Introduce agents designed to modulate cytokine production in favour of anti-inflammatory cytokines.

Each of these three approaches has been tested in the EAE model and awaits development for treatment of multiple sclerosis.

Transforming growth factor-β and interleukin-10

In addition to the clear immune suppressive effect of IFN-β, two additional cytokines have been shown to modulate the inflammation associated with EAE in rodent models.

Transforming growth factor-β is an important immunosuppressive agent. It inhibits the proliferation and function of B cells, cytotoxic T cells and natural killer cells, inhibits cytokine production among lymphocytes, and antagonizes the effects of TNF-α. The potent anti-inflammatory properties of TGF-β are supported by the observation that inactivation of the gene for TGF-β1 in mice leads to multifocal inflammatory disease (Shull et al., 1992). Treatment of mice with either TGF-β1 or TGF-β2 reduced clinical severity and the number of relapses in a model of chronic relapsing EAE (CR-EAE). Mice treated with either cytokine were protected from inflammation and demyelination in the CNS (Racke et al., 1993).

Interleukin-10 inhibits antigen-dependent cytokine production and T cell proliferation by down-regulating constitutive and INF-γ-induced expression of Class II MHC molecules on the surface of monocytes and macrophages. It also inhibits INF-γ-induced cytokine production from macrophages (de Waal Malefyt et al., 1991). In the rat model of EAE, there is evidence that IL-10 expression is up-regulated in the CNS during the recovery phase of disease. With this in mind, Rott et al. demonstrated that IL-10 suppressed EAE, prevented inflammatory cell infiltration in the CNS but supported a humoral response to MBP on systemic administration during the initiation phase of EAE (Rott et al., 1994). This cytokine therefore serves an immunomodulating function switching from a T_h1 (pro-inflammatory) to a T_h2 (pro-humoral) immune response.

Interleukin-12

Interleukin-12 is a key cytokine in the differentiation of T_h1 lymphocytes and, not surprisingly, encourages the development of encephalitogenic T cells (Waldburger et al., 1996). Antibodies directed against this cytokine were shown to completely prevent EAE in a cell transfer model in mice (Leonard et al., 1995).

Tumour necrosis factor-α

Tumour necrosis factor-α is produced by both T cells and macrophages, and is a potent mediator in inflammation, fever and toxic shock. Tumour necrosis factor-α activates vascular endothelium and increases vascular permeability. This cytokine has been a rational target for immune intervention with monoclonal antibodies in rheumatoid arthritis (Elliot et al., 1993). Baker and colleagues have used either a TNF-specific antibody or bivalent p55 and p75 TNF-receptor–immunoglobulin fusion proteins to inhibit TNF activity in the chronic relapsing model of EAE in the Biozzi AB/H mouse (Baker et al., 1994). A therapeutic effect was revealed when antibody was given after the onset of disease. Although disease activity resumed after withdrawal of treatment with either antibody or fusion protein, this study confirmed the central role of TNF-α and T_h1 lymphocyte-mediated responses in this animal model of multiple sclerosis.

Rolipram

Rolipram is a selective type IV phosphodiesterase inhibitor. This drug can suppress the production of TNF-α, lymphotoxin-α and, to a lesser extent, IFN-γ in human and rat leukocytes. In one study, Rolipram was an effective treatment for EAE and reduced TNF-α production by both human and rat T cell lines (Sommer *et al.*, 1995). In a further study, the drug was capable of suppressing disease induced by passive transfer with encephalitogenic T cell lines (Jung *et al.*, 1996). This latter study did not reveal a significant effect on either TNF-α production by T cells or the progression of an active form of disease. The drug did, however, affect TNF-α production by macrophages and consistently reduced inflammatory infiltration in the CNS. Overall the encouraging effects of Rolipram warrant further clinical investigation in multiple sclerosis.

Metalloproteinase inhibitors

A number of pharmaceutical companies are now investigating the use of metalloproteinase (MMP) inhibitors for treatment of inflammatory diseases. Metalloproteinases of both T lymphocytes and macrophages facilitate secretion of TNF-α, by cleavage of the membrane bound form. An inhibitor of MMPs blocks release of the 17 kDa polypeptide form of TNF-α and also prevents shedding of the 80 kDa TNF receptor (Crowe *et al.*, 1995). Since TNF-α plays an important role in inflammatory, autoimmune diseases such as multiple sclerosis there is every likelihood that such inhibitors will provide relief from symptoms.

Metalloproteinases may also play an important role in tissue invasion (Goetzl *et al.*, 1996). Following $\beta 1$ integrin- or vascular cell adhesion molecule (VCAM)-1-dependent stimulation by cytokines and inflammatory mediators, T cells secrete the gelatinases MMP-2 and -9. It is therefore reasonable to speculate that MMP inhibitors may influence T cell migration across the blood–brain barrier, as well as modulating TNF activity.

Adhesion molecules

Adhesion molecules such as E-selectin, VCAM-1 and intercellular adhesion molecule (ICAM)-1 are induced by cytokines on the endothelial surface, and are important for the adhesion of neutrophils, lymphocytes and monocytes. T cell adhesion to the brain microvascular endothelium and migration into the brain parenchyma is a primary event in the development of multiple sclerosis. This is mediated by the very late antigen (VLA)-4 on the surface of the T cell which interacts with its receptor, VCAM-1. Antibodies to the α_4 chain of VLA-4 block adhesion of lymphocytes and monocytes to inflamed brain endothelium and prevent development of EAE in rodent models (Yednock *et al.*, 1992).

The relevance of these observations to humans has been suggested by studies in patients with multiple sclerosis. In cryosections of multiple sclerosis brain, expression of VCAM-1 was found on both the endothelium of vessels surrounding multiple sclerosis plaques and in perivascular sites reminiscent of pericytes. Interestingly, in a cell binding assay conducted *in vitro*, T cell adhesion to TNF-α-stimulated endothelial cells was dependent on both VLA-4 and leukocyte function-associated antigen (LFA)-1, the receptor for ICAM-1. Cell adhesion to TNF-α-stimulated pericytes was, however, dominated by VLA-4 (Verbeek *et al.*, 1995). Furthermore, immunohistochemical staining for VCAM-1/VLA-4 was found to associate with active chronic multiple sclerosis lesions while ICAM-1/LFA-1 was observed more uniformly in lesions of all ages (Cannella and Raine, 1995). The drugs currently under development for blocking VLA-4 are expected to reduce the inflammatory burden in multiple sclerosis.

Towards more specific forms of immunotherapy in multiple sclerosis

There is clearly a need to increase the specificity of therapeutic approaches in autoimmune disease (Figure 4.1). Recent approaches have aimed at either the TCR or the antigen being recognized by pathogenic T lymphocytes.

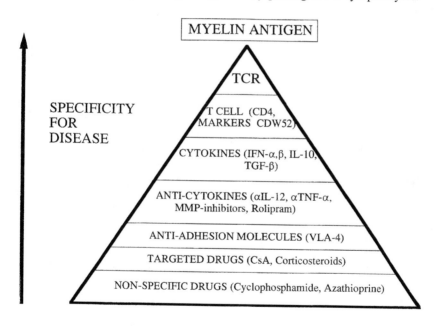

Figure 4.1. The specificity triangle of therapy for multiple sclerosis.

The T cell receptor

Since the discovery of the TCR over a decade ago there has been enormous effort put into finding a possible link between genetic susceptibility to autoimmune diseases and the TCR. Such a search in multiple sclerosis was triggered by the finding of limited heterogeneity in TCR usage in the animal model EAE (Acha-Orbea *et al.*, 1988). Limitation of the disease in the H-2^u mouse to practically a single V$_\beta$ type (V$_\beta$8.2) allowed the use of antibodies directed to the TCR to both prevent and treat disease. A different approach was developed by Irun Cohen and colleagues (Ben-Nun et al., 1981; Cohen, 1986). They developed a number of strategies for attenuating the encephalitogenic activity of T cells and found that injection of the T cells as a vaccine would suppress the induction of EAE.

Application of this approach in various diseases in humans has not led to significant changes in disease profile although Zhang and Raus have shown that the proliferation of MBP-reactive T cells could be altered following administration of MBP-specific T cell vaccine in multiple sclerosis patients (Zhang et al., 1993). Based on the assumption that the T cell vaccine effect might result from the presentation of a peptide derived from the TCR idiotype of the vaccine, Vandenbark et al. (1989) have demonstrated the successful prevention of EAE by prior administration of peptides derived from the TCR of known encephalitogenic cells. A possible mechanism for this effect, which gives hope for future application to multiple sclerosis, has come from a recent series of experiments using a naked DNA vaccine designed to express the V_β protein of a T cell clone (Waisman et al., 1996). Intramuscular administration of the DNA led to protection from EAE and an elevation in the production of cytokines consistent with the induction of T_h2 cells.

Support for this mode of treatment in multiple sclerosis patients comes from the Vandenbark group (Vandenbark et al., 1996). This group identified a TCR peptide from the $V_\beta5.2$ sequence which had been associated with disease in two independent studies (Kotzin et al., 1991; Oksenberg et al., 1993b). A peptide vaccine was injected into multiple sclerosis patients and evoked peptide-reactive T cells in patients with progressive multiple sclerosis. Vaccine responders had a reduced MBP response and remained clinically stable throughout one year of therapy. Non-responding patients displayed an increase in their MBP response over this same period and progressed clinically. Peptide-specific T cells were shown to produce IL-10, a T_h2 cytokine, providing a possible rationale for the efficacy of this approach in patients. Taken together these results indicate that modulation of the immune response to a peptide antigen associated with disease, in this case a TCR peptide, can regulate the immune response in a bystander fashion without deleterious side effects. Further experimental work continues (Gold et al., 1997; Wilson et al., 1997); the results of early clinical trials do begin to offer some support for this approach (Vandenbark et al., 1997).

Antigen-specific immunotherapy of multiple sclerosis

Since multiple sclerosis is most probably initiated and propagated by inflammatory T cells, it is reasonable to target these cells by modifying their response to antigen. Antigen-specific immunotherapy would clearly be the most specific form of intervention and hopefully will be applicable with the least risk of hazardous side effects.

The various approaches to immunotherapy with antigen have been clarified in experimental animal studies and reveal three mechanisms. One pathway for antigen-specific unresponsiveness is activation-induced cell death (AICD). This occurs as a consequence of repeated stimulation with high concentrations of antigen. In $CD4^+$ T cells, AICD is largely mediated by Fas–Fas ligand interactions and is augmented by IL-2 (Critchfield *et al.*, 1994). Somewhat disturbingly, however, it has been shown that co-administration of IL-2 and myelin antigen resulted in the aggravation of clinical disease, while antigen alone was sufficient to reduce clinical disease in an EAE model (Racke *et al.*, 1996). A second pathway of unresponsiveness is functional anergy which can be induced, at least among isolated T cell clones *in vitro*, by antigen recognition with deficient co-stimulation (Schwartz, 1992). Blockade of co-stimulation affects the development of T_h1 cells and is not associated with cell death. The third possible mechanism, applicable to inflammatory autoimmune conditions such as multiple sclerosis, involves modulation of the cytokine profile of T cells towards the T_h2 pro-humoral, anti-inflammatory type. It has been revealed, for example, that continuous, low-dose treatment with soluble foreign antigen converts the default T_h1 pathway towards T_h2, as shown by a reduction in the inflammatory cytokine IFN-γ with the concomitant increase in cytokines such as IL-4 and IL-5 (Guery *et al.*, 1996).

Interestingly each of these three approaches to antigen-specific modulation has been demonstrated independently in experiments aimed at inducing oral tolerance to myelin antigens. Soluble protein antigens administered via mucosal surfaces are generally tolerated by the immune system (Mowat, 1987): could the administration of self antigens be used to reinstate self-tolerance in autoimmunity? A number of groups have applied the approach of oral tolerance to EAE (Miller *et al.*, 1991; Whitacre *et al.*, 1991; Metzler and Wraith, 1996) and more recently to multiple sclerosis (Weiner *et al.*, 1993a).

The mechanism of oral tolerance depends on the dose of antigen administered. The default response to antigens encountered at mucosal surfaces is IgA production. It is therefore not unexpected that administration of myelin antigens by oral feeding can induce T cells whose cytokine profile is required to support IgA production. The switching of Ig subclass to IgA requires IL-5, a T_h2 cytokine, and TGF-β, and the administration of low-dose soluble MBP has been shown to induce CD4 cells producing such cytokines (Chen *et al.*, 1994). It appears, however, that administration of higher doses of antigen induces anergy (Gregerson *et al.*, 1993). Although the precise mechanism of anergy induction following oral administration of antigen has not been clarified, it seems probable that this results from the entry of antigen, or antigenic fragments, into the circulation. Finally, the administration of high doses of peptide antigen via the oral route can induce apoptosis among potentially autoreactive cells (Chen *et al.*, 1995).

The oral route of antigen administration has been compared with two other routes of peptide administration in a mouse model. Both intranasal deposition (Metzler and Wraith, 1993, 1996) and intraperitoneal injection of peptide antigens (Liu and Wraith, 1995) have proven more effective than the oral route of antigen administration. The intranasal route appears particularly promising in that the administration of a single peptide can modify disease induced with the complex mixture of antigens contained within whole myelin. In order to clarify the mechanism of peptide therapy intranasal administration of peptide antigens, Anderton and colleagues have tested a murine model of EAE involving immune responses to both MBP and PLP (Anderton and Wraith, 1998). In this case, administration of a single peptide from PLP inhibited the immune response to both MBP and PLP, thereby effectively preventing and treating clinical disease. This effect is reminiscent of a previous study of oral tolerance to MBP in a similar mouse model (Al-Sabbagh *et al.*, 1994). In this latter case, however, bystander regulation of the response to PLP could be accounted for by the induction of cells producing anti-inflammatory cytokines whereas the intranasal route did not lead to modulation of the immune response towards T_h2 cytokines. There are two obvious differences between these studies. First of all, the oral route of administration could be especially suited to the induction of T_h2 cells. Two recent studies of intranasal peptide administration in the non-obese diabetic mouse model have, however, demonstrated the induction of T_h2 responses (Daniel and Wegmann, 1996; Tian *et al.*, 1996). Secondly, the induction of T_h2 cells by mucosal administration might depend on the use of intact antigen or at least a peptide antigen large enough to associate with immunoglobulin. Antigen capture by cell surface immunoglobulin and the subsequent presentation of antigen by B cells is believed to favour the generation of T_h2 cells (Saoudi *et al.*, 1995).

At this point in the discussion it is worth asking, why use peptides when the whole antigen alone might work? Obviously use of the intact antigen, if effective, would overcome the necessity to identify every T cell epitope associated with each disease-associated MHC allele. Preparation of pure antigens in sufficient quantities for treatment is not straightforward and the results of trials with intact antigens in multiple sclerosis and rheumatoid arthritis have not thus far been convincing. As described above, however, there is increasing evidence in favour of the recognition of dominant epitopes from proteins such as MBP in multiple sclerosis. If it is possible to induce the same phenomenon of bystander suppression in humans as has been widely described in rodent models, it should be possible to administer an immunodominant epitope or possibly a selected cocktail of peptides, to a wide range of patients. The production of peptide antigens is relatively cheap and furthermore the use of synthetic peptides enables development of analogues for improved therapy.

Recent studies have revealed two approaches to modifying peptide antigens in order to improve their efficacy in peptide therapy. Both approaches require the definition of amino acids involved in determining either TCR or MHC interaction within a peptide antigen. Amino acid residues known to determine interaction with MHC may be modified in order to optimize interaction between the MHC molecule and its ligand (Fairchild *et al.*, 1993). Studies involving either the intraperitoneal (Liu and Wraith, 1995), intranasal (Metzler and Wraith, 1996) or intravenous (Samson and Smilek, 1995) routes of peptide administration have demonstrated a direct correlation between peptide affinity for MHC and their disease-suppressing properties. Modification of TCR interaction residues can also be used to alter immune responses in models of EAE (Karin *et al.*, 1994; Nicholson *et al.*, 1995; Brocke *et al.*, 1996). Analogues containing amino acid substitutions at TCR interaction residues can act as TCR antagonists (Sloan-Lancaster and Alleen, 1996) and hence reduce the levels of inflammatory cytokines produced by autoreactive cells. Treatment of experimental animals with such peptides in a soluble form can suppress either actively or passively induced disease EAE (Karin *et al.*, 1994;

Nicholson *et al.*, 1995; Brocke *et al.*, 1996). This approach holds great potential for improving peptide therapy in multiple sclerosis even though it may be difficult to identify analogues likely to be more effective than the natural sequence in the relatively outbred population of multiple sclerosis patients.

Conclusions: the specificity pyramid in immunotherapy of multiple sclerosis

This review of current and future immunotherapies for multiple sclerosis has emphasized the advantages and disadvantages of different approaches while giving some background to the likely mechanism of their action. There is a general rule: the more specific the approach for immune elements involved in disease, the less likely it is to give deleterious side effects. The immunotherapies described in this article can therefore be viewed as a pyramid of specificity up which we are all trying to climb. It is believed that the antigen is the most specific target for immune intervention and it is for this reason that this component of the trimolecular complex involved in T cell activation appears at the top of the pyramid. It should be stressed, however, that, with the possible exception of oral tolerance, none of the possible antigen-specific means of intervention have been tested. Until these are available we are forced to slide back down the slope and adopt the next best approach. A number of cell specific approaches are now in clinical trial and may find general use within the next few years. Let us hope that, as further developments are made, we can soon reach the peak of the pyramid and adopt more specific approaches to immune intervention in multiple sclerosis.

References

Acha-Orbea, H., Mitchell, D. J., Timmermann, L., Wraith, D. C., Tausch, G. S., Waldor, M. K., *et al.* (1988) Limited heterogeneity of T cell receptors from lymphocytes mediating autoimmune encephalomyelitis allows specific immune intervention. *Cell*, **54**, 263–273.

Achiron, A., Rotstein, Z., Noy, S., Mashiach, S., Dulitzky, M. and Achiron, R. (1996) Intravenous immunoglobulin treatment in the prevention of childbirth associated acute exacerbations in multiple sclerosis – a pilot study. *J. Neurol.*, **243**, 25–28.

Achiron, A., Gabbay, U., Gilad, R., HassinBaer, S., Barak, Y., Gornish, M., *et al.* (1998) Intravenous immunoglobulin treatment in multiple sclerosis – effect on relapses. *Neurology*, **50**, 398–402.

Al-Sabbagh, A., Miller, A., Santos, L. M. B. and Weiner, H. L. (1994) Antigen-driven tissue-specific suppression following oral tolerance: orally administered myelin basic protein suppresses proteolipid protein-induced experimental autoimmune encephalomyelitis in the SJL mouse. *Eur. J. Immunol.*, **24**, 2104–2109.

Anderton, S. M. and Wraith, D. C. (1998) Hierarchy in the ability of T cell epitopes to induce peripheral tolerance to antigens from myelin. *Eur. J. Immunol.*, **28**, 1251–1261.

Arnon, R. and Teitelbaum, D. (1994) Immunospecific drug design prospects for treatment of autoimmune diseases. *Therap. Immunol.*, **1**, 65–70.

Arnon, R., Sela, M. and Teitelbaum, D. (1996) New insights into the mechanism of action of copolymer 1 in experimental allergic encephalomyelitis and multiple sclerosis. *J. Neurology*, **243**, s8–s13.

Baker, D., O'Neill, J. K., Gschmeissner, S. E., Wilcox, C. E., Butter, C. and Turk, J. L. (1990) Induction of chronic relapsing experimental allergic encephalomyelitis in Biozzi mice. *J. Neuroimmunol.*, **28**, 261–267.

Baker, D., Butler, D., Scallon, B. J., O'Neill, J. K., Turk, J. L. and Feldmann, M. (1994) Control of established experimental allergic encephalomyelitis by inhibition of tumor necrosis factor (TNF) activity within the central nervous system using monoclonal antibodies and TNF receptor-immunoglobulin fusion proteins. *Eur. J. Immunol.*, **24**, 2040–2048.

Beck, J., Rondot, P. and Catinot, L. (1988) Increased production of interferon gamma and tumor necrosis factor precedes clinical manifestation in multiple sclerosis: do cytokines trigger off exacerbations? *Acta Neurol. Scand.*, **78**, 318–323.

Beck, R. W. (1995) The optic neuritis treatment trial: three-year follow-up results [letter]. *Arch. Ophthalmol.* **113**, 136–137.

Beck, R. W., Cleary, P. A., Trobe, J. D., Kaufman, D. I., Kupersmith, M. J., Paty, D. W., *et al.* (1993) The effect of corticosteroids for acute optic neuritis on the subsequent development of multiple sclerosis. *N. Engl. J. Med.*, **329**, 1764–1769.

Ben-Nun, A., Wekerle, H. and Cohen, I. R. (1981) Vaccination against autoimmune encephalomyelitis with T-lymphocyte line cells reactive against myelin basic protein. *Nature*, **292**, 60–61.

Brocke, S., Gijbels, K., Allegretta, M., Ferber, I., Piercy, C., Blankenstein, T., *et al.* (1996) Treatment of experimental encephalomyelitis with a peptide analogue of myelin basic protein. *Nature*, **379**, 343–346.

Burt, R. K., Burns, W. H. and Miller, S. D. (1997) Bone marrow transplantation for multiple sclerosis: returning to Pandora's box. *Immunol. Today*, **18**, 559–561.

Cannella, B. and Raine, C. S. (1995) The adhesion molecule and cytokine profile of multiple sclerosis lesions. *Ann. Neurol.*, **37**, 424–435.

Carrigan, D. R., Harrington, D. and Knox, K. K. (1996) Subacute leukoencephalitis caused by CNS infection with human herpesvirus-6 manifesting as acute multiple sclerosis. *Neurology*, **47**, 145–148.

Carter, J. L., Hafler, D. A., Dawson, D. M., Orav, J. and Weiner, H. L. (1988) Immunosuppression with high-dose i.v. cyclophosphamide and ACTH in progressive multiple sclerosis: cumulative 6-year experience in 164 patients. *Neurology*, **38**, 9–14.

Challoner, P. B., Smith, K. T., Parker, J. D., MacLeod, D. L., Coulter, S. N, Rose, T. M., *et al.* (1995) Plaque-associated expression of human herpesvirus 6 in multiple sclerosis. *Proc. Natl Acad. Sci. USA*, **92**, 7440–7444.

Chen, Y., Kuchroo, V. K., Inobe, J.-I., Hafler, D. A. and Weiner, H. L. (1994) Regulatory T cell clones induced by oral tolerance: suppression of autoimmune encephalomyelitis. *Science*, **265**, 1237–1240.

Chen, Y., Inobe, J. I., Marks, R., Gonnella, P., Kuchroo, V. K. and Weiner, H. L. (1995) Peripheral deletion of antigen-reactive T cells in oral tolerance. *Nature*, **376**, 177–180.

Cohen, I. R. (1986) Regulation of autoimmune disease: physiological and therapeutic. *Immunol. Rev.*, **94**, 5–21.

Comi, G., Rodegher, M., Colombo, B., Martinelli, V., Fossati, V. and Filippi, M. (1997) Low-dose total body irradiation in chronic progressive multiple sclerosis: a double blind, controlled, randomized phase II study. *Neurology* **48**, 45004.

Confavreux, C., Saddier, P., Grimaud, J., Moreau, T., Adeleine, P. and Aimard, G. (1996) Risk of cancer from azathioprine therapy in multiple sclerosis: a case-control study. *Neurology* **46**, 1607–1612.

Cook, S. D., Devereux, C., Troiano, R., Wolansky, L., Guarnaccia, J., Haffty, B., *et al.* (1997) Modified total lymphoid irradiation and low dose corticosteroids in progressive multiple sclerosis. *J. Neurol. Sci.*, **152**, 172–181.

Critchfield, J. M., Racke, M. K., Zuniga-Pflucker, J. C., Cannella, B., Raine, C. S., Goverman, J., *et al.* (1994) T cell deletion in high antigen dose therapy of autoimmune encephalomyelitis. *Science*, **263**, 1139–1143.

Crowe, P. D., Walter, B. N., Mohler, K. M., OttenEvans, C., Black, R. A. B. and Ware, C. F. (1995) A metalloprotease inhibitor blocks shedding of the 80–kD TNF receptor and TNF processing in T lymphocytes. *J. Exp. Med.*, **181**, 1205–1210.

Daniel, D. and Wegmann, D. R. (1996) Protection of nonobese diabetic mice from diabetes by intranasal or subcutaneous administration of insulin peptide B-(923). *Proc. Natl Acad. Sci. USA*, **93**, 956–960.

de Waal Malefyt, R., Yssel, H., Roncarlo, M. G., Spits, H. and de Vries, J. E. (1991) Interleukin-10. *Curr. Opin. Immunol.*, **4**, 314–320.

Duquette, P., Despault, L., Knobler, R. L., Lublin, F. D., Kelley, L., Francis, G. S., *et al.* (1995) Interferon beta-1b in the treatment of multiple sclerosis: final outcome of the randomized controlled trial. *Neurology*, **45**, 1277–1285.

Durelli, L., Bongioanni, M. R., Ferrero, B., Ferri, R., Imperiale, D., Bradac, G. B., *et al.* (1996) Interferon alpha-2a treatment of relapsing-remitting multiple sclerosis: disease activity resumes after stopping treatment. *Neurology*, **47**, 123–129.

Elliot, M. J., Maini, R. N., Feldmann, M., Long-Fox, A., Charles, P., Katsikis, P., *et al.* (1993) Treatment of rheumatoid arthritis with chimeric monoclonal antibody to tumor necrosis factor a. *Arthritis Rheum.*, **36**, 1681–1690.

European Study Group on Interferon β1b in secondary progressive MS (1998) *Lancet*, **352**, 1491–1497.

Fairchild, P. J., Wildgoose, R., Atherton, E., Webb, S. and Wraith, D. C. (1993) An autoantigenic T cell epitope forms unstable complexes with class II MHC: a novel route for escape from tolerance induction. *Int. Immunol.*, **5**, 1151–1158.

Faulds, D. and Benfield, P. (1994) Interferon beta-1b in multiple sclerosis: an initial review of its rationale for use and therapeutic potential. *Clin. Immunother.*, **1**, 79–87.

Faulds, D., Goa, K. L. and Benfield, P. (1993) Cyclosporin: a review of its pharmacodynamic and pharmacokinetic properties, and therapeutic use in immunoregulatory disorders. *Drugs*, **45**, 953–1040.

Fazekas, F., Deisenhammer, F., Strasser, F. S., Nahler, G. and Mamoli, B. (1997) Randomized placebo-controlled trial of monthly intravenous immunoglobulin therapy in relapsing-remitting multiple sclerosis. Austrian Immunoglobulin in Multiple Sclerosis Study Group. *Lancet*, **349**, 589–593.

Filippi, M., Campi, A., Mammi, S., Martinelli, V., Locatelli, T., Scotti, G., *et al.* (1995) Brain magnetic resonance imaging and multimodal evoked potentials in benign and secondary progressive multiple sclerosis. *J. Neurol. Neurosurg. Psychiat.*, **58**, 31–37.

Francis, G. S., Freedman, M. S. and Antel, J. P. (1997) Failure of intravenous immunoglobulin to arrest progression of multiple sclerosis: a clinical and MRI based study. *Multiple Sclerosis* **3**, 370–376.

Fritz, R. B., Skeen, M. J., Chou, C. H. J. and McFarlin, D. E. (1985) Major histocompatibility complex linked control of the immune response to myelin basic protein. *J. Immunol.*, **134**, 2328–2332.

Goetzl, E. J., Banda, M. J. and Leppert, D. (1996) Matrix metalloproteinases in immunity. *J. Immunol.*, **156**, 1–4.

Gold, D. P., Smith, R. A., Golding, A. B., Morgan, E. E., Dafashy, T., Nelson, J., *et al.* (1997) Results of a phase I clinical trial of a T cell receptor vaccine in patients with multiple sclerosis. 2. Comparative analysis of TCR utilization in CSF T cell populations before and after vaccination with a TCRV beta 6 CDR2 peptide. *J. Neuroimmunol.*, **76**, 29–38.

Goodkin, D. E., Rudick, R. A., VanderBrug, M. S., Daughtry, M. M., Schwetz, K. M., Fischer, J., *et al.* (1995) Low-dose (7.5 mg) oral methotrexate reduces the rate of progression in chronic progressive multiple sclerosis. *Ann. Neurol.* **37**, 30–40.

Goverman, J., Woods, A., Larson, L., Weiner, L. P., Hood, L. and Zaller, D. M. (1993) Transgenic mice that express a myelin basic protein-specific T cell receptor develop spontaneous autoimmunity. *Cell*, **72**, 551–560.

Gregerson, D. S., Obritsch, W. F. and Donoso, L. A. (1993) Oral tolerance in experimental autoimmune uveoretinitis. Distinct mechanisms are induced by low dose vs high dose feeding protocols. *J. Immunol.*, **151**, 5751–5761.

Guery, J.-C., Galbiati, F., Smiroldo, S. and Adorini, L. (1996) Selective development of T helper (Th)2 cells induced by continuous administration of low dose soluble proteins to normal and beta-microglobulin-deficient BALB/c mice. *J. Exp. Med.*, **183**, 485–497.

Jacobs, L. D., Cookfair, D. L., Rudick, R. A., Herndon, R. M., Richert, J. R., Salazar, A. M., *et al.* (1996) Intramuscular interferon beta-1a for disease progression in relapsing multiple sclerosis. The Multiple Sclerosis Collaborative Research Group (MSCRG) *Ann. Neurol.* **39**, 285–294.

Johnson, K. P., Brooks, B. R., Cohen, J. A., Ford, C. C., Goldstein, J., Lisak, R. P., *et al.* (1998) Extended use of glatiramer acetate (Copaxone) is well tolerated and maintains its clinical effect on multiple sclerosis relapse rate and degree of disability. *Neurology* **50**, 701–708.

Jung, S., Zielasek, J., Kollner, G., Donhauser, T., Toyka, K. and Hartung, H.-P. (1996) Preventive but not therapeutic application of Rolipram ameliorates experimental auto-immune encephalomyelitis in Lewis rats. *J. Neuroimmunol.*, **68**, 1–11.

Karin, N., Mitchell, D. J., Brocke, S., Ling, N. and Steinman, L. (1994) Reversal of experimental autoimmune encephalomyelitis by a soluble peptide variant of myelin basic protein epitope: T cell receptor antagonism and reduction of interferon gamma and tumor necrosis factor alpha production. *J. Exp. Med.*, **180**, 2227–2237.

Kotzin, B. L., Karuturi, S., Chou, Y. K., Lafferty, J., Forrester, J. M., Better, M., *et al.* (1991) Preferential T cell receptor V beta usage in myelin basic protein reactive T cell clones from patients with multiple sclerosis. *Proc. Natl Acad. Sci. USA*, **88**, 9161–9165.

Leonard, J. P., Waldburger, K. E. and Goldman, S. J. (1995) Prevention of experimental autoimmune encephalomyelitis by antibodies against interleukin 12. *J. Exp. Med.*, **181**, 381–386.

Likosky, W. H., Fireman, B., Elmore, R., Eno, G., Gale, K., Browne-Goode, G., *et al.* (1991) Intense immunosuppression in chronic progressive multiple sclerosis: the Kaiser study. *J. Neurol. Neurosurg. Psychiat.*, **54**, 1055–1060.

Liu, G. Y. and Wraith, D. C. (1995) Affinity for class II MHC determines the extent to which soluble peptides tolerize autoreactive T cells in naive and primed adult mice – implications for autoimmunity. *Int. Immunol.*, **7**, 1255–1263.

Liu, G. Y., Fairchild, P. J., Smith, R. M., Prowle, J. R., Kioussis, D. and Wraith, D. C. (1995) Low avidity recognition of self-antigen by T cells permits escape from central tolerance. *Immunity*, **3**, 407–415.

Lu, H.-T., Rilyer, J. L., Babcock, G. T., Huston, M., Stark, G. R., Boss, J. M., *et al.* (1995) Interferon beta acts downstream of IFN-gamma-induced class II transactivator messenger RNA accumulation to block major histocompatibility complex class II gene expression and requires the 48-kD DNA-binding protein, ISGF3-g. *J. Exp. Med.*, **182**, 1517–1525.

Lumsden, C. E. (1970) The neuropathology of multiple sclerosis. In *Handbook of Clinical Neurology* (Vinken, P. J. and Bruyn, G. W., eds), pp. 217–309. Amsterdam: North-Holland.

McDonald, W. I., Miller, D. H. and Barnes, D. (1992) The pathological evolution of multiple sclerosis. *Neuropathol. Appl. Neurobiol.*, **18**, 319–334.

Metzler, B. and Wraith, D. C. (1993) Inhibition of experimental autoimmune encephalomyelitis by inhalation but not oral administration of the encephalitogenic peptide: influence of MHC binding affinity. *Int. Immunol.*, **5**, 1159–1165.

Metzler, B. and Wraith, D. C. (1996) Mucosal tolerance in a murine model of experimental autoimmune encephalomyelitis. *Ann. N.Y. Acad. Sci.*, **778**, 228–243.

Miller, A., Lider, O. and Weiner, H. L. (1991) Antigen-driven bystander suppression after oral administration of antigens. *J. Exp. Med.*, **174**, 791–798.

Miller, D. H., Thompson, A. J., Morrissey, S. P., MacManus, D. G., Moore, S. G., Kendall, B. E., *et al.* (1992) High dose steroids in acute relapses of multiple sclerosis: MRI evidence for a possible mechanism of therapeutic effect. *J. Neurol. Neurosurg. Psychiat.*, **55**, 450–453.

Milligan, N. M., Newcombe, R. and Compston, D. A. S. (1987) A double blind controlled trial of high dose methylprednisolone in patients with multiple sclerosis: 1. clinical effects. *J. Neurol. Neurosurg. Psychiat.*, **50**, 511–516.

Moreau, T., Thorpe, J., Miller, D., Moseley, I., Hale, G., Waldmann, H., *et al.* (1994) Preliminary evidence from magnetic resonance imaging for reduction in disease activity after lymphocyte depletion in multiple sclerosis. *Lancet*, **344**, 298–301.

Moreau, T., Coles, A., Wing, M., Isaacs, J., Hale, G., Waldmann, H., *et al.* (1996) Transient increase in symptoms associated with cytokine release in patients with multiple sclerosis. *Brain*, **119**, 225–237.

Multiple Sclerosis Study Group (1990) Efficacy and toxicity of cyclosporine in chronic progressive multiple sclerosis: a randomized, double-blinded, placebo-controlled clinical trial. The Multiple Sclerosis Study Group. *Ann. Neurol.* **27**, 591–605.

Mowat, A. M. (1987) Regulation of immune responses to dietary proteins. *Immunol. Today*, **8**, 93–98.

Myers, L. W., Ellison, G. W., Merrill, J. E., El Hajjas, A., St Pierre, B., Hijazin, M. *et al.* (1998) Pentonifylline is not a promising treatment for multiple sclerosis. *Neurology*, **51**, 1483–1486.

Nicholson, L. B., Greer, J. M., Sobel, R. A., Lees, M. B. and Kuchroo, V. K. (1995) An altered peptide ligand mediates immune deviation and prevents autoimmune encephalomyelitis. *Immunity*, **3**, 397–405.

Nishimura, Y., Uenishi, K., Taniguchi, K., Ukai, S. and Takaishi, J. (1995) Long term intravenous immunoglobulin treatment in patients with chronic inflammatory demyelinating polyradiculoneuropathy and multiple sclerosis. *Jap. J. Nat. Med. Serv.*, **49**, 1013–1017.

Njenga, M. K., Pavelko, K. D., Baisch, J., Lin, X., David, C., Leibowitz, J., *et al.* (1996) Theiler's virus persistence and demyelination in major histocompatibility complex class II-deficient mice. *J. Virol.*, **70**, 1729–1737.

Noseworthy, J. H., Weinshenker, B. G., O'Brien, P. C., Weis, J. A., Petterson, T. M., Windebank, A. J., *et al.* (1997) Intravenous immunoglobulin does not reverse recently acquired, apparently permanent weakness in multiple sclerosis. *Ann. Neurol.*, **42**, M115.

Noseworthy, J. H., O'Brien, P., Erickson, B. J., Lee, D., Sneve, B., Ebers, G. C. *et al.* (1998) The Mayo Clinic–Canadian cooperative trial of sulfazalazine in active multiple sclerosis. *Neurology*, **51**, 1342–1352.

Oksenberg, J. R., Begovich, A. B., Erlich, H. A. and Steinman, L. (1993a) Genetic factors in multiple sclerosis. *J. Am. Med. Ass.*, **270**, 2362–2369.

Oksenberg, J. R., Panzara, M. A., Begovich, A. B., Mitchell, D., Erlich, H. A., Murray, R. S., *et al.* (1993b) Selection for T cell receptor V_β–D_β–J_β gene rearrangements with specificity for a myelin basic protein peptide in brain lesions of multiple sclerosis. *Nature*, **362**, 68.

Olsson, T., Sun, J., Hillert, J., Hojeberg, B., Ekre, H.-P., Andersson, G., *et al.* (1992) Increased numbers of T cells recognizing multiple myelin basic protein epitopes in multiple sclerosis. *Eur. J. Immunol.*, **22**, 1083.

Padula, S. J., Lingenheld, E. G., Stabach, P. R., Chou, C. J., Kono, D. H. and Clark, R. B. (1991) Identification of $V_\beta 4$–bearing T cells in SJL mice. *J. Immunol.*, **146**, 879–883.

Palace, J. and Rothwell, P. (1997) New treatments and azathioprine in multiple sclerosis. *Lancet* **350**, 261.

PRISMS (Prevention of relapses and disability by Interferon β-1a subcutaneously in multiple sclerosis) Study Group (1998) Randomised double-blend placebo-controlled study of Interferon β-1a in replapsing/remitting multiple sclerosis. *Lancet*, **352**, 1498–1504.

Racadot, E., Rumbach, L., Bataillard, M., Galmiche, J., Henlin, J. L, Truttmann, M., *et al.* (1993) Treatment of multiple sclerosis with anti-CD4 monoclonal antibody. *J. Autoimmun.*, **6**, 771–786.

Racke, M. K., Sriram, S., Carlino, J., Cannella, B., Raine, C. S. and McFarlin, D. E. (1993) Long-term treatment of chronic relapsing experimental allergic encephalomyelitis by transforming growth factor-beta2. *J. Neuroimmunol.*, **46**, 175–184.

Racke, M. K., Critchfield, J. M., Quigley, L., Cannella, B., Raine, C. S., McFarland, H. F., *et al.* (1996) Intravenous antigen administration as a therapy for autoimmune demyelinating disease. *Ann. Neurol.*, **39**, 46–56.

Rodriguez, M., Karnes, W. E., Bartleson, J. D. and Pineda, A. A. (1993) Plasma exchange in acute episodes of fulminant CNS inflammatory demyelination. *Neurology*, **43**, 1100–1104.

Roos, R. P., Wollmann, R. (1986) DA strain of Theiler's murine encephalomyelitis virus induces demyelination in nude mice. *Lab. Invest.*, **54**, 515–522.

Rott, O., Fleischer, B. and Cash, E. (1994) Interleukin-10 prevents experimental allergic encephalomyelitis in rats. *Eur. J. Immunol.*, **24**, 1434–1440.

Samson, M. F. and Smilek, D. E. (1995) Reversal of acute experimental autoimmune encephalomyelitis and prevention of relapses by treatment with a myelin basic protein peptide analogue modified to form long lived peptide–MHC complexes. *J. Immunol.*, **155**, 2737–2746.

Saoudi, A., Simmonds, S., Huitinga, I. and Mason, D. (1995) Prevention of experimental allergic encephalomyelitis in rats by targeting autoantigen to B cells: Evidence that the protective mechanism depends on changes in the cytokine response and migratory properties of the autoantigen-specific T cells. *J. Exp. Med.*, **182**, 335–344.

Schwartz, R. H. (1992) Costimulation of T lymphocytes: The role of CD28, CTLA-4, and B7/BB1 in interleukin-2 production and immunotherapy. *Cell*, **71**, 1065–1068.

Sharief, M. K. and Hentges, R. (1991) Association between TNF-alpha and disease progression in patients with multiple sclerosis. *N. Engl. J. Med.*, **325**, 467–472.

Shull, M. M, Ormsby, I., Kier, A. B., Pawlowski, S., Diebold, R. J., Yin, M., *et al.* (1992) Targeted disruption of the mouse transforming growth factor-β1 gene results in multifocal inflammatory disease. *Nature*, **359**, 693–699.

Sibley, W. A., Ebers, G. C., Panitch, H. S. and Reder, A. T. (1994) Interferon beta treatment of multiple sclerosis. Reply. *Neurology* **44**, 188–190.

Sloan-Lancaster, J. and Alleen, P. M. (1996) Altered peptide ligand-induced partial T cell activation: molecular mechanisms and role in T cell biology. *Annu. Rev. Immunol.*, **14**, 1–27.

Smith, R. M. (1995) *PhD Thesis.* University of Cambridge.

Smith, R. M., Morgan, A. and Wraith, D. C. (1994) Anti-class II MHC antibodies are able to prevent and treat EAE without APC depletion. *Immunology*, In press.

Sommer, N., Loschmann, P. A., Northoff, G. H., Weller, M., Steinbrecher, A., Steinbach, J. P., *et al.* (1995) The antidepressant Rolipram suppresses cytokine production and prevents autoimmune encephalomyelitis. *Nat. Med.*, **1**, 244–248.

Teitelbaum, D., Meshorer, A., Hirshfeld, T., Arono, R. and Sela, M. (1971) Suppression of experiment allergic encephalomyelitis by a synthetic polypeptide. *Eur. J. Immunol.*, **1**, 242–248.

The Canadian Cooperative Multiple Sclerosis Study Group (1991) The Canadian cooperative trial of cyclophosphamide and plasma exchange in progressive multiple sclerosis. *Lancet*, **337**, 441–446.

Tian, J., Atkinson, M. A., Clare-Salzer, M., Herschenfeld, A., Forsthuber, T., Lehmann, P. V., *et al.* (1996) Nasal administration of glutamate decarboxylase (GAD 65) peptides induces T_h2 responses and prevents murine insulin-dependent diabetes. *J. Exp. Med.*, **183**, 1561–1567.

Traugott, U., Reinherz, E. L. and Raine, C. S. (1983) Multiple sclerosis: distribution of T cell subsets within active chronic lesions. *Science*, **219**, 308–310.

Vandenbark, A. A., Hashim, G. and Offner, H. (1989) Immunization with a synthetic T cell receptor V-region peptide protects against experimental autoimmune encephalomyelitis. *Nature*, **341**, 541–544.

Vandenbark, A. A., Chou, Y. K., Whitham, R., Mass, M., Buenafe, A., Liefeld, D., *et al.* (1996) Treatment of multiple sclerosis with T cell receptor peptides: results of a double-blind pilot trial. *Nat. Med.*, **2**, 1109–1115.

Vandenbark, A. A., Chou, Y. K., Whitman, R., Mass, R., Buenafe, A., Liefeld, D., *et al.* (1997) Treatment of multiple sclerosis with T cell receptor peptides: Results of a double-blind pilot trial (vol. 2, p. 1109, 1996). *Nature Medicine* **3**, 240.

Van Oosten, B. W., Lai, M., Hodgkinson, S., Barkhof, F., Miller, D. H., Moseley, I. F., *et al.* (1997) Treatment of multiple sclerosis with the monoclonal anti-CD4 antibody cM-T412: results of a randomized, double-blind, placebo-controlled, MR-monitored phase II trial. *Neurology*, **49**, 351–357.

Verbeek, M. M., Westphal, J. R., Ruiter, D. J. and De-Waal, R. M. W. (1995) T lymphocyte adhesion to human brain pericytes is mediated via very late antigen-4/vascular cell adhesion molecule-1 interactions. *J. Immunol.*, **154**, 5876–5884.

Waisman, A., Ruiz, P. J., Hirschberg, D. L., Gelman, A., Oksenberg, J. R., Brocke, S., *et al.* (1996) Suppressive vaccination with DNA encoding a variable region gene of the T cell receptor prevents autoimmune encephalomyelitis and activates T_h2 immunity. *Nat. Med.*, **2**, 899–905.

Waldburger, K. E., Hastings, R. C., Schaub, R. G., Goldman, S. J. and Leonard, J. P. (1996)

Adoptive transfer of experimental allergic encephalomyelitis after *in vitro* treatment with recombinant interleukin-12: preferential expansion of interferon-gamma-producing cells and increased expression of macrophage-associated inducible nitric oxide synthase as immuno-modulatory mechanisms. *Am. J. Pathol.*, **148**, 375–382.

Warren, K. G., Catz, I. and Steinman, L. (1995) Fine specificity of the antibody response to myelin basic protein in the central nervous system in multiple sclerosis: the minimal B cell epitope and a model of its features. *Proc. Natl Acad. Sci. USA*, **92**, 11061–11065.

Weiner, H. L., Mackin, G. A., Matsui, M., Orav, E. J., Khoury, S. J., Dawson, D. M., *et al.* (1993a) Double-blind pilot trial of oral tolerization with myelin antigens in multiple sclerosis. *Science*, **259**, 1321–1324.

Weiner, H. L., Mackin, G. A., Orav, E. J., Hafler, D. A., Dawson, D. M., Lapierre, Y., *et al.* (1993b) Intermittent cyclophosphamide pulse therapy in progressive multiple sclerosis: final report of the Northeast Cooperative Multiple Sclerosis Treatment Group. *Neurology* **43**, 910–918.

Whitacre, C. C, Gienapp, I. E., Orosz, C. G. and Bitar, D. M. (1991) Oral tolerance in experimental autoimmune encephalomyelitis. III. Evidence for clonal anergy. *J. Immunol.*, **147**, 2155–2163.

Wilson, D. B., Golding, A. B., Smith, R. A., Dafashy, T., Nelson, J., Smith, R. M., *et al.* (1997) Results of a phase I clinical trial of a T cell receptor peptide vaccine in patients with multiple sclerosis. 1. Analysis of T cell receptor utilization in CSF cell populations. *J. Neuroimmunol.*, **76**, 15–28.

Wraith, D. C., McDevitt, H. O., Steinman, L. and Acha-Orbea, H. (1989) T cell recognition as the target for immune intervention in autoimmune disease. *Cell*, **57**, 709.

Wucherpfennig, K. W., Zhang, J., Witek, C., Matsui, M., Modabber, Y., Ota, K., *et al.* (1994) Clonal expansion and persistence of human T cells specific for an immunodominant myelin basic protein peptide. *J. Immunol.*, **152**, 5581–5592.

Wucherpfennig, K. W. and Strominger, J. L. (1995) Molecular mimicry in T cell-mediated autoimmunity: viral peptides activate human T cell clones specific for myelin basic protein. *Cell*, **80**, 695–705.

Yednock, T. A., Cannon, C., Fritz, L. C., Sanchez-Madrid, F., Steinman, L. and Karin, N. (1992) Prevention of experimental autoimmune encephalomyelitis by antibodies against alpha4beta1 integrin. *Nature*, **356**, 63–66.

Yudkin, P. L., Ellison, G. W., Ghezzi, A., Goodkin, D. E., Hughes, R. A. C., McPherson, K., *et al.* (1991) Overview of azathioprine treatment in multiple sclerosis. *Lancet*, **338**, 1051–1055.

Zamvil, S., Nelson, P., Trotter, J., Mitchell, D., Knobler, R., Fritz, R., *et al.* (1985) T cell clones specific for myelin basic protein induce chronic relapsing paralysis and demyelination. *Nature*, **317**, 355–358.

Zhang, J., Medaer, R., Stinissen, P., Hafler, D. and Raus, J. (1993) MHC-restricted depletion of human myelin basic protein-reactive T cells by T cell vaccination. *Science*, **261**, 1451–1454.

Chapter 5

Paraneoplastic disorders of the central nervous system

Neil Scolding

Introduction: paraneoplastic syndrome	118
Pathology and immunology of paraneoplastic syndromes	125
The treatment of paraneoplastic disorders	131
References	132

Introduction: paraneoplastic syndrome

Paraneoplastic syndromes are a group of disorders caused by a malignancy, but not occurring as a direct physical consequence of the cancer or any metastases. The term is often used synonymously with the *remote effects of cancer* and is usually taken to exclude a range of more commonly encountered, more general or non-specific non-metastatic manifestations of malignancy, such as fever, malaise and lethargy, nutritional disorders, infection, and iatrogenic disorders. Although paraneoplastic syndromes may involve many systems (Agarwala, 1996), e.g. the skin (acanthosis nigricans, pruritus, ichthyosis, etc.), the endocrine system (ectopic ACTH, hypercalcaemia) or the blood (anaemia, coagulopathies), more often than not, the term applies to neurological disorders. Many were described first over the course of two decades by an extraordinary generation of British neurologists – Denny-Brown, Brain, Henson and Urich. Their often definitive papers, which continue routinely to be cited and remain required reading for those interested in the area, culminated in Henson and Urich's authoritative monograph, *Cancer and the Nervous System*, in 1982 (Henson and Urich, 1982).

Some might consider it presumptuous to include the neurological paraneoplastic disorders in a text devoted to immunological and inflammatory disorders; the immune basis of central nervous system (CNS) (or peripheral nervous system (PNS)) paraneoplasia has not yet been incontrovertibly proven. However, the assumption of an autoimmune aetiology is commonly accepted and the evidence is certainly no weaker than that applying to many diseases whose immunological basis is (rightly or wrongly) no longer much questioned, e.g. paraproteinaemic neuropathies. The general pathogenetic model for paraneoplastic neurological disorders is that normal neural antigens come to represent the targets of immunological damage as innocent cross-reactive bystanders during the anti-tumour immune response. Antibody-mediated damage is, at present, much more commonly invoked than cellular responses though, as will be seen, the latter have not been ignored. Disorders of the neuromuscular junction are very well described in this respect; whilst their clinical features fall outside the scope of the current text, their immunology represents a paradigm for the paraneoplastic CNS syndromes.

Thus, while myasthenia gravis obviously occurs commonly outside the context of malignancy, the 10% (or so) of cases associated with thymoma are of paraneoplastic origin. Thymic tissue expresses the α subunit of the nicotinic acetylcholine receptor against which patients' antibodies are directed (Kornstein et al., 1995); passive transfer of immunoglobulins from patients with MG induces disease in rodents (Toyka et al., 1975), and there is a clinical response to removal of the tumour and to interference with activities of the antibody by chemotherapy or plasmapheresis (Newsom-Davis et al., 1978). Similarly, in at least a proportion of patients with the Lambert–Eaton myasthenic syndrome (LEMS), antibodies directed against components of the neuromuscular junction have been identified. These impair calcium flux in vitro (Roberts et al., 1985; Lennon et al., 1995), and therefore acetylcholine release, and may be directed against voltage-gated calcium channels (Leys et al., 1991; Lennon et al., 1995; Motomura et al., 1997). Small cell lung cancer is present in 60% patients with LEMS (O'Neill et al., 1988), and the calcium channel proteins are expressed by both tumour (Vincent et al., 1989; Johnston et al., 1994) and neurological target. Passive transfer of IgG from patients with LEMS into experimental animals induces the disorder, while immunosuppressive treatments again are symptomatically (and electrophysiologically) beneficial (Newsom-Davis, Murray, 1984).

A crucial difference, however, between the CNS paraneoplasia and paraneoplastic myasthenic syndromes concerns the site of the relevant antigen: in the latter diseases, expression of the antigen on the cell surface allows antibodies easy access; in contrast, the antigens of proposed significance in CNS paraneoplasia are all intracellular – and, indeed, on the wrong side of the blood–brain barrier.

Upon this background, the paraneoplastic disorders of the CNS may now be considered. They are not common – occurring perhaps in under 1% of patients with cancer (Anderson et al., 1987) – but generally cause profound disability and discomfort. It should be noted that, while a number of classical syndromes have been described over the past three decades or so, there is not uncommonly a degree of overlap, and neurological manifestations rather rarely fall wholly and conveniently into the pure phenotype – an observation often made explicitly in the original descriptions (Brain and Wilkinson, 1965), whose remembrance can often help smooth what might otherwise appear an uncomfortably shaped case.

Subacute cerebellar degeneration

Paraneoplastic cerebellar degeneration was described some 30 years ago by Brain and Wilkinson (Brain and Wilkinson, 1965). It may occur in the context of a variety of cancers, but small cell lung cancer, ovarian, cervical and uterine malignancy, and Hodgkin's disease represent the commonest precipitants (Dalmau et al., 1992; Peterson et al., 1992). It is the case with this and all paraneoplastic disorders that the neurological manifestation may antedate presentation or diagnosis of the underlying malignancy by an interval which rarely may extend to several years – often the cancer is identified only at post-mortem examination. In less than 50% of cases has a prior diagnosis of cancer been made.

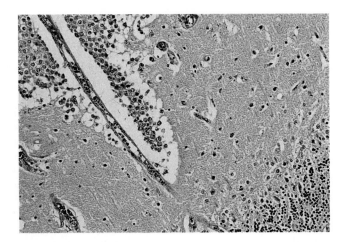

Figure 5.1 Direct cerebellar infiltration. Tempting though it may be to reach a conclusion of paraneoplasia, more prosaic (and no less serious) explanations not uncommonly emerge and must not be forgotten. This is a post-mortem study of a 51-year-old female who was referred to the author with a rapidly progressive cerebellar syndrome 6 months after removal of an infiltrating ductal breast carcinoma. The author's suspicion of paraneoplastic cerebellar syndrome was (he thought) strongly supported by wholly normal magnetic resonance imaging of the brain and upper spinal cord, normal spinal fluid (including protein, glucose and cytology) and normal isotope bone scan. Anti-neuronal antibodies were, however, absent; the patient died 2 weeks after these investigations and was found on autopsy to have malignant meningitis, with widespread infiltration of the cerebellar meninges by metastatic carcinoma of solid appearance. Quite how often direct infiltration accounts for apparently paraneoplastic neurological conditions cannot be known.

The commonest presentation is with a subacutely progressive ataxic syndrome, usually in late middle age or above (reflecting the age range of the underlying cause). What has been termed a vermis phenotype is perhaps the most typical, with prominent gait and truncal ataxia and relative sparing of the limbs: disability is profound. It has been commonly observed that in many patients the syndrome may progress to a plateau and thereafter remain stable for considerable periods, irrespective of the progression (or otherwise) of the underlying tumour (but see Figure 5.1 for a cautionary note). Nystagmus (often downbeat) is usually present. Other neurological features may be present, including sensory symptoms, dysphagia, and extensor plantar responses (Brain and Wilkinson, 1965). Magnetic resonance imaging (MRI) scanning can demonstrate cerebellar atrophy (Peterson *et al.*, 1992). Spinal fluid examination may reveal an elevated protein level; there may be a modestly raised lymphocyte count. The occasional presence of oligoclonal immunoglobulin bands completes a cerebrospinal fluid (CSF) pattern which is common to each of the paraneoplastic neurological syndromes.

Encephalomyelitis

A number of clinical phenotypes, often occurring in admixture with one another, and sharing a common underlying malignancy (small cell lung cancer), neuropathology and (often) antibody association, fall within the spectrum of encephalomyelitis (Henson et al., 1965a).

Limbic encephalitis
While the commonest underlying malignancy causing this syndrome is small cell lung cancer (Brierly et al., 1960), many other tumours have at various times also proven culpable (Henson et al., 1965; Corsellis et al., 1968). The presentation is singular, with a relatively selective subacutely progressive amnesic syndrome. Magnetic imaging can reveal abnormal T_2 high signal deep in the temporal lobes, with atrophy later apparent (Henson et al., 1965; Dirr et al., 1990). Epilepsy and psychiatric features may occasionally complicate the picture (Henson et al., 1965; Bakheit et al., 1990); accordingly, electroencephalogram changes of slow waves with or without spikes may occur.

Brainstem encephalitis
Like subacute cerebellar degeneration, this is a particularly disabling and unpleasant syndrome, with progressive vertigo, ophthalmoplegia and nystagmus, and bulbar failure (Henson et al., 1965; Reddy and Vakili, 1981; Dalmau et al., 1992). Less focal features are also commonly present, and include pyramidal and extrapyramidal signs, ataxia, autonomic failure, and a sensory neuropathy. A cerebellar presentation is well-recognised, but this is usually distinguishable clinically from *subacute cerebellar degeneration* by the additional presence of a neuropathy (see Figure 5.2) or other signs indicating more diffuse CNS involvement (and immunologically, by antibody association; see below).

Myelitis
Occurring mostly in conjunction with signs of encephalitis, this may cause multifocal wasting and weakness. The occasional finding of fasciculation may suggest amyotrophic lateral sclerosis in the absence of encephalitic features (see below), but sensory features are usually present; autonomic disturbances are also often apparent.

Necrotising myelitis, usually occurring with haematological or lung cancers, with the more profound neurological picture of a subacute paraplegia and an active CSF, is probably a distinct disorder of unrelated pathogenesis (Mancall and Rosales, 1964). *Stiff man syndrome* occurring as a paraneoplastic disorder is discussed in Chapter 6.

Subacute sensory neuronopathy

Technically outwith the scope of this text, the exclusion of subacute sensory neuronopathy would be churlish. One of the commoner paraneoplastic manifestations (Denny-Brown, 1948; Croft and Wilkinson, 1965; Hughes et al., 1996), this syndrome is often grouped with the above encephalomyeli-tides, again sharing small cell lung carcinoma as the commonest precipitant and a common antibody association (see below); in as many as 50% of cases, it co-exists with encephalitic features (Chalk et al., 1992). Autonomic failure may be prominent (Siemson and Meister, 1963; Dalmau et al., 1992). Approximately 1% of patients with small cell cancers develop clinical or

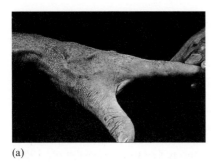
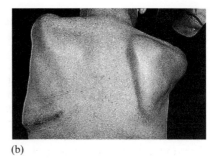

(a)   (b)

Figure 5.2 Paraneoplastic cerebellar degeneration and peripheral neuropathy. A middle-aged man presented with weight loss and a peripheral sensorimotor neuropathy with distal upper and lower limb wasting (a), and subsequently developed a rapidly progressive cerebellar syndrome. Central nervous system imaging was normal, but oligoclonal bands were present in the spinal fluid. Anti-Hu serology was positive and further investigation revealed a small cell lung cancer. Both central and peripheral symptoms deteriorated, and a superimposed mononeuritis multiplex emerged with right serratus anterior weakness and a left suprascapular nerve palsy (wasted supra- and infraspinatus) (b); the left rhomboids were also weak. The nature of the malignancy and his serology suggest the cerebellar syndrome is more likely to have been part of an otherwise subclinical encephalomyelitis with the not uncommonly associated axonal neuropathy. (With thanks to Professor D. A. S. Compston.)

electrophysiological evidence of sensory neuronopathy (Elrington *et al.*, 1991), but the disorder is also seen in breast and other cancers (Horwich *et al.*, 1977; Hughes *et al.*, 1996).

The neuronopathy is characteristically painful from the onset and accompanied by often distressing paraesthesia. The symptoms commence in the extremities and progress – sometimes very rapidly – proximally and examination reveals the not unexpected findings of distal sensory loss to all modalities, including vibration and joint position sense, with areflexia and often sensory ataxia. Electrophysiological testing reveals absent sensory action potentials with no evidence of motor disturbance (Donofrio *et al.*, 1989); the disorder is so-named (rather than *sensory neuropathy*) on histopathological grounds, the dorsal root ganglia showing changes, rather than peripheral nerve (see below). A clinically identical syndrome may occur in association with Sjögren's syndrome (Font *et al.*, 1990).

Paraneoplastic motor neuropathy and neuronopathy

The occurrence of a syndrome resembling classical motor neurone disease – of the amyotrophic lateral sclerosis phenotype, with mixed upper and lower motor neurone signs – has been intermittently reported since the first description by Brain *et al.* in 1965 (Brain *et al.*, 1965). It has, however, remained at least until recently a little controversial: the often quoted figure of up to 10% of cases of amyotrophic lateral sclerosis associated with malignancy (Norris and Engel, 1965) would certainly fall well outside most neurologists' experience.

A subacute motor neuronopathy without pyramidal signs, associated especially with lymphomatous malignancies, is a more secure entity (Schold *et al.*, 1979). The syndrome is progressive and painless, and bears some clinical resemblance with multifocal motor neuropathy with conduction block, though the latter most characteristically affects the upper limbs more than the lower, paraneoplastic motor disease mainly the reverse. The distinction more reliably is made electrophysiologically, the self-evident features of the former contrasting with the normal motor (and sensory) conduction of paraneoplastic motor neuronopathy accompanied by electro-myographic evidence of denervation. Neither upper motor neurones nor the bulbar lower motor neurones are (usually) affected. A recent case, with prominent nuchal and respiratory muscle weakness, was associated with anti-Hu antibodies and subclinical loss of cerebellar Purkinje cells (Verma *et al.*, 1996).

Clearly, the combination of this motor neuronopathy with a limited myelitis might generate the clinical picture of amyotrophic lateral sclerosis. It has been suggested that the eleven cases of cancer-related motor neurone disease described by Brain in 1965 may have represented 'burnt out paraneoplastic encephalomyelitis' (Posner, 1996). However, Younger *et al.* in 1991 reported nine patients, all with lymphoma, eight of whom had clinical features suggesting amyotrophic lateral sclerosis (Younger *et al.*, 1991). Gordon *et al.* (1997) recently reported details of 26 patients with lymphoproliferative disorders and motor neurone disease: none had motor neuropathy, 23 had 'definite or probable' upper motor neurone signs. The neurological course was altered in only two of 20 patients treated for their lymphoproliferative disease – both of whom had purely lower motor neurone disease. An association in very small numbers of patients of motor neurone disease with anti-Hu antibodies has also been recently reported, as was a possible link with breast cancer (Forsyth *et al.*, 1997).

Breast cancer may also be associated with two relatively discrete disorders, a sensorimotor neuropathy (Peterson *et al.*, 1994) and the so-called numb chin syndrome, characterized by numbness in the distribution of the mental or alveolar branches of the mandibular nerve (Horton *et al.*, 1973; Burt *et al.*, 1992; Lossos and Siegal, 1992). Other malignancies may precipitate the latter, which is thought to represent a direct effect of metastasis, rather than paraneoplasia.

Opsoclonus/myoclonus syndrome

Another profoundly disabling and distressing syndrome, wherein opsoclonic eye movements – chaotic, involuntary partial or complete saccades which are arrhythmic, continuous, and randomly directed – cause profound vertigo, nausea and anorexia, and debility, usually confining the patient to bed. The movements persist during sleep. Truncal and limb myoclonus may also be present, and central ataxia from concurrent subacute cerebellar involvement often contributes further to the picture (Anderson *et al.*, 1988). In adults, small cell lung cancer is (yet again) the commonest associated malignancy, and although a tendency to remit is described (Anderson *et al.*, 1988), the half dozen or so cases – admittedly a modest experience – seen by the current author have invariably declined relentlessly and terminally.

The syndrome was in fact first described not in adults but in children with neuroblastoma (Kinsbourne, 1962), the underlying cause in approximately 50% of children with this neurological picture (Telander *et al.*, 1989). It has

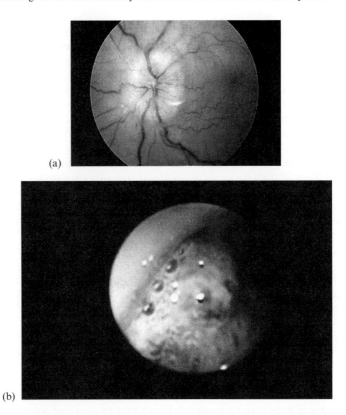

Figure 5.3 Paraneoplastic retinal degeneration and small cell lung cancer. A 71-year-old female ex-smoker was referred from the ophthalmology team with visual loss and bilateral papilloedema (a). There was no clinical or radiological evidence of direct malignant infiltration; spinal fluid analysis showed a raised protein and the presence of oligoclonal bands and further investigation – high-resolution chest computed tomography scanning followed by bronchoscopy (b) – revealed a small cell lung cancer. (With thanks to Professor D. A. S. Compston.)

also been reported in adults without cancer as a monophasic post-infectious process, usually following respiratory or gastrointestinal infection (Baringer *et al.*, 1968). In one literature survey in which the details of 58 patients with opsoclonus/myoclonus were reviewed, only 11, approximately 20%, had identified cancers, so that the clinical picture is far from the inevitable harbinger of cancer sometimes suggested.

Cancer-associated retinopathy

This syndrome again is most commonly associated with small cell lung carcinoma (Thirkill *et al.*, 1989), though other tumours may also be responsible – gynaecological malignancy and, perhaps particularly, melanoma (Kim *et al.*, 1994). Photosensitivity, night blindness, visual scotomata and retinal artery attenuation are typical features, though variations on this phenotype are well described (Jacobson *et al.*, 1990); we have seen one patient in whom (bilateral) optic disc swelling was a prominent and temporarily obfuscating feature (Figure 5.3); a small cell lung cancer was eventually identified. Visual loss is painless and may be monocular initially. Visual evoked responses usually reveal normal optic nerve function, electroretinography confirming the site of derangement.

A number of other paraneoplastic disorders may be mentioned in passing. The association of inflammatory muscle disease with malignancy has, for reasons not entirely clear, broken out of the 'neurological rarities' pigeon hole into which most paraneoplastic syndromes are consigned in most texts of internal medicine, and become part of accepted general medical knowledge. Although the association has been overstated, most accept that dermatomyositis in particular is significantly linked with cancer (Sigurgeirsson, 1992). The details of muscle disease clearly lie outside the brief of this text, as do those of paraneoplastic disorders of the neuromuscular junction, which have been briefly mentioned above. The relationships of progressive encephalomyelitis with rigidity and of stiff man syndrome with neoplasia (and with each other) are considered in Chapter 6.

Pathology and immunology of paraneoplastic syndromes

Histopathological changes in paraneoplastic disorders

The principal reason for failing to mention the pathological pictures associated with each of the described syndromes is that, anatomical target apart, the main abnormalities are strikingly similar (with a few notable exceptions which will be described). The main features were first described by Denny-Brown (Denny-Brown, 1948) and may be divided into three key groups. First, there is pronounced neuronal loss, with pyknotic changes (which would currently be interpreted as indicating apoptotic cell death), and neuronophagia. Second, there are changes indicating an inflammatory process, which include perivascular lymphocytic cuffing with parenchymal infiltration by lymphocytes and macrophages and the formation of microglial nodules; and finally there is the ubiquitous and relatively non-specific finding of astrogliosis.

Thus in paraneoplastic cerebellar degeneration these are the prominent changes in the (cerebellar) cortex (Brain and Wilkinson, 1965), where Purkinje cells are selectively lost. In encephalomyelitic syndromes, striking changes are found (according to the specific disorder) respectively in the limbic system (Corsellis et al., 1968), the brain stem (Henson et al., 1965) or the spinal cord (Mancall and Rosales, 1964), while in subacute sensory neuronopathy, the pathology is centred upon the dorsal root ganglion (Denny-Brown, 1948; Croft et al., 1967; Horwich et al., 1977). In later stages, the changes may extend proximally into the posterior columns and distally into the peripheral nerve; demyelination is a marked feature in a minority of patients. In subacute motor neuronopathy, anterior horns in the spinal cord bear the brunt of the disease process; in contrast with amyotrophic lateral sclerosis, the lateral columns are not affected (Brain and Wilkinson, 1965; Henson et al., 1965). The findings in cancer-associated retinopathy are again typical, with loss of photoreceptors and retinal ganglion cells accompanying the inflammatory changes (Grunwald et al., 1987). It should also be noted that in most of these syndromes, less pronounced findings of a similar nature may be present diffusely in the cerebral hemispheres, brain stem and spinal cord.

In paraneoplastic opsoclonus/myoclonus syndrome, the picture is a little less clear. The theoretical principle of eye movement physiology predict that the target cell is the so-called pause cell, an inhibitory interneurone putatively located in reticular formation at the level of the pons. In some patients, however, no clear abnormalities are identifiable here or indeed elsewhere (Ridley *et al.*, 1987; Anderson *et al.*, 1988); in others, the findings appear indistinguishable from those of paraneoplastic cerebellar degeneration (Ellenberger *et al.*, 1968).

The most economical interpretation of these changes would be that an immunological or inflammatory process was targeted upon certain neuronal subpopulations, resulting in death of the latter. An ambitious inference, based on the possibility that the neurones exhibit changes suggesting apoptotic cell death, might be that an unconventional mode of immunological injury was occurring – rather than more typical antibody and complement-mediated cell attack triggering lytic injury. Immunophenotypic analysis of the largely perivascular infiltrating inflammatory cells in paraneoplastic encephalomyelitis reveals a mixture of T and B lymphocytes (Graus *et al.*, 1990); Szabo *et al.* (1991) showed elegantly the presence of Hu-specific B lymphocytes in brain parenchyma of one patient.

Other possibilities must, however, be considered. In paraneoplastic motor neurone disease, a possible opportunistic infectious aetiology has been suggested. The particular association with lymphoma offers immune paresis as a contribution to this suggestion; poliomyelitis represents an obvious example of viral disease of the anterior horn cell. A lower motor neurone disorder caused by a leukaemia retrovirus in mice has been described (Gardner, 1991).

Onconeural antibodies; their nomenclature and syndrome specificity

Most – not all – of the above syndromes are associated with serum antibodies which are directed against neural antigens (Table 5.1). The extent to which the precise antigen specificity has been determined, and a pathogenetic role proven, varies, and it must be emphasized that association is not at all perfect – patients with proven cancer-associated disorders readily fitting into the above spectrum may consistently lack the 'appropriate' antibody, and conversely, antibody-positive patients who lack either the correct tumour, or the required neurology, are well-described. The nomenclature has recently been subject to discussion, advocates for the retention of the original antibody/antigen-centred terms ('anti-Yo', 'anti-Ri', etc.), based (according to common practice) on the first two letters of the original patient's surname, vying with those preferring a descriptive immunohistochemistry-based classification dictated by the target cell and pattern of reactivity (Dalmau and Posner, 1994; Lennon, 1994a,b). The issue is of great practical relevance, influencing the approach to testing samples, and diagnostic criteria. A consensus position is alleged to have emerged (Moll *et al.*, 1995), though the agreed nomenclature does not appear uniformly to have been adopted (Dalmau and Posner, 1996).

Table 5.1 The commoner central nervous system paraneoplastic disorders, tumours and antibodies

Syndrome	Tumour	Antibody
Subacute cerebellar degeneration	Breast and ovary	Anti-Yo antibodies/anti-Purkinje cell cytoplasmic antibodies (APCA)
Encephalomyelitis limbic encephalitis, subacute sensory neuronopathy; autonomic neuropathy	Small cell lung cancer	Anti-Hu antibodies/ type 1 anti-neuronal nuclear antibodies (ANNA-1)
Opsoclonus/myoclonus syndrome	Breast	Anti-Ri antibodies/type 2 anti-neuronal nuclear antibodies (ANNA-2)
Cancer-associated retinopathy	Small cell lung cancer	Recoverin antibodies
Cancer-associated retinopathy	Melanoma	Anti-bipolar retinal cell antibodies

See text for details.

Anti-Yo antibodies/anti-Purkinje cell cytoplasmic antibodies (APCA)
These antibodies are found in many patients with paraneoplastic cerebellar degeneration – almost invariably those with an underlying breast or gynaecological malignancy, rather than those with small cell lung cancer (Greenlee and Brashear, 1983; Jaeckle *et al.*, 1985; Anderson *et al.*, 1988; Smith *et al.*, 1988; Peterson *et al.*, 1992). There are isolated case reports of cerebellar degeneration with anti-Yo antibodies in men (Felician *et al.*, 1995). They are polyclonal IgG antibodies, commonly found in higher concentration in the CSF than in serum, implying intrathecal synthesis or concentration (Furneaux *et al.*, 1990).

A number of antigens for which anti-Yo/APCA are specific have been cloned, including PCD-AA, CDR62 and CDR3, all DNA-binding proteins which direct gene transcription, of the leucine zipper family (Fathallah *et al.*, 1991; Sakai *et al.*, 1990). Others appear to have similar transcription-regulatory function, acting instead through zinc finger binding activity (Sato *et al.*, 1991), while in yet other cases, antibodies to a protein (CDR34) abundantly expressed in cerebellar cortex and in breast and ovarian carcinoma, but of entirely unknown function, are found (Dropcho *et al.*, 1987) and see also Dropcho (1995).

How or indeed if these antibodies interact with these antigens *in vivo*, and whether this interaction is responsible for Purkinje cell loss is unclear. Anti-Yo/APCA antibodies do not bind to other areas of the CNS, while they are not detected in non-paraneoplastic cerebellar degenerations (Anderson *et al.*, 1988; Smith *et al.*, 1988; Peterson *et al.*, 1992), arguing against their secondary generation triggered by (otherwise mediated) Purkinje cell damage. Anti-Yo/APCA antibody binding is, according to ultrastructural immunocytochemical studies, cytoplasmic, rather than neuronal (Rodriguez *et al.*, 1988; Hida *et al.*, 1994), which is clearly not readily reconcilable with a role in interfering with transcription. How an antibody directed against any intracellularly sited target might exert its activity also requires some explanation, although there is evidence that Purkinje cells exposed *in vivo* to specific (passively transferred) anti-Yo/APCA antibodies take up these (but not other) immunoglobulin molecules (Graus *et al.*, 1991; Greenlee *et al.*, 1995). Perplexingly, however, no cerebellar cell injury is apparent in cell culture models – and there is indeed very little evidence from any immunological system that internalised antibody can cause cell damage (Naparstek and Plotz, 1993). Active immunization with recombinant (Yo) protein also fails to induce cerebellar disease (Tanaka *et al.*, 1994; Sakai *et al.*, 1995), while passive transfer of Yo/APCA specific lymphocytes into immune-deficient (SCID) mice similarly fails to replicate disease (Tanaka *et al.*, 1995).

Anti-Hu antibodies/type 1 anti-neuronal nuclear antibodies (ANNA-1)
These antibodies are predominantly associated with paraneoplastic syndromes precipitated by small cell lung cancer, particularly the various encephalomyelitides and subacute sensory neuronopathy (Graus *et al.*, 1985; Anderson *et al.*, 1988; Dalmau *et al.*, 1992) – syndromes which may, of course, occur together.

As with all onconeural antibodies, anti-Hu antibodies cannot safely be regarded as a diagnostic test. In particular, absence of antibody by no means excludes the diagnosis. One recent study of 16 patients with limbic encephalitis and small cell lung cancer, for example, showed that only half had the expected anti-Hu antibody (Alamowitch *et al.*, 1997). Nevertheless, clinically and diagnostically useful information may emerge: a suspected paraneoplastic cerebellar degeneration, perhaps with additional evidence of extra-cerebellar involvement, and with anti-Hu antibodies (rather than anti-Yo), is far more likely to have small cell lung cancer than gynaecological malignancy (see, e.g. Mason *et al.*, 1997).

Anti-Hu antibodies are also polyclonal IgG antibodies and, in common with anti-Yo/APCA, appear to be synthesized within the CNS (Furneaux *et al.*, 1990; Vega *et al.*, 1994). Ubiquitous staining of neuronal nuclei by anti-Hu/ANNA-1 is described, not only throughout the brain and spinal cord, but also of sensory neurones of the dorsal root ganglia and of autonomic ganglia (Dick *et al.*, 1988; Altermatt *et al.*, 1991). A number of antigens have been identified using molecular cloning techniques: HuC, HuD, Hel-N1 and Hel-N2 share sequence homology with each other and with a family of RNA binding proteins thought to be important in post-transcriptional gene processing (Szabo *et al.*, 1991; Dropcho and King, 1994; Sakai *et al.*, 1994); they are expressed in small cell lung cancer cells (King and Dropcho, 1996). Hel-N1 has been shown to bind to the mRNA molecules encoding the immediate early genes c-*fos* and c-*myc* and to a number of growth factors including granulocyte-macrophage colony stimulating factor (Levine *et al.*, 1993).

Small cell lung cancers almost invariably express anti-Hu/ANNA-1 antigen (Budde-Steffen *et al.*, 1988; Kiers *et al.*, 1991; Dalmau *et al.*, 1992), particularly (and perhaps exclusively) HuD (Sekido *et al.*, 1994). Detectable expression occurs regardless of whether or not the tumour has triggered neurological paraneoplasia; one suggestion is that antibody production only occurs in those cases wherein the tumour co-expresses MHC Class I antigens (Doyle *et al.*, 1985; Manley *et al.*, 1995). B lymphocytes are prominent in the perivascular inflammatory infiltrates found in patients with paraneoplastic encephalomyelitis (Jean *et al.*, 1994b), while deposits of IgG are demonstrable within neurones (Graus *et al.*, 1990; Dalmau *et al.*, 1991); complement components are not prominent (Jean *et al.*, 1994). Complement-dependent and -independent lysis of rodent cerebellar neurones by anti-Hu antibodies has been demonstrated (Greenlee *et al.*, 1993); others have shown internalization of antibody by neurones (Hormigo and Lieberman, 1994b), while yet other groups failed to find consistent *in vitro* cytotoxicity against neurones (Dick *et al.*, 1988; Hormigo *et al.*, 1994a; Jean *et al.*, 1994). In parallel with those experiments concerning anti-Yo/APCA described above, attempts to develop animal models of anti-Hu/ANNA-1–related disease by injecting antibody have repeatedly failed (Dick *et al.*, 1988).

Very recently and of considerable interest, cell surface expression of anti-Hu related antigens by small cell lung cancer cells has been reported (Tora *et al.*, 1997), with obvious and important implications for pathogenesis.

Anti-Ri antibodies/type 2 anti-neuronal nuclear antibodies (ANNA-2)
Although some patients with opsoclonus and ataxia in the context of breast cancer have anti-Purkinje cell antibodies (anti-Hu) (Peterson *et al.*, 1992), more typically, patients with paraneoplastic opsoclonus/myoclonus have antibodies known as anti-Ri or ANNA-2 (Budde-Steffen *et al.*, 1988; Luque *et al.*, 1991). These may be identified in serum and CSF – again, with evidence suggesting synthesis within the CNS (Luque *et al.*, 1991) – and are not generally found in paraneoplastic opsoclonus/myoclonus associated with small cell lung cancer; furthermore, whilst they react with breast tumour tissue from patients with opsoclonus, they are non-reactive with malignant breast tissue not associated with opsoclonus (Luque *et al.*, 1991). Some patients with anti-Ri/ANNA-2 exhibit the neurological picture not of opsoclonus-myoclonus, but of progressive encephalomyelitis with rigidity (Casado *et al.*, 1994).

Anti-Ri/ANNA-2 antibodies stain neuronal nuclei throughout the CNS in a pattern identical to ANNA-1; they are distinguished by the absence of staining of neurones in autonomic and dorsal root ganglia, and in the gut plexi (Graus *et al.*, 1993). Immunoblots prepared from human neuronal extracts indicate that ANNA-2 reacts with multiple bands. Cloning a cDNA library (from human cerebellum) with ANNA-2 has generated one protein, christened Nova (Buckanovich *et al.*, 1993). Nova is expressed exclusively in the CNS, throughout development and is largely restricted to neuronal nuclei (Buckanovich *et al.*, 1993, 1996). Its sequence, in common with anti-Hu/ANNA-1, suggests a role in translation or transcription and binding to RNA has been clearly shown; this is inhibited by anti-Ri/ANNA-2 (Buckanovich *et al.*, 1996), which recognizes specific RNA targets (Buckanovich and Darnell, 1997). Other Nova genes have also been identified (see Darnell, 1996).

No anti-neuronal antibodies have thus far been identified in childhood paraneoplastic opsoclonus and neuroblastoma. The presence of mononuclear cell infiltrates within the tumour (Telander *et al.*, 1989), the steroid-responsive of neuroblastoma-associated opsoclonus (Pranzatelli, 1992) and the improvement in prognosis in patients with neuroblastoma conferred by the presence of opsoclonus (Altman and Baehner, 1976; Musarella *et al.*, 1984) are all consistent with a tumour-specific autoimmune reaction underlying the neurological disorder.

Recoverin antibodies and cancer-associated retinopathy
Antibodies directed against the calcium-binding protein recoverin are found in patients with paraneoplastic retinal degeneration (Polans *et al.*, 1991; Thirkill *et al.*, 1992). Recoverin is located within photoreceptor cells in the retina and is important in light/dark adaptation (Polans *et al.*, 1995). Expression in tumour tissue from a patient with cancer-associated retinopathy was found (Polans *et al.*, 1995), while the presence of retinal deposits of immunoglobulin, together with loss of ganglion cells, on immunohistopathological study of patients with cancer associated retinopathy (Grunwald *et al.*, 1987) provides further evidence for an autoimmune basis to the disorder. In marked contrast to the various paraneoplastic antibodies and antigens described above, an animal model of cancer-associated retinopathy has been described: Lewis rats injected with a synthetic peptide fragment of recoverin develop photoreceptor cell degeneration (Polans *et al.*, 1995); apoptotic death of retinal cells *in vivo* caused by anti-recoverin antibodies has now been reported (Adamus *et al.*, 1997).

Paraneoplastic retinal degeneration precipitated by melanoma is clinically distinct (Kim *et al.*, 1994). Serum antibodies are associated; they are directed not against recoverin but against bipolar retinal neurones (Weinstein *et al.*, 1994). Antibodies directed against optic nerve cells are also described (Thirkill *et al.*, 1989) and, more recently, serum antibodies directed against enolase have been demonstrated in patients with retinopathy associated with a variety of malignancies (Adamus *et al.*, 1996). Both enolase and recoverin were found to be expressed in a cell line generated from small cell lung cancer tissue removed from a patient with retinopathy (Yamaji *et al.*, 1996).

Other antibodies
Recently, antibodies to a subpopulation of glial cells, reportedly oligodendrocytes, have been reported in 11 out of 45 patients with (mostly, i.e. 10 of the 11 cases) CNS paraneoplasia – cerebellar degeneration, limbic encephalitis and encephalomyelitis associated with various cancers (Honnorat *et al.*, 1996). Their significance remains to be established.

Cell-mediated immunity in paraneoplastic disorders
Paraneoplastic anti-neuronal antibodies have assumed an important diagnostic role of great practical help in investigating patients. There has properly persisted, however, some degree of scepticism concerning their potential pathogenetic contribution; a small but significant body of evidence implicating the T cell has emerged.

In addition to B cells, macrophages and T lymphocytes are prominent in the lesions of paraneoplastic encephalomyelitis (Graus *et al.*, 1990; Jean *et al.*, 1994). $CD4^+$ and $CD8^+$ cells are present. Neither Class I nor Class II MHC is detectable on the surface of neurones, however (Graus *et al.*, 1990). Significantly, tumour specific killer cells have been reported in patients with paraneoplastic cerebellar degeneration (Albert *et al.*, 1998).

The treatment of paraneoplastic disorders

A variety of therapeutic strategies have been adopted in the management of patients with neurological paraneoplasia, and isolated case reports and small, uncontrolled series describing striking treatment responses are not difficult to find in the literature – the author has witnessed a severely amnesic patient with small cell lung cancer and limbic encephalitis improve in a clear, substantial, and carefully documented way following treatment of the lung tumour. Notwithstanding these experiences, the great majority of patients with paraneoplastic diseases of the CNS do not recover neurologically; their disability may become static rather than continuing to progress, but their overall prognosis depends on that of the underlying malignancy. Symptomatic treatment therefore assumes great importance (Brady, 1996).

Successful treatment of the tumour is the most obvious and logical approach to management (Paone and Jeyasingham, 1980; Batson et al., 1992); cure of the cancer should cure the neurology, in time. Despite occasional reports of responding patients (Paone and Jeyasingham, 1980), relatively large series of patients have been studied, however, without providing support for this proposal (Graus and Delattre, 1995; Grisold et al., 1995). Moreover, it has been suggested that the common course of most paraneoplastic disorders reaching a plateau after a period of subacute progression (which course may, incidentally help to explain an apparent response to well-timed interventions) most likely suggests the acquisition of irreversible neuronal damage (Dropcho, 1995). Nevertheless, it has recently been shown that the presence of anti-Hu antibodies in small cell lung cancer patients *without* paraneoplastic neurological disease appears to correlate clearly with a much improved response to treatment (Graus et al., 1997).

It is less rational to adopt an immunotherapeutic treatment directed not against the tumour, but towards immune mediators which are no more than putatively responsible for the neurological syndrome; the strikingly high cost of many of these therapies renders this approach the more difficult to justify. However, the extreme and unremitting distress, discomfort and disability caused by many paraneoplastic disorders, and the absence of any other useful treatments (even palliative) must help to explain attempts to leave no possible therapeutic avenue unexplored. The well-documented response of paraneoplastic LEMS to plasmapheresis provides some support for this approach (Newsom and Murray, 1984).

Thus immunotherapies both conventional and novel have been exhibited and studied in this arena. Steroids may be of use in paediatric opsoclonus/myoclonus (Boltshauser et al., 1979), and it has been suggested that adult opsoclonus/myoclonus may be a more benign disease, and more commonly steroid-responsive, than other paraneoplastic disorders (Dropcho et al., 1993). However, those with much experience have not found immunosuppression to be successful in other situations (Dalmau and Posner, 1996), and the possible adverse effects of inadvertently suppressing anti-tumour immune surveillance and reactivity mitigate against non-specific immunosuppression.

Apparently immunoglobulin-specific approaches, such as plasma exchange and intravenous immunoglobulin, have also been studied. Isolated case reports or small series attest to the possible merits of both intravenous immunoglobulin (Counsell et al., 1994) and plasma exchange (Weissman and

Gottschall, 1989), but in larger series, no significant improvement has emerged (Graus and Delattre, 1995). Vega *et al.* (1994) treated 18 patients suffering anti-Hu related paraneoplastic disorders with intravenous immunoglobulin and found no benefit in seriously affected patients; similarly, in a study of 22 patients with a variety of antibody-associated paraneoplastic disorders, no significant evidence of benefit was found (Uchuya *et al.*, 1996); the same applies in respect of plasma exchange. Protein A immunoadsorptive columns have also been used in small numbers of patients (Cher *et al.*, 1995; Nitschke *et al.*, 1995).

References

Adamus, G., Aptsiauri, N., Guy, J., Heckenlively, J., Flannery, J. and Hargrave, P. A. (1996) The occurrence of serum autoantibodies against enolase in cancer-associated retinopathy. *Clin. Immunol. Immunopathol.*, **78**, 120–129.

Adamus, G., Machnicki, M. and Seigel, G. M. (1997) Apoptotic retinal cell death induced by antirecoverin autoantibodies of cancer-associated retinopathy. *Invest. Ophthalmol. Vis. Sci.*, **38**, 283–291.

Agarwala, S. S. (1996) Paraneoplastic syndromes. *Med. Clin. North Am.*, **80**, 173–184.

Alamowitch, S., Graus, F., Uchuya, M., Rene, R., Bescansa, E. and Delattre, J. Y. (1997) Limbic encephalitis and small cell lung cancer. Clinical and immunological features. *Brain*, **120**, 923–928.

Albert, M. L., Darnell, J. C., Bendes, A., Francesco, L. M., Bhardwaj, N. and Darnell, R. B. (1998). Tumorspecific killer cells in paraneoplastic cerebellar degeneration. *Nature Medicine*, **4**, 1321–1324.

Altermatt, H. J., Rodriguez, M., Scheithauer, B. W. and Lennon, V. A. (1991) Paraneoplastic anti-Purkinje and type I anti-neuronal nuclear autoantibodies bind selectively to central, peripheral, and autonomic nervous system cells. *Lab. Invest.*, **65**, 412–420.

Altman, A. J. and Baehner, R. L. (1976) Favorable prognosis for survival in children with coincident opso-myoclonus and neuroblastoma. *Cancer*, **37**, 846–852.

Anderson, N. E., Budde, S. C., Rosenblum, M. K., Graus, F., Ford, D., Synek, B. J., *et al.* (1988) Opsoclonus, myoclonus, ataxia, and encephalopathy in adults with cancer: a distinct paraneoplastic syndrome. *Med. Baltimore*, **67**, 100–109.

Anderson, N. E., Cunningham, J. M. and Posner, J. B. (1987) Autoimmune pathogenesis of paraneoplastic neurological syndromes. *Crit. Rev. Neurobiol.*, **3**, 245–299.

Anderson, N. E., Rosenblum, M. K., Graus, F., Wiley, R. G. and Posner, J. B. (1988) Autoantibodies in paraneoplastic syndromes associated with small-cell lung cancer. *Neurology*, **38**, 1391–1398.

Bakheit, A. M., Kennedy, P. G. and Behan, P. O. (1990) Paraneoplastic limbic encephalitis: clinico-pathological correlations. *J. Neurol. Neurosurg. Psychiat.*, **53**, 1084–1088.

Baringer, J. R., Sweeney, V. P. and Winkler, G. F. (1968) An acute syndrome of ocular oscillations and truncal myoclonus. *Brain*, **91**, 473–480.

Batson, O. A., Fantle, D. M. and Stewart, J. A. (1992) Paraneoplastic encephalomyelitis. Dramatic response to chemotherapy alone. *Cancer*, **69**, 1291–1293.

Boltshauser, E., Deonna, T. and Hirt, H. R. (1979) Myoclonic encephalopathy of infants or 'dancing eyes syndrome'. Report of 7 cases with long-term follow-up and review of the literature (cases with and without neuroblastoma). *Helv. Paediatr. Acta*, **34**, 119–133.

Brady, A. M. (1996) Management of painful paraneoplastic syndromes. *Hematol. Oncol. Clin. North Am.*, **10**, 801–809.

Brain, L. and Wilkinson, M. (1965) Subacute cerebellar degeneration associated with neoplasms.

Brain, **88**, 465–478.

Brain, L., Croft, P. B. and Wilkinson, M. (1965) Motor neurone disease as a manifestation of neoplasm (with a note on the course of classical motor neurone disease). *Brain*, **88**, 479–500.

Brierly, J. B., Corsellis, J. A., Hierons, L. and Nevin, S. (1960) Subacute encephalitis of later adult life mainly affecting the limbic areas. *Brain*, **83**, 357–368.

Buckanovich, R. J. and Darnell, R. B. (1997) The neuronal RNA binding protein Nova-1 recognizes specific RNA targets *in vitro* and *in vivo*. *Mol. Cell Biol.*, **17**, 3194–3201.

Buckanovich, R. J., Posner, J. B. and Darnell, R. B. (1993) Nova, the paraneoplastic Ri antigen, is homologous to an RNA-binding protein and is specifically expressed in the developing motor system. *Neuron*, **11**, 657–672.

Buckanovich, R. J., Yang, Y. Y. and Darnell, R. B. (1996) The onconeural antigen Nova-1 is a neuron-specific RNA-binding protein, the activity of which is inhibited by paraneoplastic antibodies. *J. Neurosci.*, **16**, 1114–1122.

Budde-Steffen, C., Anderson, N. E., Rosenblum, M. K. and Posner, J. B. (1988) Expression of an antigen in small cell lung carcinoma lines detected by antibodies from patients with paraneoplastic dorsal root ganglionpathy. *Cancer Res.*, **48**, 430–434.

Burt, R. K., Sharfman, W. H., Karp, B. I. and Wilson, W. H. (1992) Mental neuropathy (numb chin syndrome). A harbinger of tumor progression or relapse (see comments). *Cancer*, **70**, 877–881.

Casado, J. L., Gil, P. A., Graus, F., Arenas, C., Lopez, J. M. and Alberca, R. (1994) Anti-Ri antibodies associated with opsoclonus and progressive encephalomyelitis with rigidity. *Neurology*, **44**, 1521–1522.

Chalk, C. H., Windebank, A. J., Kimmel, D. W. and McManis, P. G. (1992) The distinctive clinical features of paraneoplastic sensory neuronopathy. *Can. J. Neurol. Sci.*, **19**, 346–351.

Cher, L. M., Hochberg, F. H., Teruya, J., Nitschke, M., Valenzuela, R. F., Schmahmann, J. D., *et al.* (1995) Therapy for paraneoplastic neurologic syndromes in six patients with protein A column immunoadsorption. *Cancer*, **75**, 1678–1683.

Corsellis, J. A., Goldberg, G. J. and Norton, A. R. (1968) 'Limbic encephalitis' and its association with carcinoma. *Brain*, **91**, 481–496.

Counsell, C. E., McLeod, M. and Grant, R. (1994) Reversal of subacute paraneoplastic cerebellar syndrome with intravenous immunoglobulin. *Neurology*, **44**, 1184–1185.

Croft, P. B., Urich, H. and Wilkinson, M. (1967) Peripheral neuropathy of sensorimotor type associated with malignant disease. *Brain*, **90**, 31–66.

Croft, P. B. and Wilkinson, M. (1965) The incidence of carcinomatous neuromyopathy in patients with various types of carcinoma. *Brain*, **88**, 427–434.

Dalmau, J., Furneaux, H. M., Cordon, C. C. and Posner, J. B. (1992) The expression of the Hu (paraneoplastic encephalomyelitis/sensory neuronopathy) antigen in human normal and tumor tissues. *Am. J. Pathol.*, **141**, 881–886.

Dalmau, J., Furneaux, H. M., Rosenblum, M. K., Graus, F. and Posner, J. B. (1991) Detection of the anti-Hu antibody in specific regions of the nervous system and tumor from patients with paraneoplastic encephalomyelitis/sensory neuronopathy. *Neurology*, **41**, 1757–1764.

Dalmau, J., Graus, F., Rosenblum, M. K. and Posner, J. B. (1992) Anti-Hu-associated paraneoplastic encephalomyelitis/sensory neuronopathy. A clinical study of 71 patients. *Med. Baltimore*, **71**, 59–72.

Dalmau, J. and Posner, J. B. (1994) Neurologic paraneoplastic antibodies (anti-Yo; anti-Hu; anti-Ri): the case for a nomenclature based on antibody and antigen specificity (comment) (see comments). *Neurology*, **44**, 2241–2246.

Dalmau, J. and Posner, J. B. (1996) Neurological paraneoplastic syndromes. *Springer Semin. Immunopathol.*, **18**, 85–95.

Darnell, R. B. (1996) Onconeural antigens and the paraneoplastic neurologic disorders: at the intersection of cancer, immunity, and the brain. *Proc. Natl Acad. Sci. USA*, **93**, 4529–4536.

Denny-Brown, D. (1948) Primary sensory neuropathy with muscular changes associated with carcinoma. *J. Neurol. Neurosurg. Psychiat.*, **11**, 73–87.

Dick, D. J., Harris, J. B., Falkous, G., Foster, J. B. and Xuereb, J. H. (1988) Neuronal anti-nuclear antibody in paraneoplastic sensory neuronopathy. *J. Neurol. Sci.*, **85**, 1–8.

Dirr, L. Y., Elster, A. D., Donofrio, P. D. and Smith, M. (1990) Evolution of brain MRI abnormalities in limbic encephalitis. *Neurology*, **40**, 1304–1306.

Donofrio, P. D., Alessi, A. G., Albers, J. W., Knapp, R. H. and Blaivas, M. (1989) Electrodiagnostic evolution of carcinomatous sensory neuronopathy. *Muscle Nerve*, **12**, 508–513.

Doyle, A., Martin, W. J., Funa, K., Gazdar, A., Carney, D., Martin, S. E., *et al.* (1985) Markedly decreased expression of class I histocompatibility antigens, protein, and mRNA in human small-cell lung cancer. *J. Exp. Med.*, **161**, 1135–1151.

Dropcho, E. J. (1995) Autoimmune central nervous system paraneoplastic disorders: mechanisms, diagnosis, and therapeutic options. *Ann. Neurol.*, **37 (Suppl 1)**, S102–S113.

Dropcho, E. J., Chen, Y. T., Posner, J. B. and Old, L. J. (1987) Cloning of a brain protein identified by autoantibodies from a patient with paraneoplastic cerebellar degeneration. *Proc. Natl Acad. Sci. USA*, **84**, 4552–4556.

Dropcho, E. J. and King, P. H. (1994) Autoantibodies against the Hel-N1 RNA-binding protein among patients with lung carcinoma: an association with type I anti-neuronal nuclear antibodies. *Ann. Neurol.*, **36**, 200–205.

Dropcho, E. J., Kline, L. B. and Riser, J. (1993) Antineuronal (anti-Ri) antibodies in a patient with steroid-responsive opsoclonus/myoclonus. *Neurology*, **43**, 207–211.

Ellenberger, C., Campa, J. F. and Netsky, M. G. (1968) Opsoclonus and parenchymatous degeneration of the cerebellum. The cerebellar origin of an abnormal ocular movement. *Neurology*, **18**, 1041–1046.

Elrington, G. M., Murray, N. M., Spiro, S. G. and Newsom Davis, J. (1991) Neurological paraneoplastic syndromes in patients with small cell lung cancer. A prospective survey of 150 patients. *J. Neurol. Neurosurg. Psychiat.*, **54**, 764–767.

Fathallah, S. H., Wolf, S., Wong, E., Posner, J. B. and Furneaux, H. M. (1991) Cloning of a leucine-zipper protein recognized by the sera of patients with antibody-associated paraneoplastic cerebellar degeneration. *Proc. Natl Acad. Sci. USA*, **88**, 3451–3454.

Felician, O., Renard, J. L., Vega, F., Creange, A., Chen, Q. M., Bequet, D., *et al.* (1995) Paraneoplastic cerebellar degeneration with anti-Yo antibody in a man. *Neurology*, **45**, 1226–1227.

Font, J., Valls, J., Cervera, R., Pou, A., Ingelmo, M. and Graus, F. (1990) Pure sensory neuropathy in patients with primary Sjogren's syndrome: clinical, immunological, and electromyographic findings. *Ann. Rheum. Dis.*, **49**, 775–778.

Forsyth, P. A., Dalmau, J., Graus, F., Cwik, V., Rosenblum, M. K. and Posner, J. B. (1997) Motor neuron syndromes in cancer patients (see comments). *Ann. Neurol.*, **41**, 722–730.

Furneaux, H. F., Reich, L. and Posner, J. B. (1990) Autoantibody synthesis in the central nervous system of patients with paraneoplastic syndromes. *Neurology*, **40**, 1085–1091.

Gardner, M. B. (1991). Retroviral leukemia and lower motor neuron disease in wild mice: natural history, pathogenesis, and genetic resistance. *Adv. Neurol.* **56**, 473–479.

Gordon, P. H., Rowland, L. P., Younger, D. S., Sherman, W. H., Hays, A. P., Louis, E. D., *et al.* (1997) Lymphoproliferative disorders and motor neuron disease: an update. *Neurology*, **48**, 1671–1678.

Graus, F., Cordon, C. C. and Posner, J. B. (1985) Neuronal antinuclear antibody in sensory neuronopathy from lung cancer. *Neurology*, **35**, 538–543.

Graus, F., Dalmou, J., Rene, R., Tora, M., Malats, N., Verschuuren, J. J., *et al.* (1997) Anti-Hu antibodies in patients with small-cell lung cancer: association with complete response to therapy and improved survival. *J. Clin. Oncol.*, **15**, 2866–2872.

Graus, F., Delattre, J. Y. (1995) Immune modulation of paraneoplastic neurologic disorders. *Clin. Neurol. Neurosurg.*, **97**, 112–116.

Graus, F., Illa, I., Agusti, M., Ribalta, T., Cruz, S. F. and Juraez, C. (1991) Effect of intraventricular injection of an anti-Purkinje cell antibody (anti-Yo) in a guinea pig model. *J. Neurol. Sci.*, **106**, 82–87.

Graus, F., Ribalta, T., Campo, E., Monforte, R., Urbano, A. and Rozman, C. (1990) Immunohistochemical analysis of the immune reaction in the nervous system in paraneoplastic encephalomyelitis (see comments). *Neurology*, **40**, 219–222.

Graus, F., Rowe, G., Fueyo, J., Darnell, R. B. and Dalmau, J. (1993) The neuronal nuclear antigen recognized by the human anti-Ri autoantibody is expressed in central but not peripheral nervous system neurons. *Neurosci. Lett.*, **150**, 212–214.

Greenlee, J. E. and Brashear, H. R. (1983) Antibodies to cerebellar Purkinje cells in patients with paraneoplastic cerebellar degeneration and ovarian carcinoma. *Ann. Neurol.*, **14**, 609–613.

Greenlee, J. E., Parks, T. N. and Jaeckle, K. A. (1993) Type IIa ('anti-Hu') antineuronal antibodies produce destruction of rat cerebellar granule neurons *in vitro*. *Neurology*, **43**, 2049–2054.

Greenlee, J. E., Burns, J. B., Rose, J. W., Jaeckle, K. A. and Clawson, S. (1995) Uptake of systemically administered human anticerebellar antibody by rat Purkinje cells following blood–brain barrier disruption. *Acta Neuropathol. Berl.*, **89**, 341–345.

Grisold, W., Drlicek, M., Liszka, S. U. and Wondrusch, E. (1995) Anti-tumour therapy in paraneoplastic neurological disease. *Clin. Neurol. Neurosurg.*, **97**, 106–111.

Grunwald, G. B., Kornguth, S. E., Towfighi, J., Sassani, J., Simmonds, M. A., Housman, C. M., et al. (1987) Autoimmune basis for visual paraneoplastic syndrome in patients with small cell lung carcinoma. Retinal immune deposits and ablation of retinal ganglion cells. *Cancer*, **60**, 780–786.

Henson, R. A., Hoffman, H. L. and Urich, H. (1965) Encephalomyelitis with carcinoma. *Brain*, **88**, 449–464.

Henson, R. A. and Urich, H. (1982) *Cancer and the Nervous System*. London: Blackwell Scientific.

Hida, C., Tsukamoto, T., Awano, H. and Yamamoto, T. (1994) Ultrastructural localization of anti-Purkinje cell antibody-binding sites in paraneoplastic cerebellar degeneration. *Arch. Neurol.*, **51**, 555–558.

Honnorat, J., Antoine, J. C., Derrington, E., Aguera, M. and Belin, M. F. (1996) Antibodies to a subpopulation of glial cells and a 66 kDa developmental protein in patients with paraneoplastic neurological syndromes. *J. Neurol. Neurosurg. Psychiat.*, **61**, 270–278.

Hormigo, A., Dalmau, J., Rosenblum, M. K., River, M. E. and Posner, J. B. (1994a) Immunological and pathological study of anti-Ri-associated encephalopathy. *Ann. Neurol.*, **36**, 896–902.

Hormigo, A. and Lieberman, F. (1994b) Nuclear localization of anti-Hu antibody is not associated with *in vitro* cytotoxicity. *J. Neuroimmunol.*, **55**, 205–212.

Horton, J., Means, E. D., Cunningham, T. J., Olson, K. B. (1973) The numb chin in breast cancer. *J. Neurol. Neurosurg. Psychiat.*, **36**, 211–216.

Horwich, M. S., Cho, L., Porro, R. S. and Posner, J. B. (1977) Subacute sensory neuropathy: a remote effect of carcinoma. *Ann. Neurol.*, **2**, 7–19.

Hughes, R., Sharrack, B. and Rubens, R. (1996) Carcinoma and the peripheral nervous system. *J. Neurol.*, **243**, 371–376.

Jacobson, D. M., Thirkill, C. E. and Tipping, S. J. (1990) A clinical triad to diagnose paraneoplastic retinopathy. *Ann. Neurol.*, **28**, 162–167.

Jaeckle, K. A., Graus, F., Houghton, A., Cardon, C. C., Nielsen, S. L. and Posner, J. B. (1985) Autoimmune response of patients with paraneoplastic cerebellar degeneration to a Purkinje cell cytoplasmic protein antigen. *Ann. Neurol.*, **18**, 592–600.

Jean, W. C., Dalmau, J., Ho, A. and Posner, J. B. (1994) Analysis of the IgG subclass distribution and inflammatory infiltrates in patients with anti-Hu-associated paraneoplastic encephalomyelitis. *Neurology*, **44**, 140–147.

Johnston, I., Lang, B., Leys, K. and Newsom Davis, J. (1994) Heterogeneity of calcium channel autoantibodies detected using a small-cell lung cancer line derived from a Lambert-Eaton myasthenic syndrome patient. *Neurology*, **44**, 334–338.

Kiers, L., Altermatt, H. J. and Lennon, V. A. (1991) Paraneoplastic anti-neuronal nuclear IgG autoantibodies (type I) localize antigen in small cell lung carcinoma. *Mayo Clin. Proc.*, **66**, 1209–1216.

Kim, R. Y., Retsas, S., Fitzke, F. W., Arden, G. B. and Bird, A. C. (1994) Cutaneous melanoma-associated retinopathy. *Ophthalmology*, **101**, 1837–1843.

King, P. H. and Dropcho, E. J. (1996) Expression of Hel-N1 and Hel-N2 in small-cell lung carcinoma. *Ann. Neurol.*, **39**, 679–681.

Kinsbourne, M. (1962) Myoclonic encephalopathy of infants. *J. Neurol. Neurosurg. Psychiat.*, **25**, 271–276.

Kornstein, M. J., Asher, O. and Fuchs, S. (1995) Acetylcholine receptor alpha-subunit and myogenin mRNAs in thymus and thymomas. *Am. J. Pathol.*, **146**, 1320–1324.

Lennon, V. A. (1994a) Paraneoplastic autoantibodies: the case for a descriptive generic nomenclature (see comments). *Neurology*, **44**, 2236–2240.

Lennon, V. A. (1994b) The case for a descriptive generic nomenclature: clarification of immunostaining criteria for PCA-1, ANNA-1, and ANNA-2 autoantibodies (letter; see comments). *Neurology*, **44**, 2412–2415.

Lennon, V. A., Kryzer, T. J., Griesmann, G. E., O'Suilleabhain, P. E., Windebank, A. J., Woppmann, A., *et al.* (1995) Calcium-channel antibodies in the Lambert–Eaton syndrome and other paraneoplastic syndromes. *N. Engl. J. Med.*, **332**, 1467–1474.

Levine, T. D., Gao, F., King, P. H., Andrews, L. G. and Keene, J. D. (1993) Hel-N1: an autoimmune RNA-binding protein with specificity for 3' uridylate-rich untranslated regions of growth factor mRNAs. *Mol. Cell Biol.*, **13**, 3494–3504.

Leys, K., Lang, B., Johnston, I. and Newsom Davis, J. (1991) Calcium channel autoantibodies in the Lambert–Eaton myasthenic syndrome. *Ann. Neurol.*, **29**, 307–314.

Lossos, A. and Siegal, T. (1992) Numb chin syndrome in cancer patients: etiology, response to treatment, and prognostic significance (see comments). *Neurology*, **42**, 1181–1184.

Luque, F. A., Furneaux, H. M., Ferziger, R., Rosenblum, M. K., Wray, S. H., Schold, S. C., *et al.* (1991) Anti-Ri: an antibody associated with paraneoplastic opsoclonus and breast cancer. *Ann. Neurol.*, **29**, 241–251.

Mancall, E. L. and Rosales, R. K. (1964) Necrotising myelopathy associated with visceral carcinoma. *Brain*, **87**, 639–664.

Manley, G. T., Smitt, P. S., Dalmau, J., Posner, J. B. (1995) Hu antigens: reactivity with Hu antibodies, tumor expression, and major immunogenic sites. *Ann. Neurol.*, **38**, 102–110.

Mason, W. P., Graus, F., Lang, B., Honnorat, J., Delattre, J. Y., Valldeoriola, F., *et al.* (1997) Small-cell lung cancer, paraneoplastic cerebellar degeneration and the Lambert–Eaton myasthenic syndrome. *Brain*, **120**, 1279–1300.

Moll, J. W., Antoine, J. C., Brashear, H. R., Delattre, J., Drlicek, M., Dropcho, E. J., *et al.* (1995) Guidelines on the detection of paraneoplastic anti-neuronal-specific antibodies: report from the Workshop to the Fourth Meeting of the International Society of Neuro-Immunology on paraneoplastic neurological disease, held October 22–23, 1994, in Rotterdam, The Netherlands. *Neurology*, **45**, 1937–1941.

Motomura, M., Lang, B., Johnston, I., Palace, J., Vincent, A. and Newsom Davis, J. (1997) Incidence of serum anti-P/O-type and anti-N-type calcium channel autoantibodies in the Lambert–Eaton myasthenic syndrome. *J. Neurol. Sci.*, **147**, 35–42.

Musarella, M. A., Chan, H. S., Deboer, G., Gallie, B. L. (1984) Ocular involvement in neuroblastoma: prognostic implications. *Ophthalmology*, **91**, 936–940.

Naparstek, Y. and Plotz, P. H. (1993) The role of autoantibodies in autoimmune disease. *Annu. Rev. Immunol.*, **11**, 79–104.

Newsom Davis, J. and Murray, N. M. (1984) Plasma exchange and immunosuppressive drug treatment in the Lambert–Eaton myasthenic syndrome. *Neurology*, **34**, 480–485.

Newsom Davis, J., Pinching, A. J., Vincent, A. and Wilson, S. G. (1978) Function of circulating antibody to acetylcholine receptor in myasthenia gravis: investigation by plasma exchange. *Neurology*, **28**, 266–272.

Nitschke, M., Hochberg, F. and Dropcho, E. (1995) Improvement of paraneoplastic opsoclonus-myoclonus after protein A column therapy (letter). *N. Engl. J. Med.*, **332**, 192.

Norris, F. H. and Engel, W. K. (1965) Carcinomatous amyotrophic lateral sclerosis. In *The Remote Effects of Cancer on the Nervous System* (Brain, W. R. and Norris, F. H., eds), pp. 24–34. New York: Grune and Stratton.

O'Neill, J. H., Murray, N. M. and Newsom Davis, J. (1988) The Lambert–Eaton myasthenic syndrome. A review of 50 cases. *Brain*, **111**, 577–596.

Paone, J. F. and Jeyasingham, K. (1980) Remission of cerebellar dysfunction after pneumonectomy for bronchogenic carcinoma. *N. Engl. J. Med.*, **302**, 156.

Peterson, K., Rosenblum, M. K., Kotanides, H. and Posner, J. B. (1992) Paraneoplastic cerebellar degeneration. I. A clinical analysis of 55 anti-Yo antibody-positive patients. *Neurology*, **42**, 1931–1937.

Peterson, K., Forsyth, P. A. and Posner, J. B. (1994) Paraneoplastic sensorimotor neuropathy associated with breast cancer. *J. Neurooncol.*, **21**, 159–170.

Polans, A. S., Buczylko, J., Crabb, J. and Palczewski, K. (1991) A photoreceptor calcium binding protein is recognized by autoantibodies obtained from patients with cancer-associated retinopathy. *J. Cell Biol.*, **112**, 981–989.

Polans, A. S., Witkowska, D., Haley, T. L., Amundson, D., Baizer, L. and Adamus, G. (1995) Recoverin, a photoreceptor-specific calcium-binding protein, is expressed by the tumor of a patient with cancer-associated retinopathy. *Proc. Natl Acad. Sci. USA*, **92**, 9176–9180.

Posner, J. B. (1996) Paraneoplastic syndromes. In *Neurology in Clinical Practice* (Marsden, C. D., Fenichel, G. M., Daroff, F. and Bradley, G., eds), pp. 1165–1172. London: Butterworth-Heinemann.

Pranzatelli, M. R. (1992) The neurobiology of the opsoclonus/myoclonus syndrome. *Clin. Neuropharmacol.*, **15**, 186–228.

Reddy, R. V., Vakili, S. T. (1981) Midbrain encephalitis as a remote effect of a malignant neoplasm. *Arch. Neurol.*, **38**, 781–782.

Ridley, A., Kennard, C., Scholtz, C. L., Buttner, E. J., Summers, B. and Turnbull, A. (1987) Omnipause neurons in two cases of opsoclonus associated with oat cell carcinoma of the lung. *Brain*, **110**, 1699–1709.

Roberts, A., Perera, S., Lang, B., Vincent, A. and Newsom Davis, J. (1985) Paraneoplastic myasthenic syndrome IgG inhibits $^{45}Ca^{2+}$ flux in a human small cell carcinoma line. *Nature*, **317**, 737–739.

Rodriguez, M., Truh, L. I., O'Neill, B. P. and Lennon, V. A. (1988) Autoimmune paraneoplastic cerebellar degeneration: ultrastructural localization of antibody-binding sites in Purkinje cells. *Neurology*, **38**, 1380–1386.

Sakai, K., Mitchell, D. J., Tsukamoto, T. and Steinman, L. (1990) Isolation of a complementary DNA clone encoding an autoantigen recognized by an anti-neuronal cell antibody from a patient with paraneoplastic cerebellar degeneration (published erratum appears in *Ann Neurol.*, **30**(5), 738). *Ann. Neurol.*, **28**, 692–698.

Sakai, K., Gofuku, M., Kitagawa, Y., Ogasawara, T., Hirose, G., Yamazaki, M., *et al.* (1994) A hippocampal protein associated with paraneoplastic neurologic syndrome and small cell lung carcinoma. *Biochem. Biophys. Res. Commun.*, **199**, 1200–1208.

Sakai, K., Gofuku, M., Kitagawa, Y., Ogasawara, T., Hirose, G. (1995) Induction of anti-Purkinje cell antibodies *in vivo* by immunizing with a recombinant 52-kDa paraneoplastic cerebellar degeneration-associated protein. *J. Neuroimmunol.*, **60**, 135–141.

Sato, S., Inuzuka, T., Nakano, R., Fujita, N., Matsubara, N., Sakimura, K., *et al.* (1991) Antibody to a zinc finger protein in a patient with paraneoplastic cerebellar degeneration. *Biochem. Biophys. Res. Commun.*, **178**, 198–206.

Schold, S. C., Cho, E. S., Somasundaram, M. and Posner, J. B. (1979) Subacute motor neuronopathy: a remote effect of lymphoma. *Ann. Neurol.*, **5**, 271–287.

Sekido, Y., Bader, S. A., Carbone, D. P., Johnson, B. E. and Minna, J. D. (1994) Molecular analysis of the HuD gene encoding a paraneoplastic encephalomyelitis antigen in human lung cancer cell lines. *Cancer Res.*, **54**, 4988–4992.

Siemson, J. K. and Meister, L. (1963) Bronchogenic carcinoma with severe orthostatic hypotension. *Ann. Intern. Med.*, **58**, 669–672.

Sigurgeirsson, B. (1992) Skin disease and malignancy. An epidemiological study. *Acta Derm. Venereol. Suppl. Stockh.*, **178**, 1–110.

Smith, J. L., Finley, J. C. and Lennon, V. A. (1988) Autoantibodies in paraneoplastic cerebellar degeneration bind to cytoplasmic antigens of Purkinje cells in humans, rats and mice and are of multiple immunoglobulin classes. *J. Neuroimmunol.*, **18**, 37–48.

Szabo, A., Dalmau, J., Manley, G., Rosenfeld, M., Wong, E., Henson, J., *et al.* (1991) HuD, a paraneoplastic encephalomyelitis antigen, contains RNA-binding domains and is homologous to Elav and Sex-lethal. *Cell*, **67**, 325–333.

Tanaka, K., Tanaka, M., Onodera, O., Igarashi, S., Miyatake, T. and Tsuji, S. (1994) Passive transfer and active immunization with the recombinant leucine-zipper (Yo) protein as an attempt to establish an animal model of paraneoplastic cerebellar degeneration. *J. Neurol. Sci.*, **127**, 153–158.

Tanaka, K., Tanaka, M., Igarashi, S., Onodera, O., Miyatake, T. and Tsuji, S. (1995) Trial to establish an animal model of paraneoplastic cerebellar degeneration with anti-Yo antibody. 2. Passive transfer of murine mononuclear cells activated with recombinant Yo protein to paraneoplastic cerebellar degeneration lymphocytes in severe combined immunodeficiency mice. *Clin. Neurol. Neurosurg.*, **97**, 101–105.

Telander, R. L., Smithson, W. A. and Groover, R. V. (1989) Clinical outcome in children with acute cerebellar encephalopathy and neuroblastoma. *J. Pediatr. Surg.*, **24**, 11–14.

Thirkill, C. E., Fitzgerald, P., Sergott, R. C., Roth, A. M., Tyler, N. K. and Keltner, J. L. (1989) Cancer-associated retinopathy (CAR syndrome) with antibodies reacting with retinal, optic-nerve, and cancer cells (see comments). *N. Engl. J. Med.*, **321**, 1589–1594.

Thirkill, C. E., Tait, R. C., Tyler, N. K., Roth, A. M. and Keltner, J. L. (1992) The cancer-associated retinopathy antigen is a recoverin-like protein. *Invest. Ophthalmol. Vis. Sci.*, **33**, 2768–2772.

Tota, M., Graus, F., De, B. C. and Real, F. X. (1997) Cell surface expression of paraneoplastic encephalomyelitis/sensory neuronopathy-associated Hu antigens in small-cell lung cancers and neuroblastomas. *Neurology*, **48**, 735–741.

Toyka, K. V., Brachman, D. B., Pestronk, A. and Kao, I. (1975) Myasthenia gravis: passive transfer from man to mouse. *Science*, **190**, 397–399.

Uchuya, M., Graus, F., Vega, F., Rene, R. and Delattre, J. Y. (1996) Intravenous immunoglobulin treatment in paraneoplastic neurological syndromes with antineuronal autoantibodies. *J. Neurol. Neurosurg. Psychiat.*, **60**, 388–392.

Vega, F., Graus, F., Chen, Q. M., Poisson, M., Schuller, E., Delattre, J. Y. (1994) Intrathecal synthesis of the anti-Hu antibody in patients with paraneoplastic encephalomyelitis or sensory neuronopathy: clinical-immunologic correlation. *Neurology*, **44**, 2145–2147.

Verma, A., Berger, J. R., Snodgrass, S. and Petito, C. (1996) Motor neuron disease: a paraneoplastic process associated with anti-hu antibody and small-cell lung carcinoma. *Ann. Neurol.*, **40**, 112–116.

Vincent, A., Lang, B. and Newsom Davis, J. (1989) Autoimmunity to the voltage-gated calcium channel underlies the Lambert–Eaton myasthenic syndrome, a paraneoplastic disorder. *Trends. Neurosci.*, **12**, 496–502.

Weinstein, J. M., Kelman, S. E., Bresnick, G. H. and Kornguth, S. E. (1994) Paraneoplastic retinopathy associated with antiretinal bipolar cell antibodies in cutaneous malignant melanoma. *Ophthalmology*, **101**, 1236–1243.

Weissman, D. E. and Gottschall, J. L. (1989) Complete remission of paraneoplastic sensorimotor neuropathy: a case associated with small-cell lung cancer responsive to chemotherapy, plasma exchange, and radiotherapy. *J. Clin. Apheresis*, **5**, 3–6.

Yamaji, Y., Matsubara, S., Yamadori, I., Sato, M., Fujita, T., Fujita, J., *et al.* (1996) Characterization of a small-cell-lung-carcinoma cell line from a patient with cancer-associated retinopathy. *Int. J. Cancer*, **65**, 671–676.

Younger, D. S., Rowland, L. P., Latov, N., Hays, A. P., Lange, D. J., Sherman, W., *et al.* (1991) Lymphoma, motor neuron diseases, and amyotrophic lateral sclerosis (see comments). *Ann. Neurol.*, **29**, 78–86.

Chapter 6

Stiff man syndrome

Neil Scolding

Introduction	139
Stiff muscles	139
The stiff man syndrome	141
Pathophysiology and treatment	141
The immunology of the stiff man syndrome	142
The stiff man syndrome, progressive encephalomyelitis with rigidity and cancer	143
References	145

Introduction

It might be considered generous to permit a disorder as uncommon as the stiff man (or person) syndrome an exclusive chapter, be it ever so small. An autoimmune origin is, however, the current best guess, but the disorder cannot conveniently be pushed into more specific categories or, therefore, chapters. Thus, while stiff man syndrome may be associated with diabetes mellitus, the majority of cases are not: it is not a complication of conventional organ-specific autoimmune disease. Similarly, stiff man syndrome as an apparent paraneoplastic disorder is reported, but the great majority of cases do not occur in the context of malignancy.

It appears to be a disorder unique among central nervous system (CNS) diseases – a primary, non-malignant immune-mediated process caused by antibodies directed against a specific subpopulation of (spinal) neurones. If this suggested aetiology should be proven correct, then myasthenia gravis (although outside the CNS) might prove to be its closest neurological relative.

Stiff muscles

Stiffness on examination of muscles occurs in an enormous number of disorders – including the whole spectrum of pyramidal or extrapyramidal disease, as well as more specific disorders such as tetanus, congenital syndromes such as Schwarz–Jampel disease (contractured, stiff, hyper-trophied, myotonic muscles associated with cranio-facial abnormalities) and the myotonic disorders (Table 6.1). In the great majority, the nature of the stiffness and the context in which the sign occurs, and the associated neurological and general clinical findings, are sufficient to exclude or confirm a movement disorder or pyramidal tract lesion disorder as the cause of the stiffness.

Table 6.1 Causes and differential diagnosis of stiff muscles

Disorders in which stiffness is the principal manifestation
  Stiff man syndrome
  Neuromyotonia
  Progressive encephalomyelitis with rigidity
  Schwarz–Jampel syndrome
  Tetanus
  Strychnine poisoning

Disorders in which other signs may predominate
  Pyramidal disorders
  Extrapyramidal disease
  Neuroleptic malignant syndrome
  Malignant hyperthermia (during anaesthesia)

Stiff muscles occurring as a primary disorder, wherein the stiffness is itself the principal (or sole) symptom and/or sign, and is caused by continuous muscle unit activity, is much less common and can be more difficult to assess diagnostically (Table 6.1). It occurs in perhaps three major conditions – tetanus, neuromyotonia and the stiff man syndrome. Other clinical features, e.g. stiffness at rest, slow relaxation, spasms (spontaneous or exertional) and percussion irritability of muscle, can provide very helpful diagnostic cues. Tetanus – again, usually apparent from the clinical context – causes stiffness at rest and spontaneous and exertional muscle spasms (as does strychnine poisoning). Hypothyroidism should be remembered as a cause of muscle stiffness, slow relaxation and painful muscle cramps and spasms.

The principal diagnostic differences between neuromyotonia and the stiff man syndrome are summarized in Table 6.2. Neuromyotonia has a peripheral origin in the distal axon and neuro-muscular junction, and while an autoimmune origin has been postulated, falls outside the remit of the current text.

Table 6.2 Differential diagnosis of stiff man syndrome and neuromyotonia

Stiff man syndrome	*Neuromyotonia* *(Isaac's syndrome, armadillo syndrome)*
Usually fourth to fifth decade	Mostly affects children and young adults
Proximal/axial stiffness	Stiffness usually more distal
Startle/action-triggered painful cramps; neurocutaneous reflexes also trigger cramps	Exercise-induced painful cramps
No myokymia	Myokymia, especially exercise-induced
Axial posturing – hyperlordosis, spinal ridging/furrows	Posturing is usually peripheral – carpopedal spasm, toe-walking
Contractures and tendon rupture seen	
No other signs, no myotonia	Slow relaxation
Normal sensorium	Excess sweating
	Psychotic episodes
Abolished by sleep, by general and spinal anaesthesia	Persists during sleep, general and spinal anaesthesia
Tizanidine, benzodiazepines, baclofen help	Phenytoin, carbamazepine help
L-dopa preparations worsen	

The stiff man syndrome

The stiff man syndrome was first described (and so-named) by Moersch and Woltman in 1956 (Moersch and Woltman, 1956). (Louis Rowland has suggested the eponymous epithet might avoid offence to women and children with the disorder. Perhaps Moersch–Woltperson Syndrome would be best.) These authors described 14 patients from the Mayo practice with rigidity of muscles, mainly but not exclusively axial, and painful muscle cramps.

It is usually of adult onset, affecting men and women equally, and develops and progresses slowly over months and years. Patients commonly complain of aching discomfort, slowness and stiffness. There may be painful spasms, often noise, startle or action induced, and these can be very severe – tendon and muscle rupture may occur. Walking may become clumsy and unsteady, and awkwardness and restriction of upper limb movements may also be noticed. There is no disturbance of sphincter function.

Examination of the limbs reveals normal power and tendon reflexes, downgoing plantar responses, and no abnormalities either of sensation or (barring spasms) coordination. However, axial and abdominal wall rigidity is apparent, and there may be proximal limb muscle stiffness, agonists and antagonists acting simultaneously. The understandable temptation at this juncture to assume an hysterical origin for the patient's symptoms should be resisted as more positive features are sought. Asymmetrical contraction of the paraspinal muscles causes a characteristic lordotic and often scoliotic posture, an important diagnostic feature (Figure 6.1). Spasms may be induced by the examiner by manoeuvres indicated above and occasionally during the elicitation of cutaneous reflexes (Meinck et al., 1984). It has recently been suggested that a subset of patients with 'stiff limb syndrome' can be defined (Baker et al., 1998).

Diabetes mellitus is present in a significant proportion – perhaps 30–40% – of patients. There is also an association with other organ-specific autoimmune diseases, including thyroid disease and pernicious anaemia. Epilepsy is reported to occur in approximately 10% of cases (see below).

Imaging of the brain and spinal cord is normal. The spinal fluid is usually normal, but oligoclonal immunoglobulin bands are found in an as yet undetermined proportion of cases. Electrophysiological muscle examination is the unsurprising key to confirmation of the diagnosis, revealing continuous muscle activity despite invitation to relax, with normal motor unit morphology. ('The patient was unable to relax during the examination' should raise suspicion.) Importantly, voluntary contraction of antagonists fails to inhibit the activity in the muscle under examination. Abnormal activity – and likewise spasms – does not persist during sleep; its central origin is confirmed by its disappearance following pharmacological peripheral nerve block or spinal or general anaesthesia, in contrast to the abnormal activity demonstrable in neuromyotonic syndromes.

Pathophysiology and treatment

Meinck et al. (1984) proposed on the basis of electrophysiological and pharmacological investigation of a single patient that stiff man syndrome resulted from an imbalance between excitatory (catecholaminergic) and

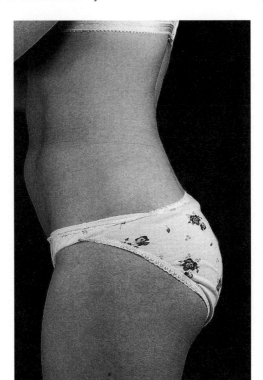

Figure 6.1 A 26-year-old female with a diagnosis of stiff man syndrome established on the basis of clinical and electrophysiological grounds exhibits the very characteristic hyperlordotic posture. She had oligoclonal bands in her spinal fluid, high titres of serum anti-glutamic acid decarboxylase antibodies and responded well to treatment with diazepam. (Courtesy Dr Jeff Cocsis, Norfolk and Norwich Hospital.)

descending inhibitory (γ-amino butyric acid or GABA-ergic) influences on spinal motor neurones. An improvement was noted with treatment either with the GABA agonists diazepam and tizanidine, or with the catecholamine antagonist clonidine.

Benzodiazepines (particularly), tizanidine, and also baclofen and occasionally sodium valproate are now used therapeutically. More recent experimental treatments have included intrathecal baclofen (Silbert *et al.*, 1995) and paraspinal botulinum toxin in small numbers of patients; as mentioned below, the place of steroids, immunosuppressants and plasmapheresis or intravenous immunoglobulin remains to be clearly established.

The immunology of the stiff man syndrome

The putative failure of GABA-ergic control over motor neurones received a boost in 1988 when Solimena *et al.* reported the presence of antibodies directed against GABA-ergic nerve terminals in both serum and spinal fluid of a patient with stiff man syndrome, diabetes mellitus and epilepsy. Evidence was presented showing that these antibodies were probably directed against glutamic acid decarboxylase (GAD), the enzyme responsible for producing GABA from glutamic acid, and that they also reacted with pancreatic islet β cells, which also contain GAD. The same group subsequently showed autoantibodies to GABA-ergic neurones to be present in 60% of patients with stiff man syndrome (Solimena et al., 1988) and antibodies to pancreatic islet cells in around 55% (one-third of their 32 patients had diabetes). Later studies indicated that the 64 kDa antigen to which antibodies are found in 80% of patients with new-onset insulin-dependent diabetes mellitus (IDDM) – and which not uncommonly arise before clinical presentation (Baekkeskov et al., 1982; Atkinson et al., 1990) – is GAD (Baekkeskov et al., 1990). Significant differences between anti-GAD antibodies present in IDDM and those in stiff man syndrome were found – though some overlap also occurs – and antibody titres are more than two orders of magnitude greater in stiff patients than in individuals with IDDM (Daw et al., 1996).

It was consequently suggested that the anti-GAD activity was responsible for the pathophysiological loss of GABA-ergic activity (Solimena and DeCamilli, 1991); the association with epilepsy, to which loss of an inhibitory GABA-ergic influence may also contribute, represents an attractive additional possible consequence of anti-GAD antibodies. Clearly, the presence of cerebrospinal fluid (CSF) oligoclonal banding supports an autoimmune aetiology, as do suggested human leukocyte antigen (HLA) associations (Williams et al., 1988).

It must be mentioned, however, that antibody-mediated disruption of GABA-ergic transmission within the spinal cord remains a best-guess hypothesis, for which some would argue that further experimental support is necessary – as Solimena et al. themselves indicate. A significant proportion of patients have no detectable anti-GAD antibody and no obvious clinical differences distinguish these individuals from stiff patients with anti-GAD antibodies. Furthermore, successful treatment with plasmapheresis and/or steroids is reported in some patients (Vicari et al., 1989), but others clearly fail to respond (Harding et al., 1989). Histopathological studies are few; some appear to show no obvious changes (Layzer, 1988), although more recent reports describe perivascular lymphocytic cuffs in the spinal cord and in the brain stem (Meinck et al., 1994).

A further difficulty is the mechanism by which antibodies might gain access to and influence an intracellular target antigen. Two isoforms of GAD are present in neuronal tissue, one soluble and one membrane bound. It is the 65 kDa form which forms the main (though not the exclusive) target in stiff man syndrome (Butler et al., 1993; Daw et al., 1996). One possibility emerges in the concentration of this isoform on the membranes of synaptic vesicles, where it may become exposed and available to antibody during exocytosis (see Ellis and Atkinson, 1996).

The stiff man syndrome, progressive encephalomyelitis with rigidity and cancer

In a small number of patients, the stiff man syndrome occurs as a paraneoplastic disorder. Breast carcinoma may be a more particular associate than other cancers (e.g. Folli *et al.*, 1993); the other usual malignant suspects have also been incriminated – small cell lung cancer (Bateman *et al.*, 1990) and lymphoma (Ferrari *et al.*, 1990). The neurological manifestations of many of such patients appears very similar to non-malignancy related stiff man syndrome (Folli *et al.*, 1993); in common with other paraneoplastic disorders, they not uncommonly antedate diagnosis of cancer.

Folli *et al.* (1993) reported the presence of antibodies to a distinct protein unrelated to GAD (for which samples were tested and found negative) in three patients with breast cancer and stiff man syndrome. In the CNS, the antibody localized to neurones and, interestingly (and like GAD antibodies), was found to be particularly concentrated at synapses; in the one sample tested, no binding to the malignant breast tissue was observed. In further studies, the target protein was shown to be homologous to the avian synaptic vesicle-associated protein amphiphysin (De Camilli *et al.*, 1993). More recent work has confirmed the relevance of this homology in mammals; localization at the node of Ranvier is also reported (Butler *et al.*, 1997).

A literature, initially unrelated to cancer, has also emerged concerning a disorder variously known as *stiff encephalomyelitis* or *progressive encephalomyelitis with rigidity* (PEWR), first described in 1971 (Whitely *et al.*, 1976; see also Moersch and Woltman, 1956). In this condition, features of the stiff man syndrome are accompanied by additional symptoms, signs, and abnormalities on investigation. Opisthotonus and opsoclonus may be found, cranial neuropathies and brain stem myoclonus are described, and there may be ataxia, diminished tendon jerks and (especially) extensor plantar responses. Electrophysiological investigation may reveal evidence of a demyelinating neuropathy (as well as stiff features), magnetic resonance imaging atrophy and signal change in the brain stem and spinal cord; and in the CSF, a pleomorphic leukocytosis. The course is substantially more aggressive, with death in 3–10 years, and autopsy shows inflammatory changes, neuronal loss particularly affecting the central grey and often more florid changes of encephalomyelitis – perivascular lymphocytic cuffing, astrogliosis and microglial reaction.

The distinct course, additional features and more florid pathology originally suggested a disorder quite separate to the stiff man syndrome, early autopsy studies of the stiff man syndrome having suggested no abnormal findings (Layzer, 1988). However, the later appreciation of inflammatory changes in 'conventional' stiff spinal cords, together with the description of serum and CSF antibodies against GAD in PEWR (Burn *et al.*, 1991), is consistent with a spectrum of (probably autoimmune) disease.

The distinction between these various disorders is blurred still further by sporadic case reports of patients with PEWR-like features and neoplasia, and by the observation that the clinical picture of some cases reported as paraneoplastic stiff man syndrome in fact more closely resemble PEWR: Bateman *et al.*'s 1990 case, for example, exhibited localized wasting and fasciculation, upper limb and ankle areflexia, complete loss of vibration sensitivity in the legs, and stiffness largely limited to the arms, with no mention of axial symptoms or signs. Similarity between the histopathological changes of PEWR and paraneoplastic CNS disease has also been noted (e.g. Roobol *et al.*, 1987).

Dropcho has recently reported a patient with small cell lung cancer, paraneoplastic encephalomyelitis and muscular rigidity resembling the stiff man syndrome: with cognitive involvement and a peripheral neuropathy, the term PEWR would not obviously be inappropriate. However, in contrast to Burn's patient with PEWR and GAD antibodies, but in common with Folli's (and other) patients with more conventional but paraneoplastic stiff man syndrome, antibodies against amphiphysin were present (Dropcho, 1996). Other patients with paraneoplastic encephalomyelitis, small cell lung cancer and anti-amphiphysin antibodies had no stiffness. Unlike Folli *et al.*, Dropcho (using reverse transcription-polymerase chain reaction) was able to demonstrate amphiphysin in both small cell lung and breast cancer tissue, though others have found it in the latter (Floyd *et al.*, 1998).

In summary, therefore, 'benign' stiff man syndrome is often associated with anti-GAD antibodies and paraneoplastic (pure) stiff man syndrome with anti-amphiphysin antibodies. PEWR unassociated with malignancy may occur with anti-GAD antibodies, while paraneoplastic PEWR again may be connected to amphiphysin antibodies. While the apparently consistent contrast in antibody specificities between non-malignant and paraneoplastic disease is of interest, too few patients have yet been described for any firm conclusions to be drawn. Moreover, though it is also striking that antibodies to either of two synaptic vesicle-associated proteins are seen in both stiff variants, a causal link remains to be proven.

References

Atkinson, M., MacLaren, N. K., Scharp, D. W., Lacy, P. E. and Riley, W. J. (1990) 64,000M autoantibodies are predictive of insulin dependent diabetes. *Lancet*, **335**, 1357–1360.

Baekkeskov, S., *et al.* (1982) Autoantibodies in newly diagnosed diabetic children with immunoprecipitate human pancreatic cells. *Nature*, **298**, 167–169.

Baekkeskov, S., Aanstoot, H.-J., Christgau, S., *et al.* (1990) The 64 kD autoantigen in insulin-dependent diabetes is the GABA-synthesising enzyme glutamic acid decarboxylase. *Nature*, **347**, 151–156.

Barker, R. A., Revesz, T., Thorn, M., Marsden, C. D. and Brown, P. (1998) Review of 23 patients affected by the stiff man syndrome: clinical subdivision into stiff trunk (man) syndrome, stiff limb syndrome, and progressive encephalomyelitis into rigidity. J. Neurol. Neurosurg. *Psychiat.*, **65**, 639–640.

Bateman, D. E., Weller, R. O. and Kennedy, P. (1990) Stiffman syndrome: a rare paraneoplastic disorder? *J. Neurol. Neurosurg. Psychiat.*, **53**, 695–696.

Burn, D. J., Ball, J., Lees, A. J., Behan, P. O. and Morgan, H. J. (1991) A case of progressive encephalomyelitis with rigidity and positive antiglutamic acid decarboxylase antibodies {corrected} {published erratum appears in J. Neurol. Neurosurg. *Psychiat.*, **54**, 1032}. *J. Neurol. Neurosurg. Psychiat.*, **54**, 449–451.

Butler, M. H., Solimena, M., Dirkx, R., Hayday, A. and De, C. P. (1993) Identification of a dominant epitope of glutamic acid decarboxylase (GAD-65) recognized by autoantibodies in stiff-man syndrome. *J. Exp. Med.*, **178**, 2097–2106.

Butler, M. H., David, C., Ochoa, G. C., Freyberg, Z., Daniell, L., Grabs, D., *et al.* (1997) Amphiphysin II (SH3P9; BIN1), a member of the amphiphysin/Rvs family, is concentrated in the cortical cytomatrix of axon initial segments and nodes of Ranvier in brain and around T tubules in skeletal muscle. *J. Cell Biol.*, **137**, 1355–1367.

Daw, K., Ujihara, N., Atkinson, M. and Powers, A. C. (1996) Glutamic acid decarboxylase autoantibodies in stiff-man syndrome and insulin-dependent diabetes mellitus exhibit similarities and differences in epitope recognition. *J. Immunol.*, **156**, 818–825.

De Camilli, P., Thomas, A., Cofiell, R., *et al.* (1993) The synaptic vesicle-associated protein amphiphysin is the 128 kD autoantigen of stiff-man syndrome with breast cancer. *J. Exp. Med.*, **178**, 2219–2223.

Dropcho, E. J. (1996) Antiamphiphysin antibodies with small-cell lung carcinoma and paraneoplastic encephalomyelitis. *Ann. Neurol.*, **39**, 659–667.

Ellis, T. M. and Atkinson, M. A. (1996) The clinical significance of an autoimmune response against glutamic acid decarboxylase. *Nat. Med.*, **2**, 148–153.

Ferrari, P., Federico, M., Grimaldi, L. M. and Silingardi, V. (1990) Stiff-man syndrome in a patient with Hodgkin's disease. An unusual paraneoplastic syndrome. *Haematologica*, **75**, 570–572.

Floyd, S., Butler, M. H., Cremona, O., David, C., Freyberg, Z., Zhang, X. *et al* (1998) Expression of amphiphysin I, an autoantigen of paraneoplastic neurological syndromes in breast cancer. *Molecular Medicine*, **4**, 29–39.

Folli, F., Solimena, M., Cofiell, R., Austoni, M., Tallini, G., Fassetta, G., *et al* (1993) Autoantibodies to a 128-kd synaptic protein in three women with the stiff-man syndrome and breast cancer. *N. Engl. J. Med.*, **328**, 546–551.

Harding, A. E., Thompson, P. D., Kocen, R. S., *et al.* (1989) Plasma exchange and immunosuppression in the stiff man syndrome. *Lancet*, **ii**, 915.

Layzer, R. B. (1988) Stiff-man syndrome – an autoimmune disease? {editorial}. *N. Engl. J. Med.*, **318**, 1060–1062.

Meinck, H. M., Ricker, K. and Conrad, B. (1984) The stiff-man syndrome: new pathophysiological aspects from abnormal exteroceptive reflexes and the response to clomipramine, clonidine, and tizanidine. *J. Neurol. Neurosurg. Psychiat.*, **47**, 280–287.

Meinck, H. M., Ricker, K., Hulser, P. J., Schmid, E., Peiffer, J. and Solimena, M. (1994) Stiff man syndrome: clinical and laboratory findings in eight patients. *J. Neurol.*, **241**, 157–166.

Moersch, F. P. and Woltman, H. W. (1956) Progressive fluctuating muscular rigidity and spasm ('stiff man syndrome'): report of a case and observations in 13 other cases. *Mayo Clin. Proc.*, **31**, 421–427.

Roobol, T. H., Kazzaz, B. A. and Vecht, C. J. (1987) Segmental rigidity and spinal myoclonus as a paraneoplastic syndrome. *J. Neurol. Neurosurg. Psychiat.*, **50**, 628–631.

Silbert, P. L., Matsumoto, J. Y., McManis, P. G., Stolpsmith, K. A., Elliott, B. A. and McEvoy, K. M. (1995) Intrathecal baclofen therapy in stiff-man syndrome: a double- blind, placebo-controlled trial. *Neurology*, **45**, 1893–1897.

Solimena, M. and De Camilli, P. (1991) Autoimmunity to glutamate decarboxylase (GAD) in stiff man syndrome and insulin-dependent diabetes. *Trends Neurosci.*, **14**, 452–457.

Solimena, M., Folli, F., Denis-Donini, S., *et al.* (1988) Autoantibodies to glutamic acid decarboxylase in a patient with stiff man syndrome, epilepsy and type 1 diabetes. *N. Engl. J. Med.*, **318**, 1012–1020.

Vicari, A. M., Folli, F. and Pozza, G. E. A. (1989) Plasmapheresis in the treatment of stiff man syndrome. *N. Engl. J. Med.*, **320**, 1499.

Whitely, A. M., Swash, M. and Urich, H. (1976) Progressive encephalomyelitis with rigidity: its relationship to 'sub-acute myoclonic spinal interneuronitis' and to the 'stiff man syndrome'. *Brain*, **99**, 27–42.

Williams, A. C., Nutt, J. G. and Hare, T. (1988) Autoimmunity in stiff-man syndrome. *Lancet*, **ii**, 22.

Chapter 7

Neurological complications of rheumatological and connective tissue disorders

Neil Scolding

Introduction	147
Rheumatoid arthritis	147
Sjögren's syndrome	150
Systemic sclerosis	152
Mixed connective tissue disease	153
Systemic lupus erythematosus	153
Seronegative arthritides	170
References	171

Introduction

Although rheumatological and connective tissue disorders may each include vasculitis within its repertoire of pathological effects, it is nosologically conventional and appropriate to distinguish the primary vasculitic disorders, such as Wegener's disease and microscopic polyarteritis, from rheumatological diseases. Additionally, many – if not most – of the consequences of these disorders arise through mechanisms wholly unrelated to vasculitis, emphasizing the importance of considering rheumatological and connective tissue disorders separately from the vasculitides (a point worth labouring, in view of the common practice in disarmingly respectable literature of using the terms 'cerebral lupus' and 'cerebral vasculitis' interchangeably).

Rheumatoid arthritis

Rheumatoid arthritis is a common disorder, affecting 1–2% of the population. The aetiology is unknown, although a genetic contribution is apparent: siblings of affected patients have an 8-fold increased risk of developing the disease (Wordsworth, 1995). It is a chronic, multisystem disease the burden of which falls upon the joints and soft tissues. Outside the musculo-skeletal system, lung complications are not uncommon, and include pulmonary nodules, pleurisy, and interstitial fibrosis and pneumonitis. Splenomegaly and hypersplenism can lead to a pancytopenia, and a systemic vasculitic process can also occur.

The Class II MHC association, specifically with human leukocyte antigen (HLA)-DR1 and -DR4 (and more recently related to a particular site – position 71 – on the DRβ chain (Hammer *et al.*, 1995)) provides one line of evidence implicating T lymphocytes mechanistically in the generation of tissue damage. T cells are prominent in the chronic inflammatory infiltrate within synovial joints; activated macrophages and plasma cells are also present (Cush and Lipsky, 1988). Once again, the nature of the initiating antigen is unknown; the usual suspects – heat shock proteins, and more indigenous molecules, such as collagen subtypes, have been incriminated (e.g. Ronnelid and Klareskog, 1995).

The role (if any) of antibodies, and specifically of the IgM antibodies recognizing IgG Fc regions which comprise rheumatoid factor, also remains to be defined (reviewed in Feldmann et al., 1996a). Rheumatoid factor IgM appears to be a normal and important component of the immune system, with essential immunoregulatory function. Pro-inflammatory cytokines are over-expressed in affected tissues, and their importance in mediating the immunological and inflammatory disturbances of rheumatoid disease is generally accepted (see Feldmann et al., 1996b). A presumed key role for tumour necrosis factor (TNF)-α helped to justify treatment trials of anti-TNF-α antibodies in rheumatoid arthritis, which so far have yielded promising results (Elliott et al., 1994; Rankin et al., 1995).

Neurological involvement is less common in this, the prototypical connective tissue disorder, than in other related diseases; furthermore, the commoner complications are either peripheral or secondary to structural abnormalities (or both). Thus an inflammatory peripheral neuropathy is well described and occurs in approximately 30% of seropositive rheumatoid cases; mononeuritis is typical, and may be accompanied by skin lesions (McCombe et al., 1991; Puechal et al., 1995). It is usually mild and conventionally the pathological change is one of segmental demyelination. A more severe and aggressive axonal polyneuropathy or mononeuritis multi-plex may be seen when rheumatoid arthritis is accompanied by a vasculitis (Weller et al., 1970). More common than either are entrapment neuropathies of conventional distribution, precipitated by inflammation and swelling of synovial tissues. Up to 50% of patients may be so affected at some stage in their disease. An autonomic neuropathy, which may be severe, has also been described (Toussirot et al., 1993).

The commonest form of central nervous system (CNS) involvement is high spinal cord compression induced by a combination of destructive changes in the cervical spine, particularly the transverse ligament of the atlas, not uncommonly resulting in subluxation, and pannus formation (Stevens et al., 1971). Recent histopathological studies have confirmed the absence of any inflammatory component to rheumatoid spinal cord disease (Henderson et al., 1993; Kauppi et al., 1996). The surgical management, often far from straightforward, is beyond the scope of this text.

Inflammatory CNS disease complicating rheumatoid arthritis is conven-tionally said to take two principal forms: vasculitis or deposition of rheumatoid nodules. The latter are usually not symptomatic (Spurlock and Richman, 1983; Jackson et al., 1984; Henderson et al., 1993); they may be found in the dura mater, where symptoms can result from pressure effects, or in the arachnoid. In the most substantial review of this area – a study of 17 previously published autopsy examinations – none was found to have parenchymal rheumatoid nodules. Isolated instances where nodules have apparently caused seizures are, however, recorded. Histologically, there is a central area of fibrinoid necrosis surrounded by pallisading histiocytes around which is found an infiltrate of giant cells, lymphocytes and plasma cells – a picture identical to that of subcutaneous rheumatoid nodules (Bathon *et al.*, 1989).

Cerebral vasculitis usually occurs in the context of multisystem vasculitic rheumatoid disease. It is not common – Scott *et al.* (1981) reviewed 50 cases of systemic rheumatoid vasculitis and found none of them to have neurological symptomatology. Only a dozen or so cases have been reported (Ramos and Mandybur, 1975). The clinical manifestations are predictably unpredictable, in keeping with cerebral vasculitis of other aetiologies (see Chapter 10), and include seizures, encephalopathy, and focal cerebral and cerebellar signs. In the two patients seen by the author, very high rheumatoid factor levels were found; neither had active arthritis or synovitis at the time of their cerebral disease (Scolding *et al.*, 1998). There is some evidence supporting the use of cyclophosphamide in rheumatoid-associated vasculitis (Luqmani *et al.*, 1994). Recently, the accepted view that rheumatoid vasculitis carried a worse prognosis than conventional non-vasculitic disease has been called into question (Mitchell *et al.*, 1986; Vollertsen *et al.*, 1986; Geirsson *et al.*, 1987).

In an excellent and informative review, Bathon *et al.* (1989) studied inflammatory CNS involvement in rheumatoid disease in 19 reported cases of well-validated disease, including one of their own.

The majority had long-standing, usually moderate-to-severely disabling seropositive disease. In the 11 whose rheumatoid factor titres were recorded, seven had values greater than 1:1000 – a proportion which might be increased to nine out of 13 cases if the current author's cases are included (Scolding *et al.*, 1998). These findings are consistent with the suggestion that rheumatoid factor/antigen immune complexes are mechanistically responsible for the vasculitic process. Of substantial practical importance is the observation that only five out of 13 (and five out of 15 including our patients) had signs of active synovitis, and only one had obvious evidence of vasculitis elsewhere (in the skin) – though at post-mortem study, four had visceral or cutaneous vasculitis. Four out of 19 (five out of 21 including our patients) had a fever.

Bathon *et al.* identified a third pattern in addition to the previously recognized vasculitis and nodule formation, non-specific meningeal inflammation with infiltration with lymphocytes and plasma cells, multinuclear giant cells and occasional areas of necrosis (Bathon *et al.*, 1989). They also noted that in over half the reported cases, combinations of all three complications – vasculitis, rheumatoid nodule formation and meningeal involvement – were apparent histopathologically. Nodules were far more likely than meningitis or vasculitis to be asymptomatic. Only two out of 11 cases had rheumatoid nodules unaccompanied by subcutaneous nodules. Spinal fluid examination usually showed a raised protein and a pleocytosis. Clinically, cranial neuropathies, headache and fever were common, as might be predicted, with or without features precipitated by the concurrent processes of vasculitis and/or rheumatoid nodules.

Unfortunately, insufficient treatment details in the previously published cases allowed Bathon *et al.* to draw no firm conclusions concerning specific treatment. The current author recommends cyclophosphamide and steroids in clearly established rheumatoid cerebral vasculitis (see Chapter 10).

Sjögren's syndrome

Sjögren's syndrome characteristically comprises a triad of (i) keratocon-junctivitis sicca and (ii) xerostomia, occurring (in approximately 50% of cases) in (iii) the context of another connective tissue, usually rheumatoid arthritis (Fox and Theofilopoulos, 1996; Manthorpe *et al.*, 1997). There is a strong HLA association (with HLA-DR3) (Pease *et al.*, 1989). The inflammatory infiltrate within affected exocrine glands is largely composed of $CD4^+$ T lymphocytes. Beyond this, the cause is unknown. Investigations seeking to identify viruses known to infect salivary glands – such as Epstein–Barr virus and cytomegalovirus – have provided some evidence of their involvement, though the case remains unproven (Venables and Rigby, 1997). Among the collagen vascular disorders, it is second only to rheumatoid arthritis in incidence. The diagnosis is confirmed by Schirmer's test (less than 5 mm wetness achieved in 5 min) or, increasingly, by the relatively straightforward procedure of minor salivary gland biopsy, which shows destruction and fibrosis of glandular tissue with a lymphocytic infiltrate (Alexander, 1992). Speckled anti-nuclear antibodies of the anti-Ro (SS-A) or anti-La (SS-B) are present in up to 75–80% of patients (see Table 7.1).

Table 7.1 Autoantibodies and their connective tissue disease associations

Immunofluorescence pattern	Antibody	Disease associations
Rim anti-nuclear antibodies	Anti-native DNA (anti-dsDNA)	Systemic lupus erythematosus (50%)
Homogeneous anti-nuclear antibodies	Anti-histone	Drug-induced lupus (97%) (n.b. low titre (< 1:320) in normals)
Speckled anti-nuclear antibodies	Anti-Ro (SS-A)	Sjögren's syndrome (75%) Systemic lupus erythematosus (30%)
	Anti-La (SS-B)	Sjögren's (60%) Systemic lupus erythematosus (15%)
	Anti-Scl-70	Systemic sclerosis (50%)
	Anti-Sm	Systemic lupus erythematosus (75%)
	Anti-RNP (Anti-U1–nRNP)	Mixed connective tissue disease (95%) Systemic lupus erythematosus (30%)
Nucleolar anti-nuclear antibodies	Anti-PM-Scl	?Identifies polymyositis/scleroderma overlap
Other organelles	Anti-centromere	Systemic sclerosis (85%)

Systemic manifestations, occurring in up to 25% of patients, include a vasculitic skin rash, interstitial nephritis, lymphadenopathy and, uncommonly, interstitial pneumonitis. There is an increased incidence of lymphoma. Conventionally, the principal neurological manifestations have been held to be peripheral, with descriptions of both a (predominantly sensory and probably vasculitic) neuropathy and of myositis. Trigeminal sensory neuropathy is also classically described (Kaltreider and Talal, 1969).

More recently, attention has been drawn to various CNS complications of the disorder, particularly by Alexander's group, quoting a frequency of up to 25% (Alexander, 1986; Spezialetti *et al.*, 1993) – though it must be said that others have consistently reported significantly lower frequencies (Binder *et al.*, 1988; Andonopoulos *et al.*, 1990). Seizures, focal stroke-like or brainstem neurological deficits may occur, as may an encephalopathy with or without an aseptic meningitis, often with raised cerebrospinal fluid (CSF) pressure, protein level and white cell count, together with oligoclonal immunoglobulin bands (Alexander, 1992). Psychiatric abnormalities, ranging from affective disorders to dementia, may occur in up to a quarter of patients (Feinglass *et al.*, 1976; Adelman *et al.*, 1986; Asherson *et al.*, 1993; Miguel *et al.*, 1994; West *et al.*, 1995). Spinal cord involvement may take the form of an acute transverse myelitis, a chronic myelopathy, or intraspinal haemorrhage.

From these widely variable neurological manifestations, Alexander and colleagues (Alexander *et al.*, 1986) have delineated a unique series of 20 patients in whom the neurological features appeared closely to resemble multiple sclerosis and indeed had led to this diagnosis in many. CNS symptoms anteceded the diagnosis of Sjögren's syndrome in 13 out of 20 cases (although sicca symptoms had often been present for many years). A relapsing–remitting course was apparent in most, though four had a chronic progressive course. Episodes of spinal cord disease, optic neuropathy, cerebellar ataxia and internuclear ophthalmoplegia all were seen, and all 20 patients met the Poser criteria for clinically definite multiple sclerosis (see p. 30). Over 50%, however, had additional features of peripheral neuropathy, myositis or undefined 'inflammatory vascular disease'. Fifteen out of 18 tested patients had abnormal brainstem, somatosensory or visual evoked potentials. Eleven out of 18 had one immunoglobulin band, three had two bands and two patients had more than two bands. Nine patients had a mild lymphocytosis in the spinal fluid. No magnetic resonance imaging (MRI) data were reported, although the same authors have reported MRI changes similar to those of multiple sclerosis in Sjögren's patients (Alexander *et al.*, 1988) – others, however, suggest that MRI changes are rather infrequent (Manthorpe *et al.*, 1992). Thirteen out of 20 patients had autoantibodies, most commonly anti-nuclear, anti-Ro or anti-La. In this report, the authors describe 'biopsy-documented vasculitis (skin in four and muscle in four)' in eight cases, though later mention that these patients had 'biopsy-documented *inflammation* (my italics) of skin or muscle (vasculitis or myositis)'; the pathological basis of the CNS disorder remains unclear.

Tesar *et al.* (1992) have described optic neuropathy with Sjögren's syndrome in three patients, two of whom had other neurological features – though some, such as bilateral third, fourth and sixth nerve palsies, were not typical of multiple sclerosis. Again, features of Sjögren's syndrome had not emerged prior to neurological presentation in two cases. Neither had oligoclonal immunoglobulin bands; all three had unequivocal Sjögren's syndrome with strongly positive anti-nuclear and anti-Ro antibodies, confirmed by salivary gland biopsy. Two patients improved with oral steroids alone, the third with steroids plus cyclophosphamide. A spectrum of autoimmune optic neuropathies has been suggested (Kupersmith *et al.*, 1988), within which that associated with Sjögren's syndrome might be included (see below, *Systemic lupus erythematosus* and also Chapter 3).

In respect of other neurological complications of Sjögren's syndrome, the pathogenesis also remains unclear. Small vessel vasculitis has been suggested as the cause of focal lesions (Molina *et al.*, 1985). Alexander's group reports the presence of anti-neuronal antibodies in cases complicated by neuropsy-chiatric features (Alexander *et al.*, 1988; Spezialetti *et al.*, 1993) and suggest these are responsible.

Steroids may be insufficient for patients with CNS complications of Sjögren's syndrome; more powerful immunosuppressants are probably more useful, though, as is so often the case, their value is yet to be proven objectively.

Systemic sclerosis

Systemic sclerosis results from the excessive deposition of collagen in the skin and other affected tissues, but perhaps particularly centred upon blood vessels (LeRoy, 1996). An immune aetiology is generally accepted (Black, 1995; White, 1996); there is an association with MHC Class II antigens (Briggs *et al.*, 1993). An inflammatory perivascular infiltrate, most marked at sites of active connective tissue deposition, is mainly composed of T cells (Prescott *et al.*, 1992). Lymphocyte-derived cytokines exhibit marked effects on fibroblast proliferation and on collagen synthesis (LeRoy, 1994, 1996), and the expansion of clones of fibroblasts actively producing collagen accompanies clinical disease progression (Kahari, 1993).

The cutaneous manifestation, scleroderma, may exist in isolation, but in the multisystem form of the disease it is accompanied by Raynaud's phenomenon, which may be severe and accompanied by distal gangrenous changes, atrophy of subcutaneous tissues, and calcinosis, telangiectasia and oesophageal strictures. Similar changes may affect the pleura and pericardia, and glomerulonephritis may be seen. Eye involvement comprises kerato-conjunctivitis, cataract and subluxation of the lens.

Neurological complications are clearly described but not common (Cerinic *et al.*, 1996). Peripheral disease predominates, and trigeminal neuropathy, often with pain, appears particularly to occur in this context (Teasdall *et al.*, 1980), Farrell reporting a frequency of 4% (Farrell and Medsger, 1982). The neuropathy may antecede symptoms of systemic sclerosis, and additional cranial nerves may also be involved. A myopathy, with elevated CPK levels, is said to occur in up to 20% of patients (Averbuch Heller *et al.*, 1992).

There are a small number of isolated case reports of angiographically diagnosed cerebral vasculitis occurring in systemic sclerosis (e.g. Estey *et al.*, 1979); none had histopathological confirmation, so that the term 'angio-pathy' might be preferable. In the majority of patients with CNS disease, an indirect link – with hypertension, hypoxia or drug treatments – or co-incidence appears the most likely explanation (Gordon and Silverstein, 1970).

Averbuch Heller *et al.*, in their series of 50 patients with progressive systemic sclerosis, draw attention to three patients (6%) with cerebrovas-cular disease (all aged 50 or over) (Averbuch Heller *et al.*, 1992). More strikingly, however, four individuals (8%), aged 22–43, suffered a myelo-pathy – cervical in three – with no (other) identifiable cause. Cerebrospinal fluid protein was modestly elevated in only a single patient; imaging of the spinal cord was normal. Interestingly, three of these patients had gastrointestinal involvement from their systemic sclerosis, though none (despite intensive investigation) had any evidence of malabsorption. A specific association of systemic sclerosis with myelopathy is therefore possible and awaits confirmation.

The management of systemic sclerosis remains very difficult (Black, 1995; Pope, 1996). There have been open studies of cyclosporin A, plasmapheresis, anti-thymocyte globulin, methotrexate, cyclophosphamide, penicillamine, and interferon-α and -γ which all have been reported as showing promise. Controlled trials have failed to confirm any benefit from penicillamine (or chlorambucil), while anti-thymocyte globulin and photopheresis (extracorporeal treatment with photoactivated methoxy-psoralen to inhibit activated T lymphocytes) have shown some benefit in small comparative or controlled trials (Black, 1995; Anonymous 1996; Pope, 1996).

Mixed connective tissue disease

In this disorder, features of scleroderma, polymyositis and systemic lupus erythematosus (SLE) coincide, and high levels of antibodies directed against extractable nuclear antigens – ribonucleoproteins (RNP) – are found (Table 7.1). Rheumatoid factor is also often present. In common with both systemic sclerosis and Sjögren's syndrome, trigeminal neuralgia and/or sensory neuropathy are described.

Central nervous system complications were not common in the original series of 25 mixed connective tissue disease (MCTD) patients (Nimelstein *et al.*, 1980) but Bennet *et al.* (1978) studied 20 patients and reported a range of neurological features in 11 (55%), including aseptic meningitis in four (20%) and seizures in two. Psychotic illnesses occurred in three and a subsequent study further emphasized the importance of neuropsychiatric disease (Bennett and O'Connell, 1980); so that the neurological features of MCTD, in common with the systemic features, appear to comprise a mixture of those found in lupus and systemic sclerosis. Stroke with small vessel vasculitis is reported in childhood MCTD (Graf *et al.*, 1993).

Systemic lupus erythematosus

Systemic lupus erythematosus is an autoimmune multisystem disease which, like many related disorders, occurs more in women than men – some authors put the ratio in adults as high as 21 : 1. Blacks are more commonly affected than whites. Fever and general malaise are accompanied by skin changes – classically, the malar butterfly rash, though various other non-specific manifestations, most typically, photosensitivity, are also described – and a largely symmetrical, non-erosive arthritis affecting large and small joints. Glomerulonephritis, pleurisy and pneumonitis, pericarditis and (so-called) Libmann–Sachs endocarditis, and haematological disorders, are among the commoner complications, the latter more specifically including thrombocytopenia, leukocytopenia and anaemia, and the generation of circulating anticoagulants. Other laboratory abnormalities include the presence of a variety of auto-antibodies, including anti-nuclear antibodies and anti-native DNA antibodies. Speckled or rarely nucleolar anti-nuclear staining may also be found, with antibody specificities illustrated in Table 7.1.

The diagnosis – particularly for research and therapeutic trial purposes – is now commonly based on the widely accepted revised diagnostic criteria (Table 7.2) suggested by the American College of Rheumatology (Tan *et al.*, 1982). The presence of any four (or more) of the listed features, "serially or simultaneously, during *any interval* of observation" (my italics) are sufficient for the diagnosis, with an estimated specificity and sensitivity of 96%.

Table 7.2 American College of Rheumatology diagnostic criteria for systemic lupus erythematosus (Tan *et al.*, 1982)

"A person shall be said to have systemic lupus erythematosus if four or more of the 11 criteria are present, serially or simultaneously, during any interval of observation" (Tan et al.*, 1982)*

- malar flush
- discoid rash
- photosensitivity
- oral ulcers
- arthritis
- serositis (pleurisy or pericarditis)
- renal disorder (proteinuria above 0.5 g/24 h or cellular casts)
- neurological disorder (seizures, psychosis; other causes excluded)
- haematological disorder (haemolytic anaemia, leukopenia or lymphopenia on two or more occasions, or thrombocytopenia)
- immunological disorder – LE cells, or anti-dsDNA or anti-Sm or persistent false positive syphilis serology
- anti-nuclear autoantibodies

Neurological sequelae

Neurological involvement in SLE is not rare – though to be more precise is not easy. Various estimates offer an incidence ranging from 25 to 75% (Adelman *et al.*, 1986; Futrell *et al.*, 1992), 50% representing a reasonable consensus figure (Lee *et al.*, 1977). Neurological *presentation,* however, is uncommon, occurring in perhaps 3% of cases (Feinglass *et al.*, 1976; Tola *et al.*, 1992). In established SLE, CNS involvement is a poor prognostic sign: a 5 year survival figure of 55% has been quoted, compared to 75% for patients without neurological features (Brick and Brick, 1989), while epidemiological studies show neurological disease to be second only to renal involvement as the cause of death, significantly excluding iatrogenic causes (Rosner *et al.*, 1982).

An enormous variety of complications can occur: any list claiming comprehensiveness would include psychiatric and cognitive disturbances, fits, myelitis, strokes and movement disorders, ataxia and brainstem abnormalities, and cranial and peripheral neuropathies (Figure 7.1). This spectrum reflects the existence of a range of aetiological mechanisms, so that cerebral lupus cannot be said to represent a single clinical or pathological entity (Kaell *et al.*, 1986). Although a number of consistent associations are apparent, such as the neurological picture associated with anti-cardiolipin

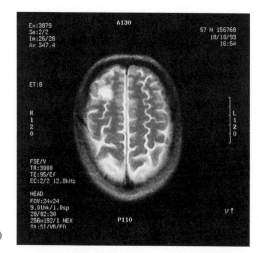

(a)

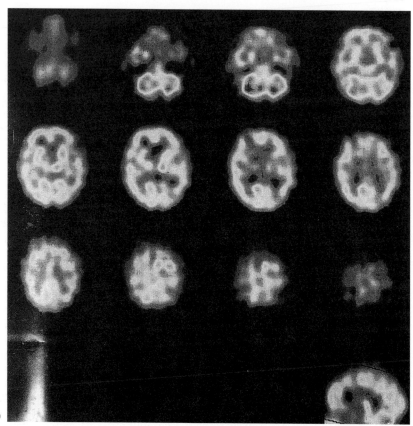

(b)

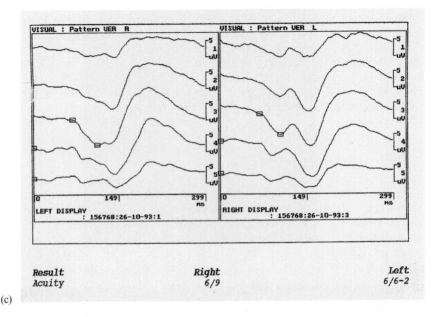

Result	Right	Left
Acuity	6/9	6/6-2

(c)

Figure 7.1 Cerebral lupus. These are investigations of a 69-year-old man with chorea, cognitive decline and a subclinical optic neuropathy; anti-nuclear serology was strongly positive, with anti-Sm antibodies and, at one stage, a thrombocytopenia. (Genetic testing for Huntington's disease revealed a normal triplet repeat number.) Magnetic resonance imaging scanning (a) showed only a single intensity lesion high in the right hemisphere, while single particle emission computed tomography images (b) indicated multiple small areas of hypoperfusion in both hemispheres, anteriorly and posteriorly. Visual evoked potential measurement (c) showed a substantially delayed potential on the right (115 versus 103 ms on the left).

antibodies (ACA), and a number of potential pathogenetic mechanisms underlying other CNS manifestations have been offered, well-substantiated and widely accepted explanations for each neurological syndrome have not emerged, so that a rational classification is not yet possible; once again, one therefore falls back on phenomenonology.

Headache

Although headache occurs very frequently in the normal population, there seems little doubt that it is commoner in patients with SLE. Its occurrence typifies the difficulty of pigeon-holing neurological aspects of SLE, inasmuch as a number of underlying causes are possible.

Migraine appears to occur with greater frequency in patients with SLE, although formal epidemiological comparisons are lacking. It was initially suggested that migraine represented a component of the anti-cardiolipin syndrome (Hughes *et al.*, 1986; see below), though more formal studies later indicated that this did not appear to be so (Montalban *et al.*, 1992) – there is no difference in the incidence of ACA between lupus patients with migraine and normal controls (Tsakiris *et al.*, 1993).

Other headache types also occur. The general increase in coagulability contributes to the increased incidence of *dural sinus thrombosis* in SLE (Vidailhet *et al.*, 1990). *Idiopathic intracranial hypertension* is also reported. *Aseptic meningitis* or meningoencephalitis both include headache in their symptomatology. Pathologically, meningeal inflammation is found in almost one-fifth of patients (Ellis and Verity, 1979). Drug-related problems, specifically *infectious meningitis* in immunocompromised patients, must not be overlooked.

Seizures

Seizures occur in 20–25% of patients with lupus, compared to 0.5–1.0% in normal populations, and therefore represent the commonest major neurological complication. They are said to be more frequent in chronic and in severe systemic disease – by the time of death, 30–50% of patients have experienced one or more seizures (Futrell *et al.*, 1992). Partial and generalized fits occur. Other clinical evidence of disease activity is frequently present, systemically, neurologically or both. Neuropsychiatric manifestations are particularly associated; the electroencephalogram is diffusely abnormal, often without unequivocal seizure activity, and a CSF pleocytosis is common. In such cases, a lupus-related encephalopathy appears to be the case.

Epilepsy may also occur in isolation. An association with the presence of high-titre IgG ACA (see below) in SLE and epilepsy has been suggested: out of 221 patients with SLE, 21 were found to have epilepsy and almost 50% of patients had ACA (Herranz *et al.*, 1994). Others have confirmed a relationship between the presence of isolated epilepsy as a complication of lupus and the presence of ACA antibodies (Liou *et al.*, 1996).

In other patients, seizures may be related to immune suppressive-related opportunistic infection or to metabolic decompensation from lupus-induced renal disease. Finally, a significant proportion of SLE-related seizures are presumed to result from old cerebral infarcts, approximately 50% of patients with fits having had past strokes (Futrell *et al.*, 1992).

There are no proper comparative trials of anti-convulsants in SLE-related seizures; it has been said that a greater incidence of drug sensitivity occurs (Futrell *et al.*, 1992).

Behavioural, cognitive and neuropsychiatric changes

While pleomorphism is the rule, rather than a characteristic or typical clinical picture, three relatively distinct patterns can be discerned: 'pure' behavioural or psychiatric illness without clouding of consciousness, dementia and an acute or subacute encephalopathy/encephalitis (organic confusional syndrome or delirium). Psychiatric disorders commonly co-exist with other signs of CNS disease (Miguel *et al.*, 1994). The difficulty in diagnostic criteria for these disorders has contributed to the widely varying estimates of their incidence, which range from around 30–75%.

Affective disorders, particularly depression, visual and auditory hallucinations, psychoses, catatonia and conversion disorders are moderately common complications of SLE, one carefully documented prospective study suggesting a prevalence of 20–25% (Hay, 1994). Recurrent, episodic symptoms are common.

Dementia is a commonly accepted complication, though rather little detailed published information is available. An incidence of cognitive changes in lupus of 55% has been suggested (Denburg et al., 1987, 1997) but an important and well-validated observation is that cognitive dysfunction in SLE is very often reversible (Hanly et al., 1997). This does not apply, however, to multi-infarct dementia, which is also described in lupus (Asherson et al., 1989; Briley et al., 1989), presumably a consequence of SLE-related cerebro- or cardiovascular complications.

Encephalopathy

An encephalopathic presentation, with clouding of consciousness with or without headache, often with seizures and usually without focal neurological signs, is also well recognized in SLE. Some have termed this entity *cerebral lupus*, though *lupus encephalopathy* is preferable. CSF examination may reveal a raised protein level and a neutrophil or lymphocyte pleocytosis. It is clearly vital in such cases to exclude infectious complications of immune suppressants or steroids, which have become a major cause of death in patients with SLE (Rosner et al., 1982). Bacterial (including mycobacterial), viral or fungal meningitis or meningo-encephalitis may be seen, and should be sought with vigour.

Stroke, the lupus anticoagulant and the primary phospholipid syndrome

Anti-cardiolipin antibodies (ACA), which may be of IgG, IgM or IgA isotype, form part of a spectrum of circulating antibodies directed against phospholipids; they are responsible for the Wasserman reaction in syphilis. It has been recognized for many years – or even decades – that 'false positive' Wasserman reaction tests are not uncommon and that individuals with such tests exhibit an increased incidence of autoimmune diseases, particularly SLE.

It has also been known for several decades that many patients with SLE possess circulating anticoagulant factors, so-called lupus anticoagulants (LA), and that the presence of these factors is paradoxically associated not with haemorrhage, but with arterial and venous thrombosis. It was subsequently shown that LA activity, detectable by prolongation of the activated partial thromboplastin time and the Russell Viper Venom time, reflected the inhibition of clot formation (*in vitro*) by certain anti-cardiolipin antibodies, and that ACA and LA positivity commonly co-existed (though not invariably, see below, *Management of central nervous system complications of lupus*, p. 168).

The thrombotic tendency in patients with SLE and LA manifests itself principally in the form of stroke and recurrent spontaneous abortion (Hughes, 1983; McCart and Farid, 1994). Intra-abdominal and deep venous thrombosis, and peripheral arterial thrombosis are also seen. Thrombocytopenia was a key additional feature.

Importantly from a practical neurological consideration, Hughes also showed that a similar clinical picture was associated with the presence of

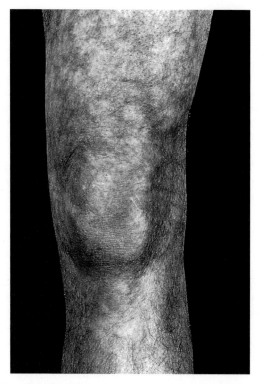

Figure 7.2 Sneddon's syndrome. A 72-year-old man developed a left hemiplegia and was found to have marked livedo reticulares. He had positive anti-cardiolipin antibody (ACA) serology. Not all patients with so-called Sneddon's syndrome have ACA.

ACA and/or LA in patients *without* serological or clinical evidence of SLE, and introduced the term 'anti-phospholipid syndrome' (APS) (see Hughes, 1983). Primary APS (i.e. APS without lupus) was shown also to include those patients described by Sneddon as having stroke in association with livedo reticulares (Figure 7.2). Not all patients with Sneddon syndrome, however, have APS – one study suggesting less than half are antibody positive, and also indicating the presence of APS in Sneddon syndrome did not correlate with severity of disease (Tourbah *et al.*, 1996). Although recurrent miscarriages and deep venous thrombosis (DVT) are still widely held to be particular associations with the primary APS, a recent European multicentre investigation has shown there to be few differences in clinical or laboratory features of primary and secondary APSs. Studying 142 patients, the only significant differences to emerge were greater incidences of autoimmune haemolytic anaemia, valvular heart disease, neutropenia, abnormal C4 levels and (most predictably of all) double-stranded DNA and extractable nuclear antigens (ENA) antibodies in patients with secondary APS (i.e. APS and lupus) (Vianna *et al.*, 1994).

Central nervous system thrombosis in patients with primary or secondary APS takes the form of completed arterial stroke or repeated transient ischaemic attacks (TIAs). (Neuroimaging studies again suggest no significant differences in the incidence of multifocal small white matter lesions, or of large vessel strokes, between patients with primary or secondary APS (Provenzale *et al.*, 1996).) Multiple strokes, and indeed multi-infarct dementia, are also seen, as is cerebral venous sinus thrombosis. Although for some years it was argued that the link between ACA and stroke might not be a true association, an epidemiologically robust study in 1993 showed conclusively that ACAs were an independent risk factor for stroke; they were found in almost 10% of stroke patients, compared to 4.3% controls, and conferred an increased risk of 2.31 after adjustment for age and other risk factors including hypertension, diabetes, smoking and heart disease (Anonymous, 1993). Controversy to some extent continues, however, recent work suggests there is no increase in the risk of second stroke in patients found to be antibody positive when tested at the time of the first event (Anonymous, 1993) – yet others suggest there is a significant risk only if there is a high titre (above 40 g/l) IgG ACA (Levine *et al.*, 1997). The background 4–5% figure for ACA positivity in healthy controls offers obvious complications for the interpretation of a positive result in individual cases.

It has also emerged that other neurological features are associated with APA. Chorea (Cervera *et al.*, 1997) is seen, with histopathological study of the small vessels showing no evidence of vasculitis, but rather of a coagulative vasculopathy (Hughson *et al.*, 1993). Recent large case controlled studies (reviewed in Levine and Brey, 1996) suggest the putative link with migraine may be factitious.

Briley *et al.* studied 25 patients with neurological features and ACA (out of a total of 80 patients found on haemostatic screening to be ACA[+]) (Briley *et al.*, 1989). Eighteen out of 25 were anti-nuclear antibody (ANA)[+], 15 with clinical evidence of a lupus-like disorder. Four distinct neurological patterns emerged. Two – multiple cerebral infarctions (in 16 patients), and vascular visual problems (six patients) including amaurosis fugax and ischaemic retinopathy – were thrombotic/vascular in nature, and might be anticipated; the authors also found six patients to have migraine.

Perhaps more interestingly, four patients suffered an *acute ischaemic encephalopathy* (Briley *et al.*, 1989). These individuals were acutely ill, with confusion and obtundation accompanied by asymmetrical hyper-reflexic quadriparesis with bilateral extensor plantar responses. Fits occurred in only one patient. In three, the encephalopathic illness occurred in the context of systemic disturbances, with dermatological manifestations (three out of three cases had livedo reticulares, with biopsies showing fibrin thrombi but no vasculitis) and mild renal failure (also three out of three). The fourth had haemolytic anaemia and a thrombocytopenia (but was ANA[-]).

All had significantly higher levels of ACA compared with the non-encephalopathic cases, while LA was present in three out of four patients. All four had thrombocytopenia, and ANA testing was positive in two, but no other features of disseminated lupus were present. Spinal fluid examination revealed an elevated protein and cell count in only one case; one other had a raised protein alone.

Two died, with post-mortem studies revealing bilateral cortical infarction, with a thrombotic vasculopathy, fibrin deposition, but no evidence of vasculitis – findings identical to the skin biopsy. The two who survived received steroids, one with azathioprine, the other with cyclophosphamide and plasmapheresis (Briley *et al.*, 1989).

It seems likely that this disorder is a closely related and (to some extent) more focal variant of the recently described *catastrophic APS*, in which there is severe multi-organ failure and a mortality of the order of 60% (Asherson and Piette, 1996). Approximately 40% are 'primary', with negative ANA testing. It is suggested that plasmapheresis is also useful in this disorder (Asherson and Piette, 1996).

Chorea and other dyskinesias

Although chorea has acquired the status of a classical neurological feature of lupus (see, e.g. Bruyn and Padberg 1984), it is found in only some 2% of cases in large series (Lusins and Szilagyi, 1975). Athetosis and ballismus are also reported, as are akinetic rigid syndromes, with or without tremor (Johnson and Richardson, 1968). In some cases, chorea may be the presenting feature of SLE, occasionally occurring as an isolated phenomenon during pregnancy and acquiring the label of 'chorea gravidarum', other manifestations of SLE emerging only later (Donaldson and Espiner, 1971). It is often of abrupt onset (consistent with a vascular origin) and can occur as hemi-chorea.

An association of chorea with ACA was suggested in early descriptions of the APS, and chorea gravidarum and oral contraceptive pill-associated chorea have also been linked to APA (Omdal and Roalso, 1992). Several studies provided further evidence of a link between chorea and APA (Cervera *et al.*, 1997; Asherson *et al.*, 1987), although in one report of 80 patients with significantly elevated ACA, 25 of whom had neurological features, none had chorea (Briley *et al.*, 1989); similarly, chorea was not recorded in any of 48 patients with neurological disease and APA (Levine *et al.*, 1990).

Transverse myelitis and systemic lupus erythematosus

Myelopathy is an established but unusual manifestation of CNS lupus (Mok *et al.*, 1998). Ellis and Verity's series (Ellis and Verity, 1979) recorded only one case in 57 autopsied patients; Johnson and Richardson (1968) found one of 24 cases to have a myelopathy, and Futrell *et al.* (1992) also found only a single case in their study of 63 patients with CNS lupus. It is usually acute or subacute and may rarely occur as the presenting feature of SLE (Andrianakos *et al.*, 1975). There is usually an elevated CSF protein and lymphocyte count, but a significantly depressed glucose level may be a slightly more useful change from a diagnostic perspective (Warren and Kredich, 1984). Contrariwise, the CSF can frequently be entirely normal (Chan and Boey, 1996). A link with ACA has been suggested (Lavalle *et al.*, 1990) but not confirmed (Mok *et al.*, 1998). Some cases of acute transverse myelopathy in lupus have been found to be primarily compressive in origin, caused by haematomata, emphasizing the (usual) importance of urgent imaging of the spinal cord in all patients. A good functional outcome is well-described (Chan and Boey, 1996).

Autoimmune optic neuropathy

In common with transverse myelitis, optic neuritis or neuropathy is recognized in neurological SLE, often included in reviews of the subject, but not common – probably substantially rarer, in fact, than cord disease. Thus, none of the total of 81 autopsied patients reported by Johnson and Richardson or by Ellis and Verity was described as having optic nerve disease, though allusion is made to isolated cases reported elsewhere (Ellis and Verity, 1979; Johnson and Richardson, 1968). Futrell *et al.* also found none of their 63 patients with CNS lupus to have optic neuritis, though six had 'visual abnormalities' (Futrell *et al.*, 1992).

Autoimmune optic neuritis or *neuropathy* is, however, reasonably well described in the ophthalmological literature. In 1982, Dutton *et al.* reported three female patients with unilateral or bilateral optic neuropathies with significantly positive anti-nuclear factors; two also had an elevated erythrocyte sedimentation rate (ESR) and CSF oligoclonal bands (Dutton *et al.*, 1982). Pain was a common feature and the visual symptoms were subacute in onset in two cases, suggesting to the authors an inflammatory, rather than a vascular cause. No patients would have met the diagnostic criteria for SLE.

Kupersmith *et al.* reported a further 14 cases, 12 women (Kupersmith *et al.*, 1988). They also found visual loss to be subacute and progressive, and commonly very severe (worst acuity less than 20/200 in most cases), but in their experience, the disorder was usually not painful. None had overt signs of systemic lupus. The ESR was elevated in only three cases. ANA testing was positive in 11; in the remaining three, ACA alone were present (IgM), while one of three ANA$^+$ patients tested for ACA also had IgM reactivity. Interestingly, biopsies of normal-appearing skin revealed immune complex deposition in five out of seven cases. Cerebrospinal fluid oligoclonal bands were present in two out of 13 cases analysed and no case had MRI changes typical of multiple sclerosis. The authors emphasized a significant response to treatment only with very high doses of intravenous steroids – 1.0–2.0 g methylprednisolone daily for 5–7 days – often followed by immunosuppressive treatment (chlorambucil, azathioprine or cyclophosphamide).

Other focal manifestations of central nervous system lupus

Focal brainstem abnormalities, cerebellar disturbances and cranial neuropathies also are seen in the context of SLE – Johnson and Richardson suggesting an incidence of around 40% in their own cases (Johnson and Richardson, 1968), though most other series have reported a lower figure perhaps of the order of 10–30%. Although peripheral cranial nerve involvement can occur, the majority of cranial neuropathies are thought to arise from brainstem disturbances, probably microvascular infarcts (Johnson and Richardson, 1968).

Systemic lupus erythematosus and multiple sclerosis: 'lupoid sclerosis'

The occurrence of neurological features which include optic neuritis (albeit rarely), subacute myelopathy, brainstem and cerebellar syndromes, and other transient neurological deficits, led to the suggestion of a possible relationship between the two disorders: the term 'lupoid sclerosis' was introduced by Fulford *et al.* (1972).

However, as pathological studies indicate (see below), primary demyelination does not form part of the wide spectrum of changes found in the larger series of patients with established CNS lupus (Ellis and Verity, 1979; Johnson and Richardson, 1968); even the syndrome of myelopathy in SLE has, as its pathological basis, not primary inflammatory demyelination but either infarction, haematoma or a vacuolar necrotic change – so-called 'subpial leukomyelopathy'. The changes are peripherally distributed and affect white more than grey matter; microscopically there is loss of axon cylinders as well as myelin (Allen *et al.*, 1979; Provenzale *et al.*, 1996). This very clear pathological difference alone is sufficient to emphasize the separateness of the two disorders and it has been suggested that those few cases reported in which systemic (lupus) disease has been accompanied by clear changes in the CNS typical of multiple sclerosis (e.g. Shepherd *et al.*, 1974), may represent the simple co-existence of two disorders, neither excessively rare (Matthews, 1991).

The clinical distinction is generally not difficult, systemic features pointing away from a primary CNS disorder. When lupus presents with exclusively neurological manifestations, and these have the character of those occurring in multiple sclerosis, a high ESR is generally the most useful pointer away from that diagnosis (Matthews, 1991). Low-titre ANA are reported in 81% of patients with multiple sclerosis (Dore *et al.*, 1982), although many neurologists might find this outside their general experience, and undue emphasis clearly cannot be placed on such a result. Most authorities suggest that further testing is warranted only with ANA titres greater than 1:160: over 95% of those with titres positive but more dilute will have no identifiable underlying disease (Homburger, 1995; Tan *et al.*, 1997). The CSF in lupus is more likely to contain a significantly elevated cell count, and rather less likely to exhibit oligoclonal immunoglobulin bands. Figures vary, and while West *et al.* report positive results in approximately 50% of patients (West *et al.*, 1995), other series have lower figures, e.g. even among those patients with autoimmune optic neuropathy, only two out of 13 had oligoclonal bands (Kupersmith *et al.*, 1988).

Magnetic resonance imaging in CNS lupus has also been studied (Miller *et al.*, 1992): abnormalities were present in only nine of 15 patients and these affected the white matter in eight. Although (mild) periventricular changes were present in five cases, multiple subcortical lesions were more common – unlike those typical of multiple sclerosis. Also, the pattern of gadolinium enhancement, which was only seen in two lesions – both large, cortical, located at a site appropriate to the neurological symptoms (i.e. clinically eloquent) and resolving rapidly in conjunction with immunosuppressive treatment – was also rather different from that seen in multiple sclerosis.

Thus, while clinical signs, CSF analysis and MRI abnormalities *may* each resemble those seen in multiple sclerosis, and each in isolation may lead to diagnostic confusion, for all to do so concurrently, with no systemic or clear laboratory evidence of SLE is most unusual, and the distinction therefore is more commonly apparent. Matthews' intimation that "there appears to be no necessity to introduce the term 'lupoid sclerosis'" seems vindicated (Matthews, 1991).

The pathogenesis and pathology of central nervous system lupus

Neither the underlying genetic contribution, nor the fundamental nature of the immunological disturbance in lupus, are fully understood (Kotzin, 1996). A monozygotic twin concordance rate of 30%, compared with 5% for dyzygotic twins or non-twin siblings, provides powerful evidence of a polygenetic component.

What is clear from the foregoing phenomenology, however, is that the enormous spectrum of neurological symptoms and signs comprising 'CNS lupus' does not represent the manifestation of a common underlying pathological process; rather, a variety of very different lupus-driven mechanisms accounts for these syndromes.

Proposed mechanisms of tissue damage in cerebral lupus are broadly and conveniently divisible into two: (i) rheological disturbances, mediated either at the vessel wall or through involvement of the coagulation system (and also including embolic phenomena), and (ii) immunological events more directly affecting the target tissue, neurones or glia, mediated by antibodies, cytokines or lymphocytes. Histopathological studies provide a useful entry point to the first of these lupus-related processes.

Cerebral lupus as a rheopathy

The principal pathological changes in brains affected by SLE are those of infarction, as first reported by Johnson and Richardson in their classic study (Johnson and Richardson, 1968). They described 'predominantly changes related to small blood vessels. Destructive and proliferative change in arterioles and capillaries were found'. They considered that the destructive changes they described, with necrosis of the vessel wall and extravasation of fibrin and red cells, together with endothelial cell proliferation and hypertrophy and the appearance of fibrin thrombi, were responsible for the numerous areas of microinfarction and the somewhat less common occurrence of macroscopic haemorrhage, but emphasized the absence of inflammatory infiltrate within the walls of affected vessels – 'a true vasculitis cannot be considered to be the fundamental vascular change' (though such was present in a small number of their cases – three out of 24). Other authors have continued with remarkable consistency to confirm that, while vasculitis can occur as a complication of lupus, it is not at all common. Johnson and Richardson went on to suggest that "the localization of vascular changes and resultant microinfarcts in the cerebral cortex and brainstem correlate well with the clinical signs in most cases" (Johnson and Richardson, 1968).

Ellis and Verity's later and larger study of 57 cases produced broadly similar results, though notably these authors drew attention to the significantly higher incidence of CNS infection in their cases, which they not unreasonably attributed to the increasing use of immune suppressive treatment (Ellis and Verity, 1979). They distinguished large infarcts – usually found within middle cerebral territory – from areas of microinfarction (widespread, but commonest in the cortex and brainstem) and again suggested that the principal lesion was microvascular injury. Platelet deposition within the walls of affected cerebral vessels is reported in CNS lupus (Ellison et al., 1993).

Multifocal fibrin deposition within injured small vessels of uncertain cause therefore accompanies and may account for much of what is seen in patients with CNS lupus, and those with APS: it has been suggested that epilepsy and brainstem manifestations, together with less well-localized manifestations such as psychiatric disease and encephalopathy, all may be attributed to this pathological change occurring focally, multifocally or diffusely (Johnson and Richardson, 1968; Briley *et al.*, 1989).

Three mechanisms underlying the microvasculopathy of CNS lupus are commonly suggested.

(i) A direct antibody-mediated effect is one possibility. Anti-cardiolipin antibodies, binding to phospholipids in the endothelial cell membrane, can increase platelet aggregation and cause local thrombosis (Brey and Coull, 1992). Jain *et al.* studied seven cases of systemic thrombotic microangiopathy in SLE (Jain *et al.*, 1994) (previously described by other authors as *thrombotic thrombocytopenic purpura (TTP) coincident with* or *complicating SLE)*. Four patients had (undescribed) CNS complications. Jain *et al.* described renal biopsy changes in two cases, with intravascular thrombus formation and intimal proliferation but no inflammatory infiltrates. They drew attention to the presence of ACA in six out of seven cases, suggesting that these might play a role in the development of small vessel disease. Despite the apparent similarity of the histopathological changes, however, Johnson and Richardson suggested that there were subtle but significant differences between the microangiopathy of CNS lupus and that of conventional TTP, implying a different mechanism (Johnson and Richardson, 1968). Furthermore, thrombocytopenia, whilst common in SLE, has not been described as a prerequisite for the development of CNS involvement and neither is the presence of ACA. Nevertheless, the similarity of the neurological manifestations, the CNS changes of multiple microinfarcts responsible, and the (at least) superficial resemblance of microscopic abnormalities suggest a degree of commonality between TTP and CNS lupus which it might be unwise to overlook.

(ii) A less direct effect of antibodies, the formation and deposition of anti-DNA antibody – antigen or ACA – cardiolipin immune complexes, has also been suggested. Deposits of immune complex are found in skin, renal glomeruli, blood vessels, and the choroid plexus of patients with lupus (Cochrane, 1971). In murine SLE, circulating immune complexes are associated with the key pathological changes of endothelial proliferation and thrombosis (Berden *et al.*, 1983). These abnormalities occurred with chronic exposure and, importantly, were not accompanied by any inflammatory change, in marked contrast to the vasculitic findings associated with more acute immune complex exposure.

(iii) Third, chronic systemic inflammation, with its associated irregularities of cytokine activity, might contribute to vasculopathy, at least in part by up-regulating adhesion molecules (Belmont *et al.*, 1994, 1996).

The cause of the microvasculopathy therefore remains rather speculative and new suggestions continue to emerge.

Hemiparetic stroke-like events and large vessel, macroscopic infarcts, together with chorea, appear less likely to be explained by microvasculopathic processes. The occurrence of stroke in SLE is significantly associated with the presence of lupus anticoagulant or ACA, i.e. secondary APS

(Futrell *et al.*, 1992). (It might be mentioned, however, that while a substantial proportion of patients with Sneddon's syndrome of livedo reticulares and stroke (Sneddon, 1965) have an underlying ACA, other explanations must explain the significant minority who do not (Kalashnikova *et al.*, 1990).) Although a contribution of ACA to microvascular injury might play an obvious role in the development of thrombotic infarction (as mentioned above), it is thought more likely that the pro-coagulant effect lies behind large vessel disease. Anti-phospholipid antibodies can bind to a variety of circulating phospholipids and plasma proteins, including prothrombin, protein C and protein S, and are therefore capable of inhibiting coagulation in a number of ways. They may also act by binding to, and blocking the function of, β_2-glycoprotein 1, which itself has a role in inhibiting platelet activation, and factor XII activation (reviewed in Esmon *et al.*, 1997a, b; Lockshin, 1997).

Libman–Sacks endocarditis, with cerebral embolization, represents an alternative cause of large vessel stroke: one autopsy-based study suggested this may occur in up to 10% of patients with CNS lupus (Devinsky *et al.*, 1988), though other series suggest this may be an atypical experience (Johnson and Richardson, 1968). An association between the presence of valvular cardiac abnormalities and ACA has been clearly demonstrated (Leung *et al.*, 1990; Nihoyannopoulos *et al.*, 1990; Nesher *et al.*, 1997).

In a recent highly informative controlled study of 69 patients with lupus, using transoesophageal echocardiography (Roldan *et al.*, 1996), valvular thickening was found in approximately 50% of patients and vegetations in 35–40%. Fascinatingly, in second evaluations of the same patients, valvular abnormalities were observed to appear, resolve or change in appearance or size during the course of the 2–3 year interval – changes appearing to be wholly unrelated to treatment. A substantial morbidity and mortality was associated with valvular disease.

Anti-brain antibodies and central nervous system lupus
Mechanistic possibilities other than vasculopathy have also been very actively pursued, perhaps in particular for psychiatric disease and other diffuse neurological abnormalities in lupus (notwithstanding the proposal that such manifestations could share a rheological explanation). Specifically, it is suggested that there may be a direct effect of autoantibodies on neurones or glia. A neuronolytic effect of antibodies might be difficult to reconcile with the transience of many neuropsychiatric features of lupus, but reversible cell injury – including glia – by sublethal concentrations of specific antibody with complement is well described (Scolding *et al.*, 1989; Morgan, 1995). Receptor blocking or stimulation provide alternative means by which specific antibodies might cause temporary functional disturbance.

Anti-neuronal antibodies are described both in serum and spinal fluid of patients with CNS lupus (Bluestein and Woods, 1982; How *et al.*, 1985; Moore and Lisak, 1995). By way of contrast with those neurone-specific antibodies associated with paraneoplastic disease (see Chapter 5) anti-neurone antibodies in lupus can, according to some authors, cause a variety of neurological defects when injected into experimental animals (Simon and Simon, 1975).

Additionally, ACA themselves may bind to neurones and astroglia (Sun *et al.*, 1992). Specific endosomal lipids have also recently been shown to represent targets for ACA (Koyabashi *et al.* 1998). Finally, anti-ribosomal P antibodies represent a third group of antibodies suggested to correlate with CNS lupus (Bonfa *et al.*, 1987; Teh *et al.*, 1993), and more specifically with psychiatric disease (Isshi and Hirohata, 1996): a clear relationship with the anti-RNP antibody *anti-Sm* was found by one group (Hirohata and Kosaka, 1994).

It has also been proposed that focal neurological deficits and seizures may share this antibody-dependent aetiology, rather than developing in relation to microinfarcts – though the various mechanisms by which antibodies might contribute to microvascular injury indicates that these diverse proposals are by no means mutually exclusive. Others have suggested, however, that antibodies to brain membrane proteins in SLE are only circumstantially linked to neurological disturbances (Hanly *et al.*, 1993).

A number of studies have, as yet another alternative, implicated antibodies directed against, and toxic to, circulating lymphocytes, in SLE, and more specifically in neuropsychiatric disease. It may be, however, that these antibodies cross-react with neuronal components and exert their alleged effect in this way (Denburg *et al.*, 1987).

Several more indirect lines of evidence implicate antibodies and suggest the involvement of humoral mechanisms of injury. There are low serum levels of complement component C4 (Petz *et al.*, 1971), and evidence of CNS complement synthesis and activation (Jongen *et al.*, 1990) and of local antibody production (demonstrated by oligoclonal immunoglobulin band detection) within the CNS. Blood–brain barrier breakdown occurs (Winfield *et al.*, 1983; Sanders *et al.*, 1998), allowing CNS access to circulating antibody; it may be precipitated by immune complex deposition (Boyer *et al.*, 1980). It should be noted, however, that in one large study, blood–brain barrier breakdown did not correlate either with the presence of serum immune complexes or indeed with CNS complications (Winfield *et al.*, 1983). Others have shown that the presence or otherwise of immune complexes in the choroid plexus also shows no correlation with clinical CNS disease (Boyer *et al.*, 1980). The potential role of antibodies therefore remains the subject of some debate, with opposing views on whether they correlate with and/or are responsible for neural damage or disturbed function (Hay and Isenberg, 1993).

Similarly, while patients with SLE and chorea do exhibit the typical and numerous microinfarcts in various sites, Johnson and Richardson pointed out that none, surprisingly, were present in the basal ganglia (Johnson and Richardson, 1968). The observation was largely confirmed by Bruyn and Padberg, who studied 10 patients with chorea and SLE, and found basal ganglia microinfarcts in only two (Bruyn and Padberg, 1984). Conversely, there is some positive evidence that chorea is associated with ACA (Asherson *et al.*, 1987) and a direct effect of these antibodies on neurones has been postulated. Cases of chorea with strokes in the context of cardiolipin antibodies do not exhibit vasculitic change in the small vessels (Hughson *et al.*, 1993), though it should be mentioned that vasculitic pathology in APS is recorded (Goldberger *et al.*, 1992). As mentioned above, chorea gravidarum and oral contraceptive pill-associated chorea have also been linked to ACA (Omdal and Roalso, 1992), while Sydenham's chorea too has been associated with anti-neuronal antibodies (Husby *et al.*, 1979).

Finally, it should be re-emphasized that secondary problems, most particularly infections, are increasingly common causes of CNS disorder in SLE; direct meningeal or parenchymal infection, or metastatic septic infiltration – perhaps least uncommonly from endocarditis – must be sought vigorously, and, as will be indicated below, are mostly far more amenable to treatment than primary CNS lupus. Metabolic derangement, usually from renal disease or, again, secondary to drugs, must also be excluded.

Management of central nervous system complications of systemic lupus erythematosus

Much has been already said concerning investigation and diagnosis. The fundamental importance of excluding as a matter of urgency secondary and/ or iatrogenic problems – drug-related, metabolic and especially infective, has been emphasized, and the diagnostic criteria for SLE have also been described above. Useful investigations in patients with SLE presenting with possible neurological complications have been mentioned in relation to the specific syndromes.

In an interesting and helpful study, West recently addressed this topic directly, and pointed out the particular value of MRI scanning (West *et al.*, 1995), as did Miller in 1992 (Miller *et al.*, 1992). (Importantly, West *et al.* also drew attention to the usefulness of skin biopsy.) Neither magnetic resonance spectroscopy (Davie *et al.*, 1995), nor positron emission tomography scanning (Sailer *et al.*, 1997) appears helpful in the diagnosis, while single photon emission computed tomography scanning may show perfusion defects which, while lacking specificity (the same appearances are seen in vasculitis, for example), may be useful in monitoring disease activity (Kodama *et al.*, 1995). Cerebral angiography is often abnormal (Weingarten *et al.*, 1997), and also may be important in excluding cerebral venous thrombosis.

Cerebrospinal fluid oligoclonal band analysis is also useful (West *et al.*, 1995), reportedly present in up to 50% of patients with CNS lupus (Winfield *et al.*, 1983; Golombek *et al.*, 1986). As mentioned above, many authorities would not consider significant any ANA titre more dilute than 1:160 (Homburger, 1995), but seeking ANA in CSF may be useful – four out of six patients with active CNS lupus exhibiting such antibodies in one study (Mevorach *et al.*, 1994).

In seeking possible APS, it should be mentioned that over 25% of patients with positive testing for one test – LA or ACA – will be negative for the other, so that individuals under investigation should always have both tests, preferably on more than a single occasion. Of the two, it is said that LA positivity carries the greater association with thrombotic complications (Ames, 1995). In ACA positive patients, although it is commonly suggested that IgM ACA is not clinically relevant, there is some evidence that elevation of either IgG or IgM ACA is associated with thrombosis, although the risk with IgM is smaller (Escalante, 1995).

Allusion has been made to the potential value of serum anti-ribosomal P antibody testing. Watanabe *et al.* (1996) found a significant correlation between anti-ribosomal P antibodies and the presence of psychiatric disease in lupus and made the additional observation that titres fell following remission, suggesting a role for such testing in monitoring disease or treatment. Anti-ribosomal P antibodies did not prove detectable in CSF (Isshi and Hirohata, 1996).

Therapy

Despite the diversity of neurological disorders associated with SLE, therapeutic efforts have fallen largely into two broad categories – secondary stroke prevention in patients with ACA and cerebral infarct or ischaemia, and the treatment of 'other' CNS complications.

It has been suggested that ACAs are a significant independent risk factor for stroke and that patients with high titre ACA who experience a thrombotic event have a substantial risk of further events (Levine *et al.*, 1997). The most effective way of attempting to prevent recurrence remains to be established, but there is anecdotal – though increasingly compelling – evidence that aspirin alone is insufficient, while moderate to high-dose warfarin therapy may confer greater protection (Rosove and Brewer, 1992). Formal trials await completion, but a moderately large retrospective study provided the firmest evidence yet of benefit from long-term warfarin treatment, keeping the international normalized ratio at 3 or higher (Brey and Levine, 1996). Similarly, the feeling amongst those with the largest experience of managing such patients is that steroids and immunosuppressive treatments are of little benefit (Khamashta and Hughes, 1994).

Whether high-level warfarinization is similarly the treatment of choice for the severe APS-related encephalopathy remains unclear; as mentioned above, most patients with this syndrome have secondary, not primary, APS, and immune suppressant therapy with or without anticoagulation might be more rational and certainly has its advocates (Asherson and Piette, 1996). Plasma exchange may be of value.

Patients with encephalopathies, psychiatric ailments, epilepsy, chorea, or other (apparently) non-stroke CNS complications of SLE present no less of a management problem. Naturally, symptomatic therapies (anti-epileptic, anti-psychotic, anti-choreic, etc.) are used wherever necessary and usually to good effect. Many of these symptoms are (often by definition) transient, so that no more than symptomatic treatment is warranted. Chorea, isolated fits, headache and some psychiatric disorders particularly fall into this category. There is some evidence that steroids may be of considerable value in treating the valvular abnormalities associated with lupus (Nesher *et al.*, 1997).

However, in more persistent or severe manifestations, the underlying disease process is treated primarily as one of brain inflammation. Thus steroids are the mainstay of treatment, as they are for systemic lupus; in cerebral disease, common practice would be to commence with a course of high-dose intravenous methylprednisolone, followed by oral steroid treatment. Cyclophosphamide (usually orally) may be exhibited for severe or steroid-resistant disease, while azathioprine is commonly used to maintain remission and spare steroids (Sharon *et al.*, 1973). This approach is obviously similar to that adopted in cerebral vasculitis (see p. 234, also for information regarding doses), which likewise lacks a firm evidence-based background, though uncontrolled studies of patients with severe neuropsychiatric lupus (Rosove and Brewer, 1992; Boumpas *et al.*, 1995; Fessler and Boumpas, 1995; Neuwelt *et al.*, 1995; Gladman, 1996) do provide support for its use. There is also, however, retrospective evidence for the efficacy and safety of weekly low doses of pulsed cyclophosphamide (500 mg) in patients with cerebral lupus but without APA (Ramos *et al.*, 1996).

Intravenous steroids and oral cyclophosphamide are also recommended for lupus myelitis (Barile and Lavalle, 1992); optic neuropathy has also been successfully treated in this way (Rosenbaum *et al.*, 1997).

The role of newer therapies, such as plasmapheresis synchronized with cyclophosphamide (Euler *et al.*, 1994, 1996; Jones, 1996) and intravenous immunoglobulin, remains to be more firmly established, though some evidence supporting intravenous immunoglobulin in acute and chronic active systemic lupus has been presented (Francioni *et al.*, 1994; De *et al.*, 1996; Schroeder *et al.*, 1996).

Seronegative arthritides

Ankylosing spondylitis

Neurological disease in the setting of ankylosing spondylitis usually reflects advanced bony disease (Matthews, 1968; Francioni *et al.*, 1994; Apple and Anson, 1995; Ramos *et al.*, 1995; De *et al.*, 1996; Schroeder *et al.*, 1996). A cauda equina syndrome is well-reported (Tullous *et al.*, 1990; Westhovens *et al.*, 1994), though unexplained and difficult to treat. Arachnoiditis may play a role (Charlesworth *et al.*, 1996). More peripherally, muscle pathology is described (Carrabba *et al.*, 1984), though this has been suggested to be a phenomenon secondary to 'pain inhibition and reduced activity' (Faus *et al.*, 1991).

An association with multiple sclerosis has been described (Khan and Kushner, 1979), though others have described unexplained abnormalities of evoked potentials in clinically normal patients with ankylosing spondylitis (Hanrahan *et al.*, 1988) and suggested caution in interpreting delayed evoked potentials when investigating possible multiple sclerosis in patients with ankylosing spondylitis. The current author is aware of no subsequent reports confirming a link between the two disorders.

Reiter's disease

The clinical triad of seronegative arthropathy, non-specific urethritis and conjunctivitis, usually following venereal or dysenteric infection, constitute Rieter's syndrome. Although this primary organ distribution is rather similar to Behçet's disease (see Chapter 10), Reiter's syndrome has achieved nothing like the same notoriety.

Neurological complications are in recent years rather uncommonly reported, but have been documented in older case studies (Oates and Hancock, 1959). As many as 25% of patients were reported to have neurological features concurrent with, or following exacerbations of, systemic disease in one large and very useful series (Good, 1974). In this study of 164 patients, peripheral symptoms and signs – radiculitis and polyneuritis – occurred as commonly as CNS disorders (both in approximately 12% of cases). Regarding the latter, aseptic meningoencephalitis is reported, some with fits, while isolated epilepsy has occurred in others. In total, seizures were recorded in 5% of patients in Good's series. Psychiatric disturbances, particularly paranoid psychosis, occurred in four patients, again during attacks of systemic disease. Cranial neuropathies and pyramidal signs were less commonly described; myelopathy is reported (Montanaro and Bennett, 1984).

A recent report suggests that cyclosporin may be of value in severe Reiter's disease (Kiyohara et al., 1997).

Psoriasis

Included as the third sero-negative arthropathy, the neurology of psoriasis is not extensive. Cord compression from cervical psoriatic spondylosis is described (Fam and Cruickshank, 1982); reports of a complicating polyneuritis (Sindrup et al., 1990) have not been substantiated by careful studies of nerve electrophysiology (Lomuto et al., 1995). Conversely, psychoneuroimmunological phenomena are invoked to explain the apparent exacerbations of skin disease precipitated by stress (Pincelli et al., 1994).

References

Anonymous (1993) Anticardiolipin antibodies and the risk of recurrent thrombo-occlusive events and death. The Antiphospholipid Antibodies in Stroke Study Group (APASS). *Neurology*, **48**, 91–94.

Anonymous (1996) Systemic sclerosis: current pathogenetic concepts and future prospects for targeted therapy (clinical conference). *Lancet*, **347**, 1453–1458.

Anonymous (1997) Anticardiolipin antibodies are an independent risk factor for first ischemic stroke. The Antiphospholipid Antibodies in Stroke Study (APASS) Group. *Neurology*, **43**, 2069–2073.

Adelman, D. C., Saltiel, E., Klinenberg, J. R. (1986) The neuropsychiatric manifestations of systemic lupus erythematosus: an overview. *Semin. Arthritis Rheum.*, **15**, 185–199.

Alexander, E. (1992) Central nervous system disease in Sjogren's syndrome. New insights into immunopathogenesis. *Rheum. Dis. Clin. North Am.*, **18**, 637–672.

Alexander, E. L. (1986) Central nervous system (CNS) manifestations of primary Sjogren's syndrome: an overview. *Scand. J. Rheumatol. Suppl.*, **61**, 161–165.

Alexander, E. L., Beall, S. S., Gordon, B., Selnes, O. A., Yannakakis, G. D., Patronas, N., et al. (1988) Magnetic resonance imaging of cerebral lesions in patients with the Sjogren syndrome. *Ann. Intern. Med.*, **108**, 815–823.

Alexander, E. L., Malinow, K., Lejewski, J. E., Jerdan, M. S., Provost, T. T. and Alexander, G. E. (1986) Primary Sjogren's syndrome with central nervous system disease mimicking multiple sclerosis. *Ann. Intern. Med.*, **104**, 323–330.

Allen, I. V., Millar, J. H., Kirk, J. and Shillington, R. K. (1979) Systemic lupus erythematosus clinically resembling multiple sclerosis and with unusual pathological and ultrastructural features. *J. Neurol. Neurosurg. Psychiat.*, **42**, 392–401.

Ames, P. R., Pyke, S., Iannaccone, L. and Brancaccio, V. (1995) Antiphospholipid antibodies, haemostatic variables and thrombosis – a survey of 144 patients. *Thromb Haemost.* **73**, 768–773.

Andonopoulos, A. P., Lagos, G., Drosos, A. A. and Moutsopoulos, H. M. (1990) The spectrum of neurological involvement in Sjögren's syndrome. *Br. J. Rheumatol.*, **29**, 21–23.

Andrianakos, A. A., Duffy, J., Suzuki, M. and Sharp, J. T. (1975) Transverse myelopathy in systemic lupus erythematosus. Report of three cases and review of the literature. *Ann. Intern. Med.*, **83**, 616–624.

Apple, D. F. J. and Anson, C. (1995) Spinal cord injury occurring in patients with ankylosing spondylitis: a multicenter study. *Orthopedics*, **18**, 1005–1011.

Asherson, R. A., Denburg, S. D., Denburg, J. A., Carbotte, R. M. and Futrell, N. (1993) Current concepts of neuropsychiatric systemic lupus erythematosus (NP-SLE). *Postgrad. Med. J.*, **69**, 602–608.

Asherson, R. A., Derksen, R. H., Harris, E. N., Bouma, B. N., Gharavi, A. E., Kater, L., *et al.* (1987) Chorea in systemic lupus erythematosus and 'lupus-like' disease: association with antiphospholipid antibodies. *Semin. Arthritis Rheum.*, **16**, 253–259.

Asherson, R. A., Khamashta, M. A., Gil, A., Vazquez, J. J., Chan, O., Baguley, E., *et al.* (1989) Cerebrovascular disease and antiphospholipid antibodies in systemic lupus erythematosus, lupus-like disease, and the primary antiphospholipid syndrome (see comments). *Am. J. Med.*, **86**, 391–399.

Asherson, R. A. and Piette, J. C. (1996) The catastrophic antiphospholipid syndrome 1996: acute multi-organ failure associated with antiphospholipid antibodies: a review of 31 patients. *Lupus*, **5**, 414–417.

Averbuch Heller, L., Steiner, I. and Abramsky, O. (1992) Neurologic manifestations of progressive systemic sclerosis. *Arch. Neurol.*, **49**, 1292–1295.

Barile, L. and Lavalle, C. (1992) Transverse myelitis in systemic lupus erythematosus – the effect of IV pulse methylprednisolone and cyclophosphamide. *J. Rheumatol.*, **19**, 370–372.

Bathon, J. M., Moreland, L. W. and Dibartolomeo, A. G. (1989) Inflammatory central nervous system involvement in rheumatoid arthritis. *Semin. Arthritis Rheum.*, **18**, 258–266.

Belmont, H. M., Abramson, S. B. and Lie, J. T. (1996) Pathology and pathogenesis of vascular injury in systemic lupus erythematosus. Interactions of inflammatory cells and activated endothelium. *Arthritis Rheum.*, **39**, 9–22.

Belmont, H. M., Buyon, J., Giorno, R. and Abramson, S. (1994) Up-regulation of endothelial cell adhesion molecules characterizes disease activity in systemic lupus erythematosus. The Shwartzman phenomenon revisited. *Arthritis Rheum.*, **37**, 376–383.

Bennett, R. M., Bong, D. M. and Spargo, B. H. (1978) Neuropsychiatric problems in mixed connective tissue disease. *Am. J. Med.*, **65**, 955–962.

Bennett, R. M. and O'Connell, D. J. (1980) Mixed connective tisssue disease: a clinicopathologic study of 20 cases. *Semin. Arthritis Rheum.*, **10**, 25–51.

Berden, J. H., Hang, L., McConahey, P. J. and Dixon, F. J. (1983) Analysis of vascular lesions in murine SLE. I. Association with serologic abnormalities. *J. Immunol.*, **130**, 1699–1705.

Binder, A., Snaith, M. L. and Isenberg, D. (1988) Sjögren's syndrome: a study of its neurological complications. *Br. J. Rheumatol.*, **27**, 275–280.

Black, C. M. (1995) The aetiopathogenesis of systemic sclerosis: thick skin–thin hypotheses. The Parkes Weber Lecture 1994. *J. R. Coll. Phys. Lond.*, **29**, 119–130.

Bluestein, H. G. and Woods, V. L. J. (1982) Antineuronal antibodies in systemic lupus erythematosus. *Arthritis Rheum.*, **25**, 773–778.

Bonfa, E., Golombek, S. J., Kaufman, L. D., Skelly, S., Weissbach, H., Brot, N., *et al.* (1987) Association between lupus psychosis and anti-ribosomal P protein antibodies. *N. Engl. J. Med.*, **317**, 265–271.

Boumpas, D. T., Austin, H. A. III, Fessler, B. J., Balow, J. E., Klippel, J. H. and Lockshin, M. D. (1995) Systemic lupus erythematosus: emerging concepts. Part 1: renal, neuropsychiatric, cardiovascular, pulmonary, and hematologic disease. *Ann. Intern. Med.*, **122**, 940–950.

Boyer, R. S., Sun, N. C., Verity, A., Nies, K. M. and Louie, J. S. (1980) Immunoperoxidase staining of the choroid plexus in systemic lupus erythematosus. *J. Rheumatol.*, **7**, 645–650.

Brey, R. L. and Coull, B. M. (1992) Antiphospholipid antibodies: origin, specificity, and mechanism of action. *Stroke*, **23**, I15–I18.

Brey, R. L. and Levine, S. R. (1996) Treatment of neurologic complications of antiphospholipid syndrome. *Lupus*, **5**, 473–476.

Brick, J. E. and Brick, J. F. (1989) Neurologic manifestations of rheumatologic disease. *Neurol.*

Clin., **7**, 629–639.

Briggs, D., Stephens, C., Vaughan, R., Welsh, K. and Black, C. (1993) A molecular and serologic analysis of the major histocompatibility complex and complement component C4 in systemic sclerosis. *Arthritis Rheum.*, **36**, 943–954.

Briley, D. P., Coull, B. M. and Goodnight, S. H. J. (1989) Neurological disease associated with antiphospholipid antibodies. *Ann. Neurol.*, **25**, 221–227.

Bruyn, G. W. and Padberg, G. (1984) Chorea and systemic lupus erythematosus. A critical review. *Eur. Neurol.*, **23**, 435–448.

Carrabba, M., Chevallard, M., Colombo, B., Dworzak, F., Mora, M. and Cornelio, F. (1984) Muscle pathology in ankylosing spondylitis. *Clin. Exp. Rheumatol.*, **2**, 139–144.

Cerinic, M. M., Generini, S., Pignone, A. and Casale, R. (1996) The nervous system in systemic sclerosis (scleroderma). Clinical features and pathogenetic mechanisms. *Rheum. Dis. Clin. North Am.*, **22**, 879–892.

Cervera, R., Asherson, R. A., Font, J., Tikly, M., Pallares, L., Chamorro, A., *et al.* (1997) Chorea in the antiphospholipid syndrome. Clinical, radiologic, and immunologic characteristics of 50 patients from our clinics and the recent literature. *Med. Baltimore*, **76**, 203–212.

Chan, K. F. and Boey, M. L. (1996) Transverse myelopathy in SLE: clinical features and functional outcomes. *Lupus*, **5**, 294–299.

Charlesworth, C. H., Savy, L. E., Stevens, J., Twomey, B. and Mitchell, R. (1996) MRI demonstration of arachnoiditis in cauda equina syndrome of ankylosing spondylitis. *Neuroradiology*, **38**, 462–465.

Cochrane, C. G. (1971) Mechanisms involved in the deposition of immune complexes in tissues. *J. Exp. Med.*, **134 (Suppl)**, 89s.

Cush, J. J. and Lipsky, P. E. (1988) Phenotypic analysis of synovial tissue and peripheral blood lymphocytes isolated from patients with rheumatoid arthritis. *Arthritis Rheum.*, **31**, 1230–1238.

Davie, C. A., Feinstein, A., Kartsounis, L. D., Barker, G. J., McHugh, N. J., Walport, M. J., *et al.* (1995) Proton magnetic resonance spectroscopy of systemic lupus erythematosus involving the central nervous system. *J. Neurol.*, **242**, 522–528.

De, V. S., Ferraccioli, G. F., Di, P. E., Bartoli, E. and Bombardieri, S. (1996) High dose intravenous immunoglobulin therapy for rheumatic diseases: clinical relevance and personal experience. *Clin. Exp. Rheumatol.*, **14 (Suppl 15)**, S85–S92.

Denburg, S. D., Carbotte, R. M. and Denburg, J. A. (1987) Cognitive impairment in systemic lupus erythematosus: a neuropsychological study of individual and group deficits. *J. Clin. Exp. Neuropsychol.*, **9**, 323–339.

Denburg, S. D., Carbotte, R. M. and Denburg, J. A. (1997) Psychological aspects of systemic lupus erythematosus: cognitive function, mood, and self-report. *J. Rheumatol.*, **24**, 998–1003.

Devinsky, O., Petito, C. K. and Alonso, D. R. (1988) Clinical and neuropathological findings in systemic lupus erythematosus: the role of vasculitis, heart emboli, and thrombotic thrombocytopenic purpura. *Ann. Neurol.*, **23**, 380–384.

Donaldson, I. M. and Espiner, E. A. (1971) Disseminated lupus erythematosus presenting as chorea gravidarum. *Arch. Neurol.*, **25**, 240–244.

Dore, D. P., Donaldson, J. O., Rothman, B. L. and Zurier, R. B. (1982) Antinuclear antibodies in multiple sclerosis. *Arch. Neurol.*, **39**, 504–506.

Dutton, J. J., Burde, R. M. and Klingele, T. G. (1982) Autoimmune retrobulbar optic neuritis. *Am. J. Ophthalmol.*, **94**, 11–17.

Elliott, M. J., Maini, R. N., Feldmann, M., Long, F. A., Charles, P., Bijl, H., *et al.* (1994) Repeated therapy with monoclonal antibody to tumour necrosis factor alpha (cA2) in patients with rheumatoid arthritis. *Lancet*, **344**, 1125–1127.

Ellis, S. G. and Verity, M. A. (1979) Central nervous system involvement in systemic lupus erythematosus: a review of neuropathologic findings in 57 cases, 1955–1977. *Semin. Arthritis Rheum.*, **8**, 212–221.

Ellison, D., Gatter, K., Heryet, A. and Esiri, M. (1993) Intramural platelet deposition in cerebral vasculopathy of systemic lupus erythematosus (see comments). *J. Clin. Pathol.*, **46**, 37–40.

Escalante, A., Brey, R. L., Mitchell, B. D. Jr and Dreiner, U. (1995) Accuracy of anticardiolipin antibodies in identifying a history of thrombosis among patients with systemic lupus erythematosus. *Am. J. Med.* **98**, 559–565.

Esmon, N. L., Smirnov, M. D. and Esmon, C. T. (1997a) Lupus anticoagulants and thrombosis: the role of phospholipids. *Haematologica*, **82**, 474–477.

Esmon, N. L., Smirnov, M. D. and Esmon, C. T. (1997b) Thrombogenic mechanisms of antiphospholipid antibodies. *Thromb. Haemost.*, **78**, 79–82.

Estey, E., Lieberman, A., Pinto, R., Meltzer, M. and Ransohoff, J. (1979) Cerebral arteritis in scleroderma. *Stroke*, **10**, 595–597.

Euler, H. H., Schroeder, J. O., Harten, P., Zeuner, R. A. and Gutschmidt, H. J. (1994) Treatment-free remission in severe systemic lupus erythematosus following synchronization of plasmapheresis with subsequent pulse cyclophosphamide. *Arthritis Rheum.*, **37**, 1784–1794.

Euler, H. H., Zeuner, R. A. and Schroeder, J. O. (1996) Plasma exchange in systemic lupus erythematosus. *Transfusion Sci.*, **17**, 245–265.

Fam, A. G. and Cruickshank, B. (1982) Subaxial cervical subluxation and cord compression in psoriatic spondylitis. *Arthritis Rheum.*, **25**, 101–106.

Farrell, D. A. and Medsger, T. A. J. (1982) Trigeminal neuropathy in progressive systemic sclerosis. *Am. J. Med.*, **73**, 57–62.

Faus, R. S., Martinez, P. S., Blanch, R. J., Benito, R. P., Duro, P. J. and Corominas, T. J. (1991) Muscle pathology in ankylosing spondylitis: clinical, enzymatic, electromyographic and histologic correlation. *J. Rheumatol.*, **18**, 1368–1371.

Feinglass, E. J., Arnett, F. C., Dorsch, C. A., Zizic, T. M. and Stevens, M. B. (1976) Neuropsychiatric manifestations of systemic lupus erythematosus: diagnosis, clinical spectrum, and relationship to other features of the disease. *Med. Baltimore*, **55**, 323–339.

Feldmann, M., Brennan, F. M. and Maini, R. N. (1996a) Rheumatoid arthritis. *Cell*, **85**, 307–310.

Feldmann, M., Brennan, F. M. and Maini, R. N. (1996b) Role of cytokines in rheumatoid arthritis. *Annu. Rev. Immunol.*, **14**, 397–440.

Fessler, B. J., Boumpas, D. T. (1995) Severe major organ involvement in systemic lupus erythematosus. Diagnosis and management. *Rheum. Dis. Clin. North Am.*, **21**, 81–98.

Fox, R. I. and Theofilopoulos, A. N. (1996) Sjögren's syndrome: Pathogenesis and prospects for therapy. *Expert Opin. Invest. Drugs*, **5**, 1127–1153.

Francioni, C., Galeazzi, M., Fioravanti, A., Gelli, R., Megale, F. and Marcolongo, R. (1994) Long-term i.v. Ig treatment in systemic lupus erythematosus. *Clin. Exp. Rheumatol.*, **12**, 163–168.

Fulford, K. W., Catterall, R. D., Delhanty, J. J., Doniach, D. and Kremer, M. (1972) A collagen disorder of the nervous system presenting as multiple sclerosis. *Brain*, **95**, 373–386.

Futrell, N., Schultz, L. R. and Millikan, C. (1992) Central nervous system disease in patients with systemic lupus erythematosus. *Neurology*, **42**, 1649–1657.

Geirsson, A. J., Sturfelt, G. and Truedsson, L. (1987) Clinical and serological features of severe vasculitis in rheumatoid arthritis: prognostic implications. *Ann. Rheum. Dis.*, **46**, 727–733.

Gladman, D. D. (1996) Prognosis and treatment of systemic lupus erythematosus. *Curr. Opin. Rheumatol.*, **8**, 430–437.

Goldberger, E., Elder, R. C., Schwartz, R. A. and Phillips, P. E. (1992) Vasculitis in the antiphospholipid syndrome. A cause of ischemia responding to corticosteroids (see comments). *Arthritis Rheum.*, **35**, 569–572.

Golombek, S. J., Graus, F. and Elkon, K. B. (1986) Autoantibodies in the cerebrospinal fluid of patients with systemic lupus erythematosus. *Arthritis Rheum.*, **29**, 1090–1097.

Good, A. E. (1974) Reiter's disease: a review with special attention to cardiovascular and neurologic sequellae. *Semin. Arthritis Rheum.*, **3**, 253–286.

Gordon, R. M. and Silverstein, A. (1970) Neurologic manifestations in progressive systemic sclerosis. *Arch. Neurol.*, **22**, 126–134.

Graf, W. D., Milstein, J. M. and Sherry, D. D. (1993) Stroke and mixed connective tissue disease. *J. Child Neurol.*, **8**, 256–259.

Hammer, J., Gallazzi, F., Bono, E., Karr, R. W., Guenot, J., Valsasnini, P., *et al.* (1995) Peptide binding specificity of HLA-DR4 molecules: correlation with rheumatoid arthritis association (see comments). *J. Exp. Med.*, **181**, 1847–1855.

Hanly, J. G., Cassell, K. and Fisk, J. D. (1997) Cognitive function in systemic lupus erythematosus: results of a 5-year prospective study. *Arthritis Rheum.*, **40**, 1542–1543.

Hanly, J. G., Walsh, N. M., Fisk, J. D., Eastwood, B., Hong, C., Sherwood, G., *et al.* (1993) Cognitive impairment and autoantibodies in systemic lupus erythematosus. *Br. J. Rheumatol.*, **32**, 291–296.

Hanrahan, P. S., Russell, A. S. and McLean, D. R. (1988) Ankylosing spondylitis and multiple sclerosis: an apparent association? *J. Rheumatol.*, **15**, 1512–1514.

Hay, E. M. (1994) Psychiatric disorder and cognitive impairment in SLE. *Lupus*, **3**, 145–148.

Hay, E. M., Isenberg, D. A. (1993) Autoantibodies in central nervous system lupus. *Br. J. Rheumatol.*, **32**, 329–332.

Henderson, F. C., Geddes, J. F. and Crockard, H. A. (1993) Neuropathology of the brainstem and spinal cord in end stage rheumatoid arthritis: implications for treatment (see comments). *Ann. Rheum. Dis.*, **52**, 629–637.

Herranz, M. T., Rivier, G., Khamashta, M. A., Blaser, K. U. and Hughes, G. R. (1994) Association between antiphospholipid antibodies and epilepsy in patients with systemic lupus erythematosus. *Arthritis Rheum.*, **37**, 568–571.

Hirohata, S. and Kosaka M. (1994) Association of anti-Sm antibodies with organic brain syndrome secondary to systemic lupus erythematosus (letter). *Lancet*, **343**, 796.

Homburger, H. A. (1995) Cascade testing for autoantibodies in connective tissue diseases. *Mayo Clin. Proc.*, **70**, 183–184.

How, A., Dent, P. B., Liao, S. K. and Denburg, J. A. (1985) Antineuronal antibodies in neuropsychiatric systemic lupus erythematosus. *Arthritis Rheum.*, **28**, 789–795.

Hughes, G. R. (1983) Thrombosis, abortion, cerebral disease, and the lupus anticoagulant (editorial). *Br. Med. J. Clin. Res. Edn.*, **287**, 1088–1089.

Hughes, G. R., Harris, N. N. and Gharavi, A. E. (1986) The anticardiolipin syndrome. *J. Rheumatol.*, **13**, 486–489.

Hughson, M. D., McCarty, G. A., Sholer, C. M. and Brumback, R. A. (1993) Thrombotic cerebral arteriopathy in patients with the antiphospholipid syndrome. *Mod. Pathol.*, **6**, 644–653.

Husby, G., Forre, O. and Williams, R. C. J. (1979) IgG subclass, variable H-chain subgroup, and light chain-type composition of antineuronal antibody in Huntington's disease and Sydenham's chorea. *Clin. Immunol. Immunopathol.*, **14**, 361–367.

Isshi, K. and Hirohata, S. (1996) Association of anti-ribosomal P protein antibodies with neuropsychiatric systemic lupus erythematosus. *Arthritis Rheum.*, **39**, 1483–1490.

Jackson, C. G., Chess, R. L. and Ward, J. R. (1984) A case of rheumatoid nodule formation within the central nervous system and review of the literature. *J. Rheumatol.*, **11**, 237–240.

Jain, R., Chartash, E., Susin, M. and Furie, R. (1994) Systemic lupus erythematosus complicated by thrombotic microangiopathy. *Semin. Arthritis Rheum.*, **24**, 173–182.

Johnson, R. T. and Richardson, E. P. (1968) The neurological manifestations of systemic lupus erythematosus. *Med. Baltimore*, **47**, 337–369.

Jones, J. V. (1996) Plasmapheresis in the treatment of systemic lupus erythematosus. *Transfusion Sci.*, **17**, 283–288.

Jongen, P. J., Boerbooms, A. M., Lamers, K. J., Raes, B. C. and Vierwinden, G. (1990) Diffuse CNS involvement in systemic lupus erythematosus: intrathecal synthesis of the 4th component of complement. *Neurology*, **40**, 1593–1596.

Kaell, A. T., Shetty, M., Lee, B. C. and Lockshin, M. D. (1986) The diversity of neurologic events in systemic lupus erythematosus. Prospective clinical and computed tomographic classification of 82 events in 71 patients. *Arch. Neurol.*, **43**, 273–276.

Kahari, V. M. (1993) Activation of dermal connective tissue in scleroderma. *Ann. Med.*, **25**, 511–518.

Kalashnikova, L. A., Nasonov, E. L., Kushekbaeva, A. E. and Gracheva, L. A. (1990) Anticardiolipin antibodies in Sneddon's syndrome. *Neurology*, **40**, 464–467.

Kaltreider, H. B. and Talal, N. (1969) The neuropathy of Sjögren's syndrome. Trigeminal nerve involvement. *Ann. Intern. Med.*, **70**, 751–762.

Kauppi, M., Sakaguchi, M., Konttinen, Y. T., Hamalainen, M. and Hakala, M. (1996) Pathogenetic mechanism and prevalence of the stable atlantoaxial subluxation in rheumatoid arthritis. *J. Rheumatol.*, **23**, 831–834.

Khamashta, M. A. and Hughes, G. R. (1994) Antiphospholipid antibodies. A marker for thrombosis and recurrent abortion. *Clin. Rev. Allergy*, **12**, 287–296.

Khan, M. A. and Kushner, I. (1979) Ankylosing spondylitis and multiple sclerosis. A possible association. *Arthritis Rheum.*, **22**, 784–786.

Kiyohara, A., Takamori, K., Niizuma, N. and Ogawa, H. (1997) Successful treatment of severe recurrent Reiter's syndrome with cyclosporine. *J. Am. Acad. Dermatol.*, **36**, 482–483.

Kodama, K., Okada, S., Hino, T., Takabayashi, K., Nawata, Y., Uchida, Y., *et al.* (1995) Single photon emission computed tomography in systemic lupus erythematosus with psychiatric symptoms. *J. Neurol. Neurosurg. Psychiat.*, **58**, 307–311.

Kotzin, B. L. (1996) Systemic lupus erythematosus. *Cell*, **85**, 303–306.

Koyabashi, T., Stang, E., Fang, K. S., de Moerloose, P., Parton, R. G. and Gruenberg, J. (1998) A lipid associated with the antiphospholipid syndrome regulates endosome structure and function. *Nature*, **392**, 193–197.

Kupersmith, M. J., Burde, R. M., Warren, F. A., Klingele, T. G., Frohman, L. P. and Mitnick, H. (1988) Autoimmune optic neuropathy: evaluation and treatment (published erratum appears in *J. Neurol. Neurosurg. Psychiat.*, **52**(5), 692). *J. Neurol. Neurosurg. Psychiat.*, **51**, 1381–1386.

Lavalle, C., Pizarro, S., Drenkard, C., Sanchez, G. J. and Alarcon, S. D. (1990) Transverse myelitis: a manifestation of systemic lupus erythematosus strongly associated with anti-phospholipid antibodies (see comments). *J. Rheumatol.*, **17**, 34–37.

Lee, P., Urowitz, M. B., Bookman, A. A., Koehler, B. E., Smythe, H. A., Gordon, D. A., *et al.* (1977) Systemic lupus erythematosus. A review of 110 cases with reference to nephritis, the nervous system, infections, aseptic necrosis and prognosis. *Quart. J. Med.*, **46**, 1–32.

Leroy, E. C. (1994) The control of fibrosis in systemic sclerosis: a strategy involving extracellular matrix, cytokines, and growth factors. *J. Dermatol.*, **21**, 1–4.

Leroy, E. C. (1996) Systemic sclerosis. A vascular perspective. *Rheum. Dis. Clin. North Am.*, **22**, 675–694.

Leung, W. H., Wong, K. L., Lau, C. P., Wong, C. K. and Liu, H. W. (1990) Association between antiphospholipid antibodies and cardiac abnormalities in patients with systemic lupus erythematosus. *Am. J. Med.*, **89**, 411–419.

Levine, S. R. and Brey, R. L. (1996) Neurological aspects of antiphospholipid antibody syndrome. *Lupus*, **5**, 347–353.

Levine, S. R., Deegan, M. J., Futrell, N. and Welch, K. M. (1990) Cerebrovascular and neurologic disease associated with antiphospholipid antibodies: 48 cases. *Neurology*, **40**, 1181–1189.

Levine, S. R., Salowich, P. L., Sawaya, K. L., Perry, M., Spender, H. J., Winkler, H. J., *et al.* (1997) IgG anticardiolipin antibody titer > 40 GPL and the risk of subsequent thrombo-occlusive events and death. A prospective cohort study. *Stroke*, **28**, 1660–1665.

Liou, H. H., Wang, C. R., Chen, C. J., Chen, R. C., Chuang, C. Y., Chiang, I. P., *et al.* (1996) Elevated levels of anticardiolipin antibodies and epilepsy in lupus patients. *Lupus*, **5**, 307–312.

Lockshin, M. D. (1997) Why do patients with antiphospholipid antibody clot? (editorial; comment). *Lupus*, **6**, 351–352.

Lomuto, M., Simone, P., Iannantuono, M., Di Viesti, P., Zarrelli, M., Ditano, G., *et al.* (1995) Myelinated nerve behavior in psoriasis. *Acta Dermatovenerologica Alpina, Panonica et Adriatica*, **4**, 3–7.

Luqmani, R. A., Watts, R. A., Scott, D. G. and Bacon, P. A. (1994) Treatment of vasculitis in rheumatoid arthritis. *Ann. Med. Intern. Paris*, **145**, 566–576.

Lusins, J. O. and Szilagyi, P. A. (1975) Clinical features of chorea associated with systemic lupus erythematosus. *Am. J. Med.*, **58**, 857–861.

McCarty, Farid G. (1994) Antiphospholipid antibodies in systemic lupus erythematosus. *Curr. Opin. Rheumatol.*, **6**, 493–500.

McCombe, P. A., Klestov, A. C., Tannenberg, A. E., Chalk, J. B. and Pender, M. P. (1991)

Sensorimotor peripheral neuropathy in rheumatoid arthritis. *Clin. Exp. Neurol.*, **28**, 146–153.

Manthorpe, R., Asmussen, K. and Oxholm, P. (1997) Primary Sjögren's syndrome: diagnostic criteria, clinical features, and disease activity. *J. Rheumatol.*, **24 (Suppl 50)**, 8–11.

Manthorpe, R., Manthorpe, T. and Sjoberg, S. (1992) Magnetic resonance imaging of the brain in patients with primary Sjogren's syndrome. *Scand. J. Rheumatol.*, **21**, 148–149.

Matthews, W. B. (1991) Differential diagnosis. In *McAlpine's Multiple Sclerosis* (Matthews, W. B., ed.), pp. 165–188. London: Churchill Livingstone.

Matthews, W. B. (1968) The neurological complications of ankylosing spondylitis. *J. Neurol. Sci.*, **6**, 561–573.

Mevorach, D., Raz, E. and Steiner, I. (1994) Evidence for intrathecal synthesis of autoantibodies in systemic lupus erythematosus with neurological involvement. *Lupus*, **3**, 117–121.

Miguel, E. C., Pereira, R. M., Pereira, C. A., Baer, L., Gomes, R. E., De S. L., et al. (1994) Psychiatric manifestations of systemic lupus erythematosus: clinical features, symptoms, and signs of central nervous system activity in 43 patients. *Med. Baltimore*, **73**, 224–232.

Miller, D. H., Buchanan, N., Barker, G., Morrissey, S. P., Kendall, B. E., Rudge, P., et al. (1992) Gadolinium-enhanced magnetic resonance imaging of the central nervous system in systemic lupus erythematosus. *J. Neurol.*, **239**, 460–464.

Mitchell, D. M., Spitz, P. W., Young, D. Y., Bloch, D. A., McShane, D. J. and Fries, J. F. (1986) Survival, prognosis, and causes of death in rheumatoid arthritis. *Arthritis Rheum.*, **29**, 706–714.

Mok, C. C., Lau, C. S., Chan, E. Y. and Wong, R. W. (1998) Acute transverse myelopathy in systemic lupus erythematosus: clinical presentation, treatment and outcome. *J. Rheumatol.*, **25**, 467–473.

Molina, R., Provost, T. T. and Alexander, E. L. (1985) Two types of inflammatory vascular disease in Sjögren's syndrome. Differential association with seroreactivity to rheumatoid factor and antibodies to Ro (SS-A) and with hypocomplementemia. *Arthritis Rheum.*, **28**, 1251–1258.

Montalban, J., Cervera, R., Font, J., Ordi, J., Vianna, J., Haga, H. J., et al. (1992) Lack of association between anticardiolipin antibodies and migraine in systemic lupus erythematosus. *Neurology*, **42**, 681–682.

Montanaro, A. and Bennett, R. M. (1984) Myelopathy in Reiter's disease. *J. Rheumatol.*, **11**, 540–541.

Moore, P. M. and Lisak, R. P. (1995) Systemic lupus erythematosus: immunopathogenesis of neurologic dysfunction. *Springer Semin. Immunopathol.*, **17**, 43–60.

Morgan, B. P. (1995) Physiology and pathophysiology of complement: Progress and trends. *Crit. Rev. Clin. Lab. Sci.*, **32**, 265–298.

Nesher, G., Ilany, J., Rosenmann, D. and Abraham, A. S. (1997) Valvular dysfunction in antiphospholipid syndrome: prevalence, clinical features, and treatment. *Semin. Arthritis Rheum.*, **27**, 27–35.

Neuwelt, C. M., Lacks, S., Kaye, B. R., Ellman, J. B. and Borenstein, D. G. (1995) Role of intravenous cyclophosphamide in the treatment of severe neuropsychiatric systemic lupus erythematosus. *Am. J. Med.*, **98**, 32–41.

Nihoyannopoulos, P., Gomez, P. M., Joshi, J., Loizou, S., Walport, M. J. and Oakley, C. M. (1990) Cardiac abnormalities in systemic lupus erythematosus. Association with raised anticardiolipin antibodies (see comments). *Circulation*, **82**, 369–375.

Nimelstein, S. H., Brody, S., McShane, D. and Holman, H. R. (1980) Mixed connective tissue disease: a subsequent evaluation of the original 25 patients. *Med. Baltimore*, **59**, 239–248.

Oates, J. K. and Hancock, J. A. H. (1959) Neurological symptoms and lesions occurring in the course of Reiter's disease. *Am. J. Med. Sci.*, **238**, 79–84.

Omdal, R. and Roalso, S. (1992) Chorea gravidarum and chorea associated with oral contraceptives – diseases due to antiphospholipid antibodies? *Acta Neurol. Scand.*, **86**, 219–220.

Pease, C. T., Shattles, W., Charles, P. J., Venables, P. J. and Maini, R. N. (1989) Clinical, serological, and HLA phenotype subsets in Sjögren's syndrome. *Clin. Exp. Rheumatol.*, **7**, 185–190.

Petz, L. D., Sharp, G. C., Cooper, N. R. and Irvin, W. S. (1971) Serum and cerebral spinal fluid complement and serum autoantibodies in systemic lupus erythematosus. *Med. Baltimore*, **50**, 259–275.

Pincelli, C., Fantini, F., Magnoni, C. and Giannetti, A. (1994) Psoriasis and the nervous system. *Acta Derm. Venereol. Suppl. Stockh.*, **186**, 60–61.

Pope, J. E. (1996) Treatment of systemic sclerosis. *Rheum. Dis. Clin. North Am.*, **22**, 893–907.

Prescott, R. J., Freemont, A. J., Jones, C. J., Hoyland, J. and Fielding, P. (1992) Sequential dermal microvascular and perivascular changes in the development of scleroderma. *J. Pathol.*, **166**, 255–263.

Provenzale, J. M., Barboriak, D. P., Allen, N. B. and Ortel, T. L. (1996) Patients with antiphospholipid antibodies: CT and MR findings of the brain. *AJR. Am. J. Roentgenol.*, **167**, 1573–1578.

Puechal, X., Said, G., Hilliquin, P., Coste, J., Job, D. C., Lacroix. C., et al. (1995) Peripheral neuropathy with necrotizing vasculitis in rheumatoid arthritis. A clinicopathologic and prognostic study of thirty-two patients. *Arthritis Rheum.*, **38**, 1618–1629.

Ramos, M. and Mandybur, T. I. (1975) Cerebral vasculitis in rheumatoid arthritis. *Arch. Neurol.*, **32**, 271–275.

Ramos, P. C., Mendez, M. J., Ames, P. R., Khamashta, M. A. and Hughes, G. R. (1996) Pulse cyclophosphamide in the treatment of neuropsychiatric systemic lupus erythematosus. *Clin. Exp. Rheumatol.*, **14**, 295–299.

Ramos, R. C., Gomez, V. A., Guzman, G. J., Jimenez, G. F., Gamez, N. J., Gonzalez, L. L., et al. (1995) Frequency of atlantoaxial subluxation and neurologic involvement in patients with ankylosing spondylitis. *J. Rheumatol.*, **22**, 2120–2125.

Rankin, E. C., Choy, E. H., Kassimos, D., Kingsley, G. H., Sopwith, A. M., Isenberg, D. A., et al. (1995) The therapeutic effects of an engineered human anti-tumour necrosis factor alpha antibody (CDP571) in rheumatoid arthritis. *Br. J. Rheumatol.*, **34**, 334–342.

Roldan, C. A., Shively, B. K., Crawford, M. H. (1996) An echocardiographic study of valvular heart disease associated with systemic lupus erythematosus. *N. Engl. J. Med.*, **335**, 1424–1430.

Ronnelid, J., Klareskog, L. (1995) Local versus systemic immunoreactivity to collagen and the collage-like region of C1q in rheumatoid arthritis and SLE. *Scand. J. Rheumatol. Suppl.*, **101**, 57–61.

Rosenbaum, J. T., Simpson, J. and Neuwelt, C. M. (1997) Successful treatment of optic neuropathy in association with systemic lupus erythematosus using intravenous cyclophosphamide. *Br. J. Ophthalmol.*, **81**, 130–132.

Rosner, S., Ginzler, E. M., Diamond, H. S., Weiner, M., Schlesinger, M., Fries, J. F., et al. (1982) A multicenter study of outcome in systemic lupus erythematosus. II. Causes of death. *Arthritis Rheum.*, **25**, 612–617.

Rosove, M. H. and Brewer, P. M. (1992) Antiphospholipid thrombosis: clinical course after the first thrombotic event in 70 patients. *Ann. Intern. Med.*, **117**, 303–308.

Sailer, M., Burchert, W., Ehrenheim, C., Smid, H. G. O. M., Haas J., Wildhagen, K., et al. (1997) Positron emission tomography and magnetic resonance imaging for cerebral involvement in patients with systemic lupus erythematosus. *J. Neurol.*, **244**, 186–193.

Sanders, M. E., Alexander, E. L., Koski, C. L., Frank, M. M. and Joiner, K. A. (1998) Detection of activated terminal complement (c5b-9) in cerebrospinal fluid from patients with central nervous system involvement of primary Sjogren's syndrome or systemic lupus erythematosus. *J. Immunol.*, **138**, 2095–2099.

Schroeder, J. O., Zeuner, R. A., Euler, H. H. and Loffler, H. (1996) High dose intravenous immunoglobulins in systemic lupus erythematosus: clinical and serological results of a pilot study. *J. Rheumatol.*, **23**, 71–75.

Scolding, N. J., Jayne, D. R., Zajicek, J. P., Meyer, P. A. R., Wraight, E. P. and Lockwood, C. M. (1998) The syndrome of cerebral vasculitis: recognition, diagnosis and management. *Quart. J. Med.*, **90**, 61–73.

Scolding, N. J., Morgan, B. P., Houston, W. A. J., Linington, C., Campbell, A. K. and Compston, D. A. S. (1989) Vesicular removal by oligodendrocytes of membrane attack complexes formed by activated complement. *Nature*, **339**, 620–622.

Scott, D. G., Bacon, P. A. and Tribe, C. R. (1981) Systemic rheumatoid vasculitis: a clinical and laboratory study of 50 cases. *Med. Baltimore*, **60**, 288–297.

Sharon, E., Kaplan, D. and Diamond, H. S. (1973) Exacerbation of systemic lupus erythematosus after withdrawal of azathioprine therapy. *N. Engl. J. Med.*, **288**, 122–124.

Shepherd, D. I., Downie, A. W. and Best, P. V. (1974) Systemic lupus erythematosus and multiple sclerosis. *Trans. Am. Neurol. Ass.*, **99**, 173–176.

Simon, J. and Simon, O. (1975) Effect of passive transfer of anti-brain antibodies to a normal recipient. *Exp. Neurol.*, **47**, 523–534.

Sindrup, S. H., Ibsen, H. H., Sindrup, J. H. and Sindrup, E. H. (1990) Psoriasis and polyneuropathy. Three case histories. *Acta Derm. Venereol.*, **70**, 443–445.

Sneddon, J. B. (1965) Cerebral-vascular lesions in livedo reticulares. *Br. J. Dermatol.*, **77**, 180–185.

Spezialetti, R., Bluestein, H. G., Peter, J. B. and Alexander, E. L. (1993) Neuropsychiatric disease in Sjögren's syndrome: anti-ribosomal P and anti-neuronal antibodies. *Am. J. Med.*, **95**, 153–160.

Spurlock, R. G. and Richman, A. V. (1983) Rheumatoid meningitis. A case report and review of the literature. *Arch. Pathol. Lab. Med.*, **107**, 129–131.

Stevens, J. C., Cartlidge, N. E., Saunders, M., Appleby, A., Hall, M. and Shaw, D. A. (1971) Atlanto-axial subluxation and cervical myelopathy in rheumatoid arthritis. *Q. J. Med.*, **40**, 391–408.

Sun, K. H., Liu, W. T., Tsai, C. Y., Liao, T. S., Lin, W. M. and Yu, C. L. (1992) Inhibition of astrocyte proliferation and binding to brain tissue of anticardiolipin antibodies purified from lupus serum. *Ann. Rheum. Dis.*, **51**, 707–712.

Tan E. M., Cohen, A. S., Fries, J. F., *et al.* (1982) The 1982 revised criteria for the classification of systemic lupus erythematosus. *Arthritis Rheum.*, **25**, 1271–1277.

Tan, E. M., Feltkamp, T. E., Smolen, J. S., Butcher, B., Dawkins, R., Fritzler, M. J., *et al.* (1997) Range of antinuclear antibodies in 'healthy' individuals. *Arthritis Rheum.*, **40**, 1601–1611.

Teasdall, R. D., Frayha, R. A., Shulman, L. E. (1980) Cranial nerve involvement in systemic sclerosis (scleroderma): a report of 10 cases. *Med. Baltimore*, **59**, 149–159.

Teh, L. S., Hay, E. M., Amos, N., Black, D., Huddy, A., Creed, F., *et al.* (1993) Anti-P antibodies are associated with psychiatric and focal cerebral disorders in patients with systemic lupus erythematosus. *Br. J. Rheumatol.*, **32**, 287–290.

Tesar, J. T., McMillan V., Molina, R. and Armstrong, J. (1992) Optic neuropathy and central nervous system disease associated with primary Sjögren's syndrome. *Am. J. Med.*, **92**, 686–692.

Tola, M. R., Granieri, E., Caniatti, L., Paolino, E., Monetti, C., Dovigo, L., *et al.* (1992) Systemic lupus erythematosus presenting with neurological disorders. *J. Neurol.*, **239**, 61–64.

Tourbah, A., Piette, J. C., Iba, Z. M., Lyon, C. O., Godeau, P. and Frances, C. (1996) The natural course of cerebral lesions in Sneddon syndrome. *Arch. Neurol.*, **54**, 53–60.

Toussirot, E., Serratrice, G. and Valentin, P. (1993) Autonomic nervous system involvement in rheumatoid arthritis. 50 cases. *J. Rheumatol.*, **20**, 1508–1514.

Tsakiris, D. A., Kappos, L., Reber, G., Marbet, G. A., Le-Floch, R. J., Roux, E., *et al.* (1993) Lack of association between antiphospholipid antibodies and migraine. *Thromb. Haemost.*, **69**, 415–417.

Tullous, M. W., Skerhut, H. E., Story, J. L., Brown, W. E. J., Eidelberg, E., Dadsetan, M. R., *et al.* (1990) Cauda equina syndrome of long-standing ankylosing spondylitis. Case report and review of the literature. *J. Neurosurg.*, **73**, 441–447.

Venables, P. J. and Rigby, S. P. (1997) Viruses in the etiopathogenesis of Sjogren's syndrome. *J. Rheumatol.*, **24 (Suppl 50)**, 3–5.

Vianna, J. L., Khamashta, M. A., Ordi, R. J., Font, J., Cervera, R., Lopez, S. A., *et al.* (1994) Comparison of the primary and secondary antiphospholipid syndrome: a European Multicenter Study of 114 patients (see comments). *Am. J. Med.*, **96**, 3–9.

Vidailhet, M., Piette, J. C., Wechsler, B., Bousser, M. G. and Brunet, P. (1990) Cerebral venous thrombosis in systemic lupus erythematosus (see comments). *Stroke*, **21**, 1226–1231.

Vollertsen, R. S., Conn, D. L., Ballard, D. J., Ilstrup, D. M., Kazmar, R. E. and Silverfield, J. C.

(1986) Rheumatoid vasculitis: survival and associated risk factors. *Med. Baltimore*, **65**, 365–375.

Warren, R. W., Kredich, D. W. (1984) Transverse myelitis and acute central nervous system manifestations of systemic lupus erythematosus. *Arthritis Rheum.*, **27**, 1058–1060.

Watanabe, T., Sato, T., Uchiumi, T. and Arakawa, M. (1996) Neuropsychiatric manifestations in patients with systemic lupus erythematosus: diagnostic and predictive value of longitudinal examination of anti-ribosomal P antibody. *Lupus*, **5**, 178–183.

Weingarten, K., Filippi, C., Barbut, D. and Zimmerman, R. D. (1997) The neuroimaging features of the cardiolipin antibody syndrome. *Clin. Imaging*, **21**, 6–12.

Weller, R. O., Bruckner, F. E. and Chamberlain, M. A. (1970) Rheumatoid neuropathy: a histological and electrophysiological study. *J. Neurol. Neurosurg. Psychiat.*, **33**, 592–604.

West, S. G., Emlen, W., Wener, M. H. and Kotzin, B. L. (1995) Neuropsychiatric lupus erythematosus: a 10-year prospective study on the value of diagnostic tests. *Am. J. Med.*, **99**, 153–163.

Westhovens, R., Verstraeten, A., Knockaert, D., Van Holsbeeck, M., Sileghem, A., Vanderschueren, D., *et al.* (1994) Cauda equina syndrome complicating ankylosing spondylitis: role of computed tomography and magnetic resonance imaging. *Clin. Rheumatol.*, **13**, 284–289.

White, B. (1996) Immunopathogenesis of systemic sclerosis. *Rheum. Dis. Clin. North Am.*, **22**, 695–708.

Winfield, J. B., Shaw, M., Silverman, L. M., Eisenberg, R. A., Wilson, H. A. and Koffler, D. (1983) Intrathecal IgG synthesis and blood–brain barrier impairment in patients with systemic lupus erythematosus and central nervous system dysfunction. *Am. J. Med.*, **74**, 837–844.

Wordsworth, P. (1995) Genes and arthritis. *Br. Med. Bull.*, **51**, 249–266.

Chapter 8

Organ-specific autoimmune and inflammatory disease and the central nervous system

Neil Scolding

Introduction   181
Inflammatory bowel disease and the brain   181
The thyroid gland   189
References   190

Introduction

The classification of systemic inflammatory and autoimmune disorders remains problematical, particularly in the absence of any clear understanding of the initiating causes of primary diseases. Pragmatically, a clinical and anatomical approach based upon the parts affected has much to offer – although this too has obvious limitations and will only serve until a system properly founded on aetiology becomes possible.

In this chapter, (central) neurological involvement in some of the classically described organ-specific autoimmune diseases will be considered. (The most significant of these in the current context, multiple sclerosis and related disorders, by nature fall into this category; they have duly and for practical purposes been privileged with their own chapters.)

Inflammatory bowel disease and the brain

Inflammatory bowel disease and multiple sclerosis

Although the term inflammatory bowel disease most commonly refers to ulcerative colitis and Crohn's disease, other disorders such as coeliac disease, Whipple's disease and tropical sprue also exhibit pathological changes of gastrointestinal inflammation, and these too deserve mention. However, before discussing the neurological aspects of specific conditions, it is worthwhile to consider the relationship between inflammatory bowel disease and multiple sclerosis.

Rang *et al.* (1982) surveyed 2579 women who had ulcerative colitis and found 10 with multiple sclerosis – much significance has been attributed to this figure, though in fact with a background prevalence of the order of 150 per 100 000 and taking a maximal female to male ratio of 3 : 1, as many as six patients with multiple sclerosis might have been expected by chance; if the

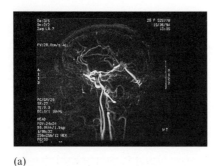
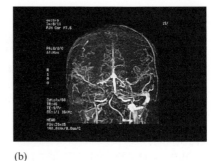

(a)   (b)

Figure 8.1 Cerebral sinus thrombosis and inflammatory bowel disease. A 25-year-old female with active ulcerative colitis developed headache, fever, seizures and focal neurological signs. Magnetic resonance analysis revealed the absence of blood flow in the sagittal (a) and the right sigmoid (b) sinuses.

fact that ulcerative colitis and multiple sclerosis share (approximately) the same age range, then a figure even higher than six could be predicted. However, a subsequent population study of approximately 1 million individuals (Minuk and Lewkonia, 1986) revealed 17 families in whom an association of multiple sclerosis and inflammatory bone disease – either Crohn's disease or ulcerative colitis – occurred. Drawing upon the unique British Columbia Multiple Sclerosis Clinic database, Sadovnick *et al.* (1989) studied 748 consecutive, unrelated patients with multiple sclerosis and found 27 instances wherein either ulcerative colitis or Crohn's disease had occurred in first degree relatives. This group estimated the frequency at which concurrence of inflammatory bowel disease and multiple sclerosis might occur by chance to be of the order of 1 per million; an excess of observed over expected cases was apparent, and concurrence of the two disorders both within families and within individuals was suggested.

The association has not been explained. The possibility of a general 'autoimmune diathesis', non-specific with regard to target tissue (or at least of limited specificity), and of acquired or inherited origin, seems unlikely, inasmuch as concurrence of multiple sclerosis with other autoimmune diseases, such as diabetes mellitus and rheumatoid arthritis, has not been substantiated. Specific immunological abnormalities common to multiple sclerosis and inflammatory bowel disease therefore seem more likely. The author has observed one remarkable patient who developed her first episode of brainstem inflammatory demyelination simultaneously with her first attack of acute bloody diarrhoea. Ulcerative colitis was confirmed on pathological grounds and her later course allowed a diagnosis of clinically definite multiple sclerosis with laboratory support to be made. Subsequently and on repeated occasions, relapses of her colitis and her multiple sclerosis occurred concurrently.

It is possible that the genetic loci predisposing to multiple sclerosis are shared with those involved in inflammatory bowel disease. Familial disease in both ulcerative colitis and Crohn's disease is well-described, but in neither case has any human leukocyte antigen (HLA) association emerged, except in those unusual cases with additional ankylosing spondylitis.

Ulcerative colitis and Crohn's disease

Although these inflammatory bowel diseases are clearly distinct pathologi-cally, clinical differentiation can be difficult. Furthermore, when occurring in familial patterns, either disease may be seen within single families. Most authors, in studying the extra-intestinal manifestations of these disorders, have adopted an inclusive approach; while differences in the frequency and type of, for example, dermatological or articular complications may occur between ulcerative colitis and Crohn's disease, the neurological associations are similar.

Approximately 3% of patients with ulcerative colitis or Crohn's disease develop neurological complications (Lossos et al., 1995). Three types of central nervous system (CNS) disease have been associated: cerebrovascular accidents, epilepsy and, in some reports, myelopathy.

Almost any type of *vascular pathology* may be seen in the context of inflammatory bowel disease. Talbot et al. (1986), in a very large study of systemic vascular complications in almost 7200 patients with either ulcerative colitis or Crohn's disease, reported venous thromboembolic disease in 61 (0.8%), arterial thromboembolism in 31 (0.4%) and one or other forms of vasculitis (including, for example, cutaneous vasculitis and lupus-related vasculitis) in 12 patients (0.17%). Overall, there was little difference in the incidence of vascular disease between Crohn's disease and ulcerative colitis. Although rare, vasculitis may involve the CNS (Nelson et al., 1986); interestingly, these authors reported that activity of the vasculitic disorder paralleled that of the bowel disease.

Arterial strokes occurred in nine patients in this series (0.12%), others reporting frequencies varying between 0.65% (Lossos et al., 1995) and up to 4% (Elsehety and Bertorini, 1997). These too appear to correlate with disease activity (Mayeux and Fahn, 1978). Cerebral sinus venous disease is also well recognized (Lossos et al., 1995), albeit infrequently (Figure 8.1) (also reviewed in Mayeux and Fahn, 1978).

It is generally accepted that a hypercoagulable state is responsible for much of the increased incidence of vascular disease, with increased platelet counts, fibrinogen levels, factor VIII and rates of thromboplastin generation having been reported (reviewed in Talbot et al., 1986). Whether dehydration plays a role – in view of the correlation with disease activity of the enteropathy – has not formally been established, but appears likely. No trials of either prophylaxis or treatment have appeared, though the risk of gastrointestinal haemorrhage militates against formal anticoagulation.

Seizures are reported to occur frequently in patients with inflammatory bowel disease – in one series, epilepsy was the commonest neurological complication, seen in almost 6% of cases (Elsehety and Bertorini, 1997). Although autoimmune phenomena involving small vessels in the CNS were postulated, others have observed that at least half the seizure disorders occurred in connection with dehydration or sepsis (Gendelman et al., 1997). Other metabolic disturbances, including electrolyte imbalances, provide a further possible explanation, but in a significant proportion of cases, no other cause is found and a primary association is possible. Focal and generalized fits occur.

In their recent study, Lossos et al. (1995) described five patients – four with Crohn's disease and one with ulcerative colitis – with a slowly progressive *myelopathy*. Aged between 21 and 71, these patients typically exhibited no sensory level, no lower motor signs, and no sphincter disturbance. Three patients showed mild elevations of cerebrospinal fluid (CSF) protein content (mean 0.75 g/l), one of whom had oligoclonal immunoglobulin bands; one, aged 68, had periventricular white matter lucencies on T_2-weighted magnetic resonance imaging (MRI), of doubtful significance; none fulfilled the diagnostic criteria of multiple sclerosis. An inflammatory origin has been postulated, although the multiplicity of systemic and metabolic abnormalities, particularly including malabsorption, in patients with inflammatory bowel disease complicates explanation of a myelopathy. Other moderately large series (Elsehety and Bertorini, 1997; Gendelman *et al.*, 1997) make no mention of myelopathy, but Ray *et al.* (1993) reported a single patient with ulcerative colitis who developed an unexplained acute cervical myelopathy.

Other isolated cases of neurological disease – confusional episodes, syncope, optic atrophy, extrapyramidal disease and cerebellar degeneration – in the context of inflammatory bowel disease are mentioned in the literature, but their rarity suggests no significant relationship (Elsehety and Bertorini, 1997; Gendelman *et al.*, 1997). Beyond the CNS and the scope of this text, but of interest nonetheless, is peripheral neuropathy, which is seen in 0.5–1.0% of cases (Lossos *et al.*, 1995a; Elsehety and Bertorini, 1997). Acute Guillain–Barré syndrome is the commonest, and since *Campylobacter* infection is linked both with exacerbations of inflammatory bowel disease (Podolsky, 1991a,b) and acute inflammatory neuropathy, an obvious common explanation suggests itself. Myopathy, sometimes of metabolic origin but mostly inflammatory, is also reported.

Whipple's disease

Whipple's disease is an uncommon disorder first described 90 years ago (Whipple, 1919). Although conventionally classified as a gastrointestinal disease, the first patient described had multisystem involvement, with an arthropathy, respiratory symptoms, anaemia, fever, erythema nodosum and severe wasting in addition to steatorrhoea and abdominal distension. It is now clearly recognized as a multisystem granulomatous disease caused by an organism only recently identified after decades of search, *Tropheryma whippelii* (Wilson *et al.*, 1991; Relman *et al.*, 1992).

Moderately large series have confirmed that the typical clinical features are essentially as described by Whipple in his original case, with prominent diarrhoea and steatorrhoea, weight loss and abdominal pain, an arthropathy, pigmentation, lymphadenopathy, and fever with general malaise (Fleming *et al.*, 1988). The diagnosis has conventionally been based upon the demonstration of the characteristic periodic acid–Schiff (PAS)-positive bacilli in the wall of the small intestine and in mesenteric lymph nodes, but may also now be confirmed by polymerase chain reaction (PCR) amplification of bacillary DNA.

Approximately 10% of patients have neurological involvement; 5% are said to present in this way (Brown *et al.*, 1990), and a wide variety of features may be seen including (probably most commonly) dementia, ophthalmoplegia (which may be supranuclear), seizures and ataxia (Finelli *et al.*, 1980; Adams *et al.*, 1987; Wroe *et al.*, 1991; Louis *et al.*, 1996). Louis' survey and analysis of published cases has confirmed this order of frequency – of 84 reported patients, cognitive changes were recorded in 71% (with episodes of encephalopathy in 50% and psychiatric abnormalities in 44%), supranuclear gaze palsy in 51%, fits in 23% and ataxia in 20% (Louis *et al.*, 1996). Pyramidal signs are common (37%). Movement disorders are well described, particularly myoclonus (25%), and so-called oculo-masticatory or oculo-facio-skeletal myorhythmia, characterized by rhythmic vergeance oscillations associated with synchronous jaw movements and reported in 20% of patients, is said to occur solely in the context of Whipple's disease (Schwartz *et al.*, 1986; Hausser *et al.*, 1988; Louis *et al.*, 1996). Hypothalamic features, including somnolence and other sleep disturbances, polydipsia, increased appetite and hypogonadism, are reported in 31% of cases (Adams *et al.*, 1987; Louis *et al.*, 1996), as is eye disease, ranging from keratitis to uveitis, papilloedema and ptosis (23%) (Finelli *et al.*, 1977; Louis *et al.*, 1996). Cranial neuropathies are seen in 25% of patients.

It is now well recognized that perhaps 20% of cases of cerebral Whipple's disease occur in the absence of gastrointestinal or indeed other systemic symptoms (Adams *et al.*, 1987; Wroe *et al.*, 1991; Louis *et al.*, 1996). It will come as no surprise to the reader to learn that in such patients, the diagnosis can be difficult. Computed tomography scanning may be normal, and MRI likewise, although the latter in other cases reveals abnormalities which are essentially non-specific, multiple high signal intensity areas on T_2-weighted images, perhaps seen particularly in the vicinity of the hypothalamus. Multiple enhancing mass lesions warranting biopsy have also been reported (Wroe *et al.*, 1991; see Figure 8.2).

Spinal fluid examination reveals an elevated protein in approximately 50% of cases; there is a raised cell count in a similar proportion (Louis *et al.*, 1996); widely varying ratios of monocytes and polymorphonucleocytes are reported. Pathognomic PAS-positive bacilli are identified in the spinal fluid in 29% of samples (Feurle *et al.*, 1979; Louis *et al.*, 1996); repeat spinal fluid examination may be necessary before organisms are identified.

A normal or non-informative small bowel biopsy does not exclude cerebral Whipple's disease – approximately 30% of reported cases (Finelli *et al.*, 1977; Feurle *et al.*, 1979). Louis *et al.* (1996), in their careful and extremely valuable review of the literature, make the important point that electron microscopy forms a vital part of this investigation – none of the 14 non-diagnostic small bowel biopsies identified in the literature had undergone electron microscopy. Lymph node biopsy can also be extremely useful – Louis *et al.* report samples of positive diagnostic value in 14 out of 15 biopsies. Again, the single non-diagnostic lymph node sample was not examined using electron microscopy; similarly, 10 out of 12 brain biopsies described in the literature were diagnostic and the two negative samples were not examined ultrastructurally (Louis *et al.*, 1996). Polymerase chain reaction analysis of blood, lymph node, spinal fluid, small bowel tissue or brain (Lynch *et al.*, 1997) is increasingly used as a diagnostic test (Cohen *et al.*, 1996).

Uniformly fatal before the introduction of antibiotics, Whipple's disease usually responds to tetracyclines, penicillin or, more commonly nowadays,

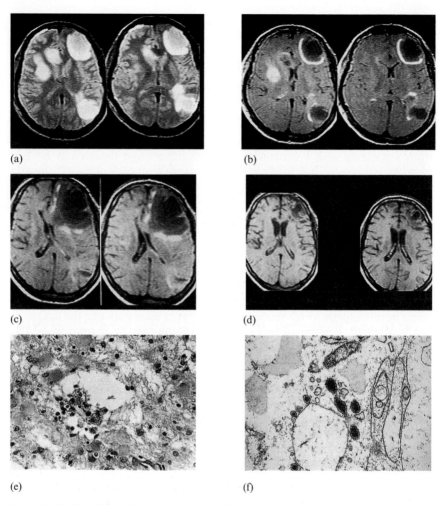

(a)   (b)

(c)   (d)

(e)   (f)

Figure 8.2 Cerebral Whipple's disease. Magnetic resonance imaging showed multiple high signal intensity lesions (a), many of which exhibited marked ring enhancement with gadolinium (b). Eight weeks later, many of these lesions – conspicuously that in the left frontal area – had enlarged considerably in size (c). After biopsy and 6 weeks' treatment (with tetracyclines followed by cotrimoxazole), there was a substantial improvement, with regression of many areas and only minimal enhancement (d). The biopsy showed PAS-positive granular material within foamy macrophages (e), ultrastructural study demonstrating the presence of bacilli within the cytoplasm (f). (Photographs kindly donated by Dr Steve Wroe, Ipswich Hospital.)

co-trimoxazole. *Tropheryma whippelii* has only very recently been cultured (Fredricks and Relman, 1997; Schoedon *et al.*, 1997), so that at present, the choice of treatment depends on experience (usually others') rather than laboratory guidance. Prompt treatment is, however, of the utmost importance in patients with neurological disease, which may (if untreated) run a profoundly aggressive and not unusually rapidly fatal course (Adams *et al.*, 1987). Relapse may occur in up to 40% of all cases (Keinath *et al.*, 1985), approximately one-third of these presenting with neurological features. In Keinath's series, the use of combined antibiotic regimes was associated with a reduced risk of relapse.

Antibiotics which are able to cross the blood–brain barrier have been recommended for the treatment of cerebral Whipple's disease, though only on empirical or anecdotal grounds (Ryser et al., 1984), Keinath et al. (1985) specifically suggesting penicillin and streptomycin (respectively in doses of 1.2 million units and 1.0 g) daily for 2 weeks, followed by oral co-trimoxazole, two tablets twice daily. In addition to its diagnostic use, PCR detection of persisting T. whippelii sequence is a valuable predictor of potential relapse – and its absence a useful indicator of therapeutic success (Ramzan et al., 1997; von Herbay et al., 1997).

The presence of PAS-positive bacilli within macrophages or microglia of CNS lesions implies strongly that CNS involvement occurs by direct infection rather than as a para-infectious inflammatory or metabolic/nutritional consequence. A Trojan Horse phenomenon, whereby bacilli gain access to the CNS parenchyma within circulating monocytes during the normal low-level passage across the blood–brain barrier (Hickey et al., 1991), may be the most likely explanation of cerebral disease. Prolonged survival and proliferation of organisms within the CNS, an environment relatively protected both from further immune policing and from circulating antibacterials, leads to later clinical recrudescence.

For the sake of completeness, it should also be mentioned that myopathy (with PAS-positive macrophages within muscle) and peripheral neuropathy are also reported, albeit rarely, in Whipple's disease.

Coeliac disease

Coeliac disease (non-tropical sprue) is an immunologically mediated disorder resulting from intolerance to dietary gluten, a protein present in wheat and many other cereals (Maki and Collin, 1997). Affected individuals develop weight loss with steatorrhoea and/or diarrhoea, with clinical evidence of malabsorption. Pathologically, the small bowel displays partial villous atrophy with loss of the surface mucosa and hyperplasia of the crypts.

In common with other enteropathies, neurological sequelae of a predictable nature may complicate coeliac disease as a direct consequence of malabsorption. An overall incidence of 10% is commonly quoted (Finelli et al., 1980). Hypokalaemia and hypocalcaemia may cause muscle weakness with a vacuolar myopathy; vitamin D deficiency may also contribute to muscle wasting. A neuropathy may occur for similar reasons, B_{12} deficiency here forming the principal culprit. Indeed, a syndrome closely resembling subacute combined degeneration of the spinal cord is described (Cooke and Smith, 1966), as is a Wernicke's-like picture. A suggested association with epilepsy has been disputed (Hanly et al., 1982).

A non-nutritional association with inflammatory muscle disease, specifically polymyositis, has been reported (Henriksson et al., 1982) and CNS complications apparently unrelated to deficiency states may also occur. Systemic and cutaneous vasculitis occurs rarely in patients with coeliac disease and two patients have been reported who developed biopsy- or necropsy-proven isolated CNS vasculitis in the context of established coeliac disease (Rush et al., 1986; Mumford et al., 1996). Neither exhibited granulomata pathologically. Both had seizures, one with ataxia and myoclonus (Ramsay–Hunt syndrome).

However, the cause of the most commonly described and distinctive CNS association, cerebellar or spino-cerebellar degeneration, with marked and usually progressive ataxia in some cases combined with brainstem eye movement disorders, remains unresolved. The clinical picture may also include myoclonus and epilepsy, and also dementia; a fatal outcome is not uncommon (Kinney *et al.*, 1982). Pathologically, there is no evidence of a vasculitic process in the large majority of cases (Kinney *et al.*, 1982; Ward *et al.*, 1985), with relatively non-specific findings of neuronal loss and gliosis in the cerebellum, in brainstem nuclei and spinal cord. Myelin loss also may be seen.

Vitamin E deficiency, which can, of course occur in malabsorption of any cause (Harding *et al.*, 1982), has been implicated, but although coeliac patients with this disorder responding to dietary treatment and vitamin supplementation are reported, vitamin E levels may be normal and gluten exclusion diets are more commonly entirely ineffective in preventing progressive neurological deterioration (Ward *et al.*, 1985). Furthermore, the onset of neurological features may occur simultaneously with or even precede gastrointestinal symptoms (Cooke and Smith, 1966; Finelli *et al.*, 1980; Kinney *et al.*, 1982), mitigating against deficiency as a cause. Finally, the retinal degeneration typical of vitamin E deficiency is not found in coeliac patients with ataxia.

It may be noted, however, that while the pathological changes of 'frank vasculitis' (not further detailed) described in a single patient with coeliac disease and Ramsay–Hunt syndrome (Mumford *et al.*, 1996) are not reported in the commoner cases of 'degenerative' spino-cerebellar disease, the clinical phenotypes are in fact clearly very similar. In fact, Kinney *et al.* (1982) mentioned that perivascular lymphocytic infiltrates were reported in five of the then 10 reported cases, raising the possibility of an immunological or inflammatory basis underlying the cerebellar disease. Pathological similarities with paraneoplastic CNS disorder have been drawn (Kinney *et al.*, 1982), supporting the hypothesis that immune responses to specific neuronal subpopulations may account for this, the commonest CNS complication of coeliac disease. The current author is not aware of studies seeking anti-neuronal antibodies in coeliac-associated cerebellar disease.

The extent to which inflammatory and immune enteropathies are associated with neurological complications is curious. Organ-specific diseases elsewhere do not, by and large, share this apparent propensity to metastasise to the brain. Primary inflammatory lung disease, for example, such as cryptogenic fibrosing alveolitis, does not spill in this way; no more do hepatobiliary diseases such as the chronic hepatititides and primary biliary cirrhosis. Inflammatory arthropathies are genuine multisystem disorders and are accorded their own chapter (see Chapter 7); likewise sarcoidosis (see Chapter 9). Primary renal disease, glomerulonephritis, tends to remain confined except when part of a systemic vasculitic disease – again dealt with separately (see Chapter 10). Autoimmune endocrine diseases commonly have neurological complications, but these are mostly unrelated to autoimmunity – stroke and neuropathy in diabetes, for example, tetany and fits in hypoparathyroidism. Stiff man syndrome has an oblique relationship to diabetes (see Chapter 6), but it is only the thyroid gland which is able to provide anything more than passing interest to the neurologist with an immunological bent.

The thyroid gland

Hyperthyroidism and myxoedema both carry neurological complications which have generally been considered direct consequences of abnormal thyroxine levels – anxiety, tremor, occasionally chorea, etc., in thyrotoxicosis, and lethargy, myopathy and dementia in hypothyroidism. Other organ-specific autoimmune diseases may co-exist, myasthenia gravis occurring in 0.35% of hyperthyroid patients, while in a large Mayo Clinic series of 153 patients with Hashimoto's thyroiditis, 23.5% had an associated autoimmune condition, such as rheumatoid arthritis, ulcerative colitis or pernicious anaemia (Becker and Ferguson, 1963).

The ophthalmoplegia of Graves' disease, whilst not strictly CNS involvement, is thought to be immunologically driven. The orbit and extraocular muscles are infiltrated with cells – lymphocytes and macrophages – together with glycosaminoglycans, resulting in restrictive muscle disease (Weetman, 1991). Circulating antibodies which react with orbital tissue, and bind to (and stimulate) thyroid-stimulating hormone receptors on thyroid cells are found (Strakosch et al., 1982a,b; Kendall Taylor et al., 1984). The orbital fibroblast, rather than the myocyte, appears to be the target, and thyroid-stimulating antibodies from patients with Graves' ophthalmopathy can also stimulate fibroblast collagen synthesis (Rotella et al., 1986). Radiotherapy and steroid treatment are equally effective in treatment (Prummel et al., 1989; Prummel and Wiersinga, 1995). An optic neuropathy may occur in the context of (usually severe) dysthyroid eye disease, due either to infiltration of the optic nerve or compression by hypertrophied muscles (Leonard et al., 1984; Dresner and Kennerdell, 1985).

Ataxia is perhaps the commonest CNS manifestation of hypothyroidism, occurring in 5–10% of patients. Pathologically there is Purkinje cell loss without evidence of inflammation, and an improvement with thyroxine treatment occurs. Although the dementia, psychiatric disturbances ('myxoedema madness') and subacute hypothermic, hypotensive coma of hypothyroidism likewise respond to (judicious) thyroxine hormone replacement (Cook and Boyle, 1986), an encephalopathy of apparently immunological, not endocrine, origin is described.

Shaw et al. (1991) reported five cases of what the authors termed Hashimoto's encephalopathy, a condition first identified by the Lord Brain (and co-authors) in 1966 (Lord Brain et al., 1966). The disorder presents classically as a relapsing encephalopathy, often associated with seizures, which may be focal or generalized. Myoclonus is often prominent (50% of cases) and stroke-like episodes are seen with a similar frequency. Tremor is common.

Imaging by computed tomography or even MRI is often normal (Shaw et al., 1991; Barker et al., 1996), as is angiography, though isotope brain scanning may show patchy uptake. Spinal fluid examination may reveal a raised protein level but typically a normal cell count. Most cases are clinically and biochemically euthyroid at presentation, but hypo- and hyperthyroid cases are reported (Shaw *et al.*, 1991; Barker *et al.*, 1996).

High titres of anti-thyroid antibodies are found, usually anti-microsomal. These plainly are fundamental to the diagnosis, but a role in pathogenesis has yet to be established – in one patient, thyroid microsomal antibodies were detected in the CSF (Shaw *et al.*, 1991). It is possible, but thus far entirely speculative, that these antibodies cross-react with brain antigens. An alternative suggestion is that they may through immune complex formation drive a putative vasculitic process (Shein *et al.*, 1986; Barker *et al.*, 1996); an association of Hashimoto's thyroiditis with vasculitis has in other tissues been reported – specifically, with giant cell arteritis (Nicholson *et al.*, 1984; Barker *et al.*, 1996) and vasculitic peripheral neuropathy. However, in the single case (thus far) of Hashimoto's encephalopathy with (post-mortem) histopathological investigation, no vasculitic changes were found – indeed the brain appeared normal (Lord Brain *et al.*, 1966).

Most patients respond well to steroid treatment; some have received further immunosuppressive therapy, such as cyclophosphamide or azathioprine.

References

Adams, M., Rhymer, P. A., Day, J., Dearmond, S. and Smuckler, E. A. (1987) Whipple's disease confined to the central nervous system. *Ann. Neurol.*, **21**, 104–108.

Barker, R., Zajicek, J. and Wilkinson, I. (1996) Thyrotoxic Hashimoto's encephalopathy {letter}. *J. Neurol. Neurosurg. Psychiat.*, **60**, 234.

Becker, K. L. and Ferguson, R. H. (1963) The connective tissue diseases and symptoms associated with Hashimoto's thyroiditis. *N. Engl. J. Med.*, **268**, 277–280.

Brown, A. P., Lane, J. C., Murayama, S. and Vollmer, D. G. (1990) Whipple's disease presenting with isolated neurological symptoms. Case report. *J. Neurosurg.*, **73**, 623–627.

Cohen, L., Berthet, K., Dauga, C., Thivart, L. and Pierrot, D. C. (1996) Polymerase chain reaction of cerebrospinal fluid to diagnose Whipple's disease {letter}. *Lancet*, **347**, 329.

Cook, D. M. and Boyle, P. J. (1986) Rapid reversal of myxedema madness with triiodothyronine {letter}. *Ann. Intern. Med.*, **104**, 893–894.

Cooke, W. T. and Smith, W. T. (1966) Neurological disorders associated with adult coeliac disease. *Brain*, **89**, 683–722.

Dresner, S. C. and Kennerdell, J. S. (1985) Dysthyroid orbitopathy. *Neurology*, **35**, 1628–1634.

Elsehety, A. and Bertorini, T. E. (1997) Neurologic and neuropsychiatric complications of Crohn's disease. *South. Med. J.*, **90**, 606–610.

Feurle, G. E., Volk, B. and Waldherr, R. (1979) Cerebral Whipple's disease with negative jejunal histology. *N. Engl. J. Med.*, **300**, 907–908.

Finelli, P. F., McEntee, W. J., Ambler, M. and Kestenbaum, D. (1980) Adult celiac disease presenting as cerebellar syndrome. *Neurology*, **30**, 245–249.

Finelli, P. F., McEntee, W. J., Lessell, S., Morgan, T. F. and Copetto, J. (1977) Whipple's disease with predominantly neuroophthalmic manifestations. *Ann. Neurol.*, **1**, 247–252.

Fleming, J. L., Wiesner, R. H. and Shorter, R. G. (1988) Whipple's disease: clinical, biochemical, and histopathologic features and assessment of treatment in 29 patients. *Mayo Clin. Proc.*, **63**, 539–551.

Fredricks, D. N. and Relman, D. A. (1997) Cultivation of Whipple bacillus: the irony and the ecstasy. *Lancet*, **350**, 1262–1263.

Gendelman, S., Present, D. and Janowitz, H. D. (1997) Neurological complications of inflammatory bowel disease. *Gastroenterology*, **82**, 1065.

Hanly, J. G., Stassen, W., Whelton, M. and Callaghan, N. (1982) Epilepsy and coeliac disease. *J.*

Neurol. Neurosurg. Psychiat., **45**, 729–730.

Harding, A. E., Muller, D. P., Thomas, P. K. and Willison, H. J. (1982) Spinocerebellar degeneration secondary to chronic intestinal malabsorption: a vitamin E deficiency syndrome. *Ann. Neurol.*, **12**, 419–424.

Hausser, H. C., Roullet, E., Robert, R. and Marteau, R. (1988) Oculo-facio-skeletal myorhythmia as a cerebral complication of systemic Whipple's disease. *Mov. Disord.*, **3**, 179–184.

Henriksson, K. G., Hallert, C., Norbby, K. and Walan, A. (1982) Polymyositis and adult coeliac disease. *Acta Neurol. Scand.*, **65**, 301–319.

Hickey, W. F., Hsu, B. L. and Kimura, H. (1991) T-lymphocyte entry into the central nervous system. *J. Neurosci. Res.*, **28**, 254–260.

Keinath, R. D., Merrell, D. E., Vlietstra, R. and Dobbins, W. O. (1985) Antibiotic treatment and relapse in Whipple's disease. Long-term follow-up of 88 patients. *Gastroenterology*, **88**, 1867–1873.

Kendall Taylor, P., Atkinson, S. and Holcombe, M. (1984) A specific IgG in Graves' ophthalmopathy and its relation to retro-orbital and thyroid autoimmunity. *Br. Med. J. Clin. Res. Edn*, **288**, 1183–1186.

Kinney, H. C., Burger, P. C., Hurwitz, B. J., Hijmans, J. C. and Grant, J. P. (1982) Degeneration of the central nervous system associated with celiac disease. *J. Neurol. Sci.*, **53**, 9–22.

Leonard, T. J., Graham, E. M., Stanford, M. R. and Sanders, M. D. (1984) Graves' disease presenting with bilateral acute painful proptosis, ptosis, ophthalmoplegia, and visual loss. *Lancet*, **ii**, 431–433.

Lord Brain, Jellinek, E. H. and Ball, K. (1966) Hashimoto's disease and encephalopathy. *Lancet*, **ii**, 512–514.

Lossos, A., River, Y., Eliakim, A. and Steiner, I. (1995) Neurologic aspects of inflammatory bowel disease. *Neurology*, **45**, 416–421.

Louis, E. D., Lynch, T., Kaufmann, P., Fahn, S. and Odel, J. (1996) Diagnostic guidelines in central nervous system Whipple's disease. *Ann. Neurol.*, **40**, 561–568.

Lynch, T., Odel, J., Fredericks, D. N., Louis, E. D., Forman, S., Rotterdam, H., *et al.* (1997) Polymerase chain reaction-based detection of *Tropheryma whippelii* in central nervous system Whipple's disease. *Ann. Neurol.*, **42**, 120–124.

Maki, M. and Collin, P. (1997) Coeliac disease. *Lancet*, **349**, 1755–1759.

Mayeux, R. and Fahn, S. (1978) Strokes and ulcerative colitis. *Neurology*, **28**, 571–574.

Minuk, G. Y. and Lewkonia, R. M. (1986) Possible familial association of multiple sclerosis and inflammatory bowel disease {letter} {see comments}. *N. Engl. J. Med.*, **314**, 586.

Mumford, C. J., Fletcher, N. A., Ironside, J. W. and Warlow, C. P. (1996) Progressive ataxia, focal seizures, and malabsorption syndrome in a 41 year old woman {clinical conference}. *J. Neurol. Neurosurg. Psychiat.*, **60**, 225–230.

Nelson, J., Barron, M. M., Riggs, J. E., Gutmann, L. and Schochet, S. S. J. (1986) Cerebral vasculitis and ulcerative colitis. *Neurology*, **36**, 719–721.

Nicholson, G. C., Gutteridge, D. H., Carroll, W. M. and Armstrong, B. K. (1984) Autoimmune thyroid disease and giant cell arteritis: a review, case report and epidemiological study. *Aust. NZ J. Med.*, **14**, 487–490.

Podolsky, D. K. (1991a) Inflammatory bowel disease (1) {see comments}. *N. Engl. J. Med.*, **325**, 928–937.

Podolsky, D. K. (1991b) Inflammatory bowel disease (2) {see comments}. *N. Engl. J. Med.*, **325**, 1008–1016.

Prummel, M. F., Mourits, M. P., Berghout, A., Krenning, E. P., Van Der Gaag, R., Koornneef, L., *et al.* (1989) Prednisone and cyclosporine in the treatment of severe Graves' ophthalmopathy {see comments}. *N. Engl. J. Med.*, **321**, 1353–1359.

Prummel, M. F. and Wiersinga, W. M. (1995) Medical management of Graves' ophthalmopathy. *Thyroid.*, **5**, 231–234.

Ramzan, N. N., Loftus, E., Burgart, L. J., Rooney, M., Batts, K. P., Wiesner, R. H., *et al.* (1997) Diagnosis and monitoring of Whipple disease by polymerase chain reaction. *Ann. Intern. Med.*, **126**, 520–527.

Rang, E. H., Brooke, B. N. and Hermon, T. J. (1982) Association of ulcerative colitis with multiple sclerosis {letter}. *Lancet*, **ii**, 555.

Ray, D. W., Bridger, J., Hawnaur, J., Waldek, S., Bernstein, R. M. and Dornan, T. L. (1993) Transverse myelitis as the presentation of Jo-1 antibody syndrome (myositis and fibrosing alveolitis) in long-standing ulcerative colitis. *Br. J. Rheumatol.*, **32**, 1105–1108.

Relman, D. A., Schmidt, T. M., MacDermott, R. P. and Falkow, S. (1992) Identification of the uncultured bacillus of Whipple's disease {see comments}. *N. Engl. J. Med.*, **327**, 293–301.

Rotella, C. M., Zonefrati, R., Toccafondi, R., Valente, W. A. and Kohn, L. D. (1986) Ability of monoclonal antibodies to the thyrotropin receptor to increase collagen synthesis in human fibroblasts: an assay which appears to measure exophthalmogenic immunoglobulins in Graves' sera. *J. Clin. Endocrinol. Metab.*, **62**, 357–367.

Rush, P. J., Inman, R., Bernstein, M., Carlen, P. and Resch, L. (1986) Isolated vasculitis of the central nervous system in a patient with celiac disease. *Am. J. Med.*, **81**, 1092–1094.

Ryser, R. J., Locksley, R. M., Eng, S. C., Dobbins, W. O., Schoenknecht, F. D. and Rubin, C. E. (1984) Reversal of dementia associated with Whipple's disease by trimethoprim-sulfamethoxazole, drugs that penetrate the blood–brain barrier. *Gastroenterology*, **86**, 745–752.

Sadovnick, A. D., Paty, D. W. and Yannakoulias, G. (1989) Concurrence of multiple sclerosis and inflammatory bowel disease {letter; comment}. *N. Engl. J. Med.*, **321**, 762–763.

Schoedon, G., Goldenberger, D., Forrer, R., Gunz, A., Dutly, F., Hochli, M., *et al.* (1997) Deactivation of macrophages with interleukin-4 is the key to the isolation of *Tropheryma whippelii*. *J. Infect. Dis.*, **176**, 672–677.

Schwartz, M. A., Selhorst, J. B., Ochs, A. L., Beck, R. W., Campbell, W. W., Harris, J. K., *et al.* (1986) Oculomasticatory myorhythmia: a unique movement disorder occurring in Whipple's disease. *Ann. Neurol.*, **20**, 677–683.

Shaw, P. J., Walls, T. J., Newman, P. K., Cleland, P. G. and Cartlidge, N. E. (1991) Hashimoto's encephalopathy: a steroid-responsive disorder associated with high anti-thyroid antibody titers – report of 5 cases. *Neurology*, **41**, 228–233.

Shein, M., Apter, A., Dickerman, Z., Tyano, S. and Gadoth, N. (1986) Encephalopathy in compensated Hashimoto thyroiditis: a clinical expression of autoimmune cerebral vasculitis. *Brain Dev.*, **8**, 60–64.

Strakosch, C. R., Joyner, D., Manley, S. W. and Wall, J. R. (1982a) The species specificity of TSH receptor binding antibodies as measured by radioreceptor study. *Clin. Endocrinol. Oxf.*, **17**, 173–179.

Strakosch, C. R., Wenzel, B. E., Row, V. V. and Volpe, R. (1982b) Immunology of autoimmune thyroid diseases. *N. Engl. J. Med.*, **307**, 1499–1507.

Talbot, R. W., Heppell, J., Dozois, R. R. and Beart, R. W. J. (1986) Vascular complications of inflammatory bowel disease. *Mayo Clin. Proc.*, **61**, 140–145.

Von Herbay, A., Ditton, H. J., Schuhmacher, F. and Maiwald, M. (1997) Whipple's disease: Staging and monitoring by cytology and polymerase chain reaction analysis of cerebrospinal fluid. *Gastroenterology*, **113**, 434–441.

Ward, M. E., Murphy, J. T. and Greenberg, G. R. (1985) Celiac disease and spinocerebellar degeneration with normal vitamin E status. *Neurology*, **35**, 1199–1201.

Weetman, A. P. (1991) Thyroid-associated eye disease: pathophysiology {see comments}. *Lancet*, **338**, 25–28.

Whipple, G. H. (1919) A hitherto undescribed disease characterised anatomically by deposits of fat and fatty acids in the intestinal and mesenteric lymphatic tissues. *Johns Hopkins Hosp. Bull.*, **18**, 382–391.

Wilson, K. H., Blitchington, R., Frothingham, R. and Wilson, J. A. (1991) Phylogeny of the Whipple's-disease-associated bacterium. *Lancet*, **338**, 474–475.

Wroe, S. J., Pires, M., Harding, B., Youl, B. D. and Shorvon, S. (1991) Whipple's disease confined to the CNS presenting with multiple intracerebral mass lesions. *J. Neurol. Neurosurg. Psychiat.*, **54**, 989–992.

Chapter 9

Sarcoidosis and the central nervous system

John Zajicek

Introduction	193
The pathogenesis of sarcoidosis	195
Clinical presentation of neurosarcoidosis	196
Making the diagnosis of neurosarcoidosis	199
Treatment and clinical course	206
References	207

Introduction

Sarcoidosis is a multisystem granulomatous disease of unknown aetiology (Newman *et al.*, 1997), which has a propensity to affect the lungs and rarely the nervous system; neurosarcoidosis may be an enigmatic diagnosis which is often entertained but rarely made with conviction. Prevalence rates for intrathoracic sarcoidosis vary from greater than 50 per 100 000, e.g. in New York African-Americans, to under 10 per 100 000 (James and Hosoda, 1994). Much higher prevalence rates were obtained when consecutive post-mortems were performed on approximately 60% of all deaths in an area of Sweden, when evidence of sarcoidosis was found in 43 individuals, only three of whom were known to have sarcoidosis during life, yielding a prevalence of 641 per 100 000 (Hagerstrand and Linel, 1963). The clinical significance of these findings is uncertain, but they suggest that the pathological process is far commoner than we recognize but this may be limited to subclinical disease in most cases. Intermediate estimates for the prevalence of systemic sarcoidosis of 10–20 per 100 000 are likely for Caucasians in London and New York.

Previous data from large series of patients with sarcoidosis have estimated that approximately 5% of such patients will have clinical involvement of the nervous system (Maycock *et al.*, 1963; Stilzbach *et al.*, 1974; Delaney, 1977; Stern *et al.*, 1985), although post-mortem studies suggest that ante-mortem diagnosis is only made in 50% with nervous system involvement (Iwai *et al.*, 1993). Conservatively we can therefore estimate that about five to 10 patients per million population will have clinical neurosarcoidosis.

The criteria upon which a clinical diagnosis of neurosarcoidosis is made have not been firmly established in the absence of positive nervous system histology; variation has existed between series of patients with the disease, although the criteria commonly accepted are a clinical picture compatible with neurosarcoidosis and histological confirmation of disease elsewhere. Conventionally it is therefore possible to make the diagnosis of neurosarcoidosis simply on the basis of a patient with an inflammatory clinical phenotype and a positive Kveim antigen skin test. Newer diagnostic techniques including magnetic resonance imaging and investigations to exclude other causes of granulomatous diseases must be encompassed in any attempt to refine such criteria further. Not surprisingly, therefore, effective means of treating the condition beyond the use of corticosteroids have not been established.

Advances in the treatment of any condition must rely on three factors:

1 The accurate assessment and diagnosis of patients.
2 An adequate knowledge of the natural history of each clinical manifestation.
3 The application of treatments which have been subjected to rigorous randomized placebo-controlled trials.

It is also preferable that this bulk of knowledge is underpinned by an adequate understanding of the pathogenesis of the condition. Because the number of patients with neurosarcoidosis is so small, the only way to obtain this information is through multicentre collaboration. In the absence of any definitive data on the management of neurosarcoidosis, this chapter will primarily be concerned with establishing the diagnosis of neurosarcoidosis and suggest treatments based on available studies from the literature, but will start with an overview on the pathogenesis of the central lesion in the disease, the sarcoid granuloma.

Table 9.1 Causes of granulomatous reactions

1. Infections	4. Inflammatory disorders
Cryptococcus	Sarcoidosis
Histoplasma	Wegener's granulomatosis
Coccidiodes	Giant cell arteritis
Blastomyces	Systemic lupus erythematosus
Aspergillus	Churg–Strauss syndrome
toxocara	Melkersson–Rosenthal syndrome
Toxoplasma	Primary angiitis of the nervous system
treponema	
Mycobacteria (TB)	
Whipple's disease	
	5. Others
	Radiotherapy
2. Chemicals	Chemotherapy
Silica	Chronic granulomatous disease of children
Beryllium	
Starch	
Zirconium	
Contrast agents	
3. Tumours	
Carcinoma	
Lymphoma	
Pinealoma	
Dysgerminoma	
Dermoid cyst	
Seminoma	
Reticulum cell sarcoma	
Malignant nasal granuloma	
Histiocytosis X	

The pathogenesis of sarcoidosis

In order that a diagnosis of sarcoidosis can be considered, non-caseating epithelioid cell granulomata must be demonstrated histologically. Numerous agents may provoke a granulomatous reaction and it is incumbent upon the clinician to try and exclude any potential provocation before accepting a diagnosis of sarcoidosis (see Table 9.1).

The predominant cell type in any granuloma is the mononuclear phagocyte, a term which includes blood-borne monocytes, tissue macrophages, brain microglia and epithelioid cells. These latter cells may amalgamate to produce giant cells. Well-formed granulomata usually contain macrophages with varying degrees of maturity, including activated and non-activated cells. Macrophages in areas of early granuloma formation express the calcium binding protein calgranulin Mac 387, which is an antigen shared by granulocytes and circulating monocytes but only a small proportion of tissue macrophages (Chilosi et al., 1990). This suggests that local recruitment from blood-borne monocytes is important in granuloma formation. Epithelioid cells retain macrophage markers within granulomata, confirming their lineage (Poulter, 1983). They also strongly express MHC Class II molecules and act as antigen-presenting cells (van der Oord et al., 1984). Epithelioid cells possess numerous well-developed cytoplasmic organelles containing material which is of intermediate electron density on electron microscopy. There is no evidence that these organelles contain fragments of microorganisms but it has been postulated that the epithelioid cells found in tuberculosis contain more prominent rough endoplasmic reticulum and fewer lysosymes, whereas the reverse may be true in sarcoidosis (Epstein, 1991).

As well as phagocytic cells, sarcoid granulomata also contain lymphocytes, reflecting their immune aetiology. Inorganic foreign body granulomata, e.g. those induced by silica, consist almost entirely of macrophages with very few lymphocytes. The inorganic material is resistant to degradation within macrophages and may induce cell death, leading to giant cell formation, but under these circumstances, there is little evidence of T cell activation and these granulomata therefore do not resemble immunologically-induced granulomata commonly found in sarcoidosis. Most lymphocytes found within sarcoid granulomata are CD4$^+$ T cells, found particularly at the centre of the lesion. CD8$^+$ cells and B cells tend to occur towards the periphery of granulomata (Modlin et al., 1984), but $\gamma\delta$ T cells may also play a role in the inflammatory process and cell numbers may be raised both systemically and locally at the site of granuloma formation (Balbi et al., 1990).

Not surprisingly, when investigators have looked at the cytokine and adhesion molecule profile within granulomata, a large array of molecules can be found. Lymphocyte function-associated molecule (LFA) and intracellular adhesion molecule (ICAM)-1 appear to be two of the major adhesion molecules expressed (Semenzato et al., 1994). Interleukin (IL)-1 and interferon (IFN)-γ are preferentially expressed at the centre of granulomata and the overall pattern of cytokine involvement is T_h1 rather than T_h2 (tumor necrosis factor-α, IL-1, IL-2). It is beyond the scope of the present chapter to provide great detail on granuloma formation and this can be found elsewhere (Semenzato *et al.*, 1994), but the end result of such granulomata is often fibrosis and scar formation which is not necessarily specific to sarcoidosis. Numerous proteins may be released which promote this process including platelet-derived growth factor, insulin-like growth factor (IGF)-1, transforming growth factor-β as well as tissue breakdown products including collagenases and free radicals.

The fundamental question concerning the driving stimulus behind granuloma formation remains extremely controversial and unanswered. Most observers would accept that there is undoubtedly an exaggerated immune response to an as yet unidentified antigen. Some argue that this is a mycobacterium, based on polymerase chain reaction (PCR) analysis of granuloma tissue (Mangiapan and Hance, 1995; Mitchell, 1997) together with the histological similarity between tuberculous and sarcoid lesions. Recent evidence implicating herpesvirus 8 has been presented (DiAlberti *et al.*, 1997).

One argument is that there is a genetic predisposition to an exaggerated response which is able to eradicate the microorganisms early and thus make identification very difficult (there is some evidence that sarcoidosis susceptibility may be inherited, as familial cases have been described and there appears to be a higher level of the disease in monozygotic rather than dizygotic twins (British Thoracic and Tuberculous Association, 1973)). Whatever the strength and weakness behind these arguments, no agent has fulfilled Koch's postulates and there is therefore insufficient evidence to firmly implicate any single agent in the pathogenesis of sarcoidosis.

Clinical presentation of neurosarcoidosis

Because nervous system sarcoidosis is relatively rare, few large series exist in the literature; the largest has been a British series of 68 patients (Zajicek *et al.*, 1999). In assessing the available data it is important to be aware of how each series has been compiled. For example, there is no prospective analysis of consecutive cases and most series will either have been compiled from patients in a sarcoidosis/chest clinic or from neurology departments. These factors have inevitably led to bias in certain directions, so that data from thoracic departments are more likely to show abnormalities on chest X-rays, whilst patients presenting to neurologists may not have had any previous evidence of systemic disease. Variation also exists in the degree to which individual clinicians pursue a diagnosis, e.g. although facial nerve paresis is a relatively common manifestation of neurosarcoidosis, 'Bell's palsy' is considered to have a generally benign clinical course and so it is not often that such cases are fully investigated to look for possible neurosarcoidosis.

Allowing for these caveats, some useful information can be obtained by comparing some of the largest series in the literature (James and Sharma, 1967; Delaney, 1977; Stern *et al.*, 1985; Oksanen, 1986; Chapelon *et al.*, 1990; Zajicek *et al.*, 1999). The total number of cases in these series is 247 and although the average percentage of cases with peripheral nerve and muscle involvement in all except the most recent series was in the order of 30%, Zajicek *et al.* (1999) found no cases with peripheral nervous system involvement. It certainly appears that such manifestations are rare in

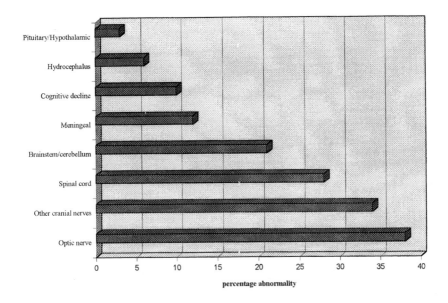

Figure 9.1 Clinical presentations of neurosarcoidosis in the 68 patients of the UK series.

peripheral nerve clinics in the UK (P. T. Thomas, personal communication) and this may reduce one's tendency to obtain a tissue diagnosis using peripheral tissue.

Of the 68 patients identified as having definite or probable neurosarcoidosis, according to criteria postulated in the British series, 53% of patients were male and 47% female. Mean age at presentation was 38.9 years (range 21–64 years). 17.7% had histological confirmation from CNS tissue in the absence of any other identifiable cause and thus fulfilled the criteria for definite neurosarcoidosis. The average length of follow-up was 4.6 years (range 2 months–18 years). Sixty-nine percent of patients were followed up for a period of greater than 18 months and it was on this group that treatment results were reported.

Clinical presentation

Thirty-eight percent of patients in the British series had sarcoidosis previously diagnosed in another organ. Most commonly this was confined to the chest or anterior uvea, but 62% of patients presented with central nervous system (CNS) involvement. Details of clinical features at presentation are summarized in Figure 9.1.

Optic nerve disease is a very common presentation of neurosarcoidosis and 38% of patients had evidence of a lesion at this site in our series, 69% with clinical evidence of unilateral and 31% bilateral disease. The characteristic picture is often an atypical optic neuritis, subacute in onset, which might recover following steroids or cause permanent visual impairment. Initial steroid sensitivity is occasionally followed by dependence, with symptoms

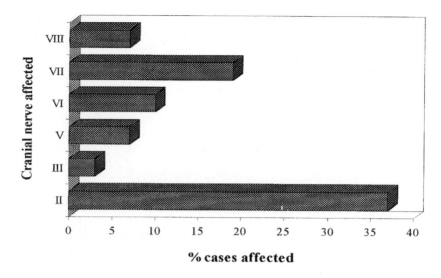

Figure 9.2 Cranial nerve involvement in the series total of 68 patients.

deteriorating below a certain dosage level. In a prognostic analysis of patients with optic nerve disease who were followed up for lengthy periods, visual acuities were available in 16 cases who were followed up for at least 18 months. Thirteen of these patients had visual acuities of 6/18 or worse in at least one eye at presentation. Over the follow-up period five patients showed a deterioration to at least 6/60, five patients improved to at least 6/9 and three patients showed no significant change from their presentation acuity. As all these patients received corticosteroid treatment, these data would suggest an approximate 40% chance of appreciable recovery over long-term follow-up with this therapy. Other series have confirmed the anterior visual pathways as a site of predilection for neurosarcoid, often second only to the facial nerve.

When investigating patients for neurosarcoidosis, a full neuro-ophthalmological workup is therefore indicated, including a search for both anterior and posterior segment disease with slit lamp examination and fluorescein angiography, as well as seeking clinical and/or visual evoked potential evidence for optic nerve disease. Unfortunately, optic nerve disease has a tendency to be severe with profound impairment of visual acuity being all too common.

Other cranial nerve palsies formed the second most common presentation in the British series in one-third of patients (see Figure 9.2). If optic nerve disease is also taken into account then 72% of patients presented with cranial nerve palsies; this compares with 59% in the combined series of 247 patients (see above). Nineteen percent of patients in the British series had facial nerve paralysis (33% in the combined series); eight of these were unilateral palsies, two were bilateral and simultaneous, two were recurrent on the same side, and there was one case of sequential palsy initially on the left and then involving the right within weeks.

Only seven patients who presented with facial nerve palsies were followed up for more than 18 months, five of whom deteriorated or died over this period and two stabilized, but there was evidence from those followed up for shorter periods of time that presenting with facial nerve paresis carried a more favourable prognosis than optic nerve or spinal cord disease. Facial nerve palsies are a classical manifestation of neurosarcoidosis and have been reported as carrying a good prognosis in previous publications (Delaney, 1977). Although sarcoidosis does not appear to feature prominently among the causes of facial nerve palsies in large series (Prescott, 1988; Keane, 1994), there has not been a large prospective analysis of such patients looking specifically for sarcoidosis. Relatively little comment can be made on the prognosis of neurosarcoidosis presenting with facial palsy based on the largest series in view of the relatively small number of patients in whom long-term follow-up data were available. There may well be a difference in prognosis depending on where the facial nerve is affected along its course. Certainly examples of cerebrospinal fluid (CSF) abnormalities in cases of apparently pure facial palsy in the British series suggest that the lesion may result from a meningitic reaction, but the classical explanation for facial palsy in neurosarcoidosis is that it is secondary to inflammation in the parotid gland, although many early authors also noted the lack of temporal correlation between parotitis and facial palsy (Wilson, 1940). More detailed prospective studies are clearly needed to assess the site and significance of such palsies.

Zajicek et al. (1999) described 28% of patients with clinical signs of spinal cord disease. In 10 patients this was clinically confined to the cord whilst nine patients also had clinical disease elsewhere in the neuraxis. Fifteen cases with spinal cord disease were followed up for more than 18 months and 11 of these deteriorated (73%), these results suggesting that such a presentation carries a poorer prognosis than certain other manifestations of neurosarcoidosis. Previous large series have reported prevalence levels of up to 10% (James and Sharma, 1967; Stern et al., 1985; Oksanen, 1986). Syndromes ranged from intramedullary tumour-like presentations to meningitic-radicular syndromes (reviewed in Zajicek, 1990).

Brainstem and/or cerebellar presentations occurred in 21% of patients in the British series, who principally exhibited limb or gait ataxia and eye movement abnormalities such as failure of vertical gaze. There was one instance of central vomiting. Ten percent of cases presented with cognitive decline and 12% with a meningitic illness in the series at presentation. Details of other presentations are shown in Figure 9.1.

Making the diagnosis of neurosarcoidosis

A confident diagnosis of neurosarcoidosis is often difficult, particularly when the clinician is presented with an isolated CNS disorder which has an inflammatory 'flavour'. The nervous system is a relatively uncommon site for the disease to manifest and as a consequence, investigation to establish a diagnosis has centred on searching for histological confirmation in other organs. Clinical criteria for making the diagnosis of neurosarcoidosis based upon clinical certainty have been postulated (Zajicek et al., 1997); thus in order to fulfil conditions for definite disease the patient must have an appropriate clinical syndrome with positive nervous system histology in the absence of any other cause. Probable disease has then been defined according to various indirect indicators of disease as outlined in Table 9.2. A rigorous definition of neurosarcoidosis is necessary for a number of reasons. Most important among these is the possibility of alternative explanations for neurological syndromes in patients with suspected systemic sarcoidosis. Particular difficulty arises with clinical phenotypes resembling multiple sclerosis with optic nerve, spinal cord or brainstem disease; other diseases may also exhibit clinical features similar to those of neurosarcoidosis and these include Lyme disease (with facial nerve palsies and root irritation syndromes), Wegener's granulomatosis (with meningeal involvement), Behçet's disease, meningeal carcinomatosis, tuberculosis and lymphomatosis.

Table 9.2 Proposed criteria for the diagnosis of neurosarcoidosis

Definite	Clinical presentation suggestive of neurosarcoidosis with exclusion of other possible diagnoses and the presence of positive nervous system histology.
Probable	Clinical syndrome suggestive of neurosarcoidosis with laboratory support for central nervous system inflammation (elevated levels of cerebrospinal fluid protein and/or cells, the presence of oligoclonal bands and/or magnetic resonance imaging evidence compatible with neurosarcoidosis) and exclusion of alternative diagnoses together with evidence for systemic sarcoidosis (either through positive histology, including Kveim test, *and/or* at least two indirect indicators from Gallium scan, chest imaging and serum ACE).
Possible	Clinical presentation suggestive of neurosarcoidosis with exclusion of alternative diagnoses where the above criteria are not met.

A greater precision in diagnostic definition not only allows for accurate prospective analysis of prognostic indicators and better assessment and validation of indirect indicators of disease, but also enables therapeutic trials to be conducted in a meaningful fashion. However, biopsy of CNS tissue is required to make a definite diagnosis of neurosarcoidosis according to these criteria. When the patient is seriously ill with rapidly progressive disease in several parts of the neuraxis it is important to achieve a diagnosis as quickly as possible in order that appropriate therapy can be commenced and under these circumstances guided stereotactic or open biopsy is often performed, either of meninges and/or of parenchymal lesions. With less severe disease and/or a more gradual course, it is often more appropriate to perform indirect investigations to look for systemic disease and treat accordingly (see below).

Retrospective analysis of the usefulness of biopsy to assess the specificity and sensitivity of any other single investigation inevitably introduces bias, as biopsy is undertaken selectively, e.g. on mass lesions, where the possibility of neoplasia has been raised, in patients with severe and rapidly progressive disease or in cases where histology is relatively easy to obtain. The site of lesions (which influences the decision to biopsy) will also influence the clinical presentation – for example cortical lesions may be more likely to present with epilepsy and be biopsied, thus interpretation of the clinical presentation of this group of patients must be cautious. Another major difficulty with interpreting data from these patients is the incomplete data available, as investigations are often halted once tissue diagnosis is achieved. Establishing the diagnosis of neurosarcoidosis is often difficult and the only way to acquire firm evidence for the value of any single investigation is to perform a prospective study using appropriate investigations in all patients, especially those in whom a definite histological diagnosis has been obtained. The understandable tendency not to perform further investigations once the diagnosis has been obtained has limited our knowledge on the usefulness of non-invasive methods for investigating neurosarcoidosis.

Most patients being investigated for neurosarcoidosis have a chest radiograph and at presentation in the British series 31% were abnormal. This compares with 65% abnormality in the combined series and probably again reflects referral bias (see above). The most common abnormality was bilateral hilar lymphadenopathy, seen in 28% of patients, 6% of whom had some pulmonary abnormality in addition. There were two cases of pulmonary shadowing in the absence of obvious lymphadenopathy. Previous studies utilizing chest computed tomography (CT) suggest it may assist in targeting transbronchial biopsy. Subclinical thoracic disease is present in most cases of extrathoracic sarcoidosis (Wallaert et al., 1986; Ohara et al., 1993).

The most useful investigation continues to be the Kveim antigen skin test, which was positive in 85% of patients who were tested in the British series. This compares favourably with rates of positivity in other patients with systemic sarcoidosis (Scadding and Mitchell, 1985). The usefulness of this test compared to tissue diagnosis by other means has previously been assessed (Mitchell et al., 1980). That study reviewed the procedures by which histological confirmation was obtained in 79 patients with a final diagnosis of sarcoidosis. Transbronchial lung biopsy was performed in 42 cases and showed sarcoid-type granulomata in 37. Kveim tests were performed in 44 and were interpreted as being positive in 19 and equivocal in 11. Thus whilst rates of granulomatous 'positive' Kveim test responses are usually lower than those obtained by appropriate tissue biopsy, a positive Kveim test can be regarded as comparable to that of finding granulomata in a biopsy of a site remote from that principally affected and compared with other positive tissue biopsies, it has the advantage of an added degree of selectivity for sarcoidosis appropriate to a carefully validated Kveim test suspension.

Material for the Kveim test performed in British patients is prepared from human sarcoid spleen by the Public Health Laboratory Service, under a product licence approved by the UK Medicines Commission. Before a spleen can be accepted for processing, the utmost care is used to ensure that there is minimum possibility of an infectious risk. The test suspension is validated alongside a reference suspension of known potency and selectivity to maintain the expected proportion of positive reactions among patients with sarcoidosis and a negligible number (1.3–3%) among others. No untoward or unexpected clinical findings have been reported after Kveim testing over 20 years, and this is in keeping with earlier international studies in which 3244 individuals in 37 countries have been given one or more Kveim tests with no adverse effects (Stilzbach, 1966). Recent questions concerning safety of the test and particularly the idea that it may transfer sarcoidosis, have been vigorously refuted (DuBois *et al.*, 1993); it has yet, however, to gain approval by the US Food and Drugs Administration (Newman *et al.*, 1997). The major problem with the Kveim test lies in the 4–6 week time interval required to elapse before biopsy can be performed. This period may be crucial in intervening in the disease process, particularly when lesions occur in clinically critical sites. Concomitant use of corticosteroids may reduce systemic granuloma formation including the site of Kveim antigen insertion and this is a likely explanation for negative Kveim results observed in cases of biopsy proven disease. All seven of the Kveim negative patients in the British series were being treated with systemic corticosteroids. Hence, although the Kveim test is an invaluable aid in the diagnosis of neurosarcoidosis, up to 3% may be false positive and negative results may occur with concomitant corticosteroid therapy.

The usefulness of performing 'blind' biopsies from other organs, including liver and lung, in patients with suspected neurosarcoidosis, is uncertain. Whilst tissue diagnosis from sites outside the nervous system has previously been considered sufficient to establish the diagnosis of neurosarcoidosis in the context of an appropriate clinical syndrome, we would still only consider this as evidence of systemic disease which by itself is insufficient to be certain of neurological involvement by granulomatous tissue.

Cerebrospinal fluid abnormalities are common in neurosarcoidosis and were present in over 80% of cases at presentation in the British series. The most common abnormality was an elevation in protein, sometimes to very high levels. Forty-five percent of cases demonstrated a CSF lymphocytosis, with occasional rare neutrophils and monocytes. Fifty-five percent of patients had CSF oligoclonal bands: one-third of these cases provided evidence for systemic synthesis and two-thirds fulfilled the criteria for local synthesis. Only three of this latter group of patients had normal CSF protein levels, which may be a way of helping to distinguish them from those patients with multiple sclerosis.

The significance of raised CSF angiotensin converting enzyme (ACE) levels in the context of elevated protein concentrations or CSF cell counts remains uncertain. It is likely that their usefulness may be principally confined to that small number of patients where levels are raised out of proportion to the protein concentration, when the CSF does not contain large numbers of inflammatory cells, and the serum ACE is not elevated. The best estimate would be an ACE index analogous to the IgG index (CSF/serum ACE divided by CSF/serum albumin). Serum ACE was elevated in 23.5% of patients in the British series. Other biochemical indices were unhelpful in establishing a diagnosis, serum calcium was normal in all cases and erythrocyte sedimentation rate was elevated in 6% of cases.

Whole body gallium scanning remains a useful indicator of systemic disease, which although again is a relatively non-specific measure, adds diagnostic probability to a case. [67]Ga citrate is taken up at sites of active sarcoidosis and also by other inflammatory and malignant diseases, including tuberculosis and lymphomas, but the pattern of uptake among patients with active sarcoidosis is well recognized. Accordingly, as a component of the investigations relevant to the diagnosis of extrathoracic sarcoidosis it can be very helpful although constrained by the limitations

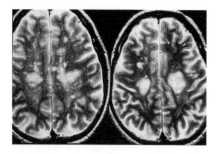
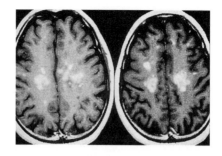

(a)   (b)

Figure 9.3 An example of multiple magnetic resonance imaging (MRI) white matter lesions and meningeal enhancement in a 27-year-old man of middle-eastern extraction who originally developed bilateral anterior uveitis which responded to treatment with steroid eye drops. A year later he developed gradually increasing weakness of his legs with urinary symptoms, impotence and an abdominal sensory level. Cerebrospinal fluid at the time showed 19 lymphocytes and a protein of 0.7 g/l. Kveim test was positive and myelogram demonstrated an expansion of the thoracic cord. Cranial T_2-weighted MRI (a) revealed multiple areas of high signal intensity, predominantly in the white matter, although some also involved the cortex. There was also abnormal high signal on T_2-weighted images within the cord at the mid-thoracic level. He was commenced on oral prednisolone after a course of intravenous therapy which improved his leg spasticity somewhat but attempts to reduce the dose to less than 30 mg/day led to a worsening of his symptoms. His disease slowly progressed over the course of the next 9 years, but clinically appeared to be confined to the spinal cord. Magnetic resonance imaging 7 years after the onset of his neurological disease (b) again demonstrated numerous areas of high signal within the white matter, many of which were periventricular and a high proportion of which enhanced with gadolinium as shown above. There was also abnormal enhancement of the meninges covering the temporal lobes, but no basal enhancement. On sagittal T_2-weighted fast spin echo images there was an area of high signal of the cord opposite T_5 and T_6, which had changed little since the original examination.

imposed by subjective interpretation. In a consecutive unpublished series of 42 such patients a definite pattern of uptake was obtained in 18 (42%), whilst the pattern of uptake was considered equivocal in eight and negative in 16. In the British series, 45% of patients in whom this investigation was performed proved to have increased uptake which was usually in the salivary glands or chest.

Magnetic resonance imaging (MRI) has greatly aided the investigation of patients with inflammatory brain disease and has consistently proved to be more sensitive than CT. Magnetic resonance imaging or CT scans were available for review in 44 patients in the British series, eight of whom fulfilled the proposed criteria for definite neurosarcoidosis. The T_2-weighted cranial MRIs of 37 patients (seven definite), were reviewed along with gadolinium-enhanced T_1-weighted scans in 29 patients; 11 patients had spinal MRI. Cranial CT was carried out in 20 patients, with contrast enhancement in 15. Seven patients had brain CT without MRI.

The most common abnormality on MRI was multiple white matter lesions, which were present in 16, 43% of the patients whose scans were reviewed; an example of this is shown in Figure 9.3. Meningeal enhancement occurred in 11 out of 29 (38%) of cases studied and four out of seven (57%) of the definite cases. Figures 9.4 and 9.5 illustrate meningeal enhancement.

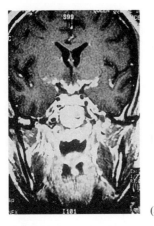
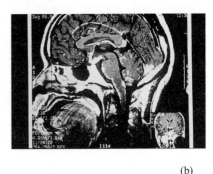

(a)   (b)

Figure 9.4 An example of meningeal involvement in a 32-year-old man who presented with blurred vision in his right eye, with subsequent weight loss, cerebrospinal fluid lymphocytosis and protein above 2 g/l. Panels (a) and (b) show sagittal and coronal T_1-weighted gadolinium-enhanced brain magnetic resonance images with extensive leptomeningeal enhancement, especially in the basal meninges, and including the optic chiasm and the upper cervical meninges.

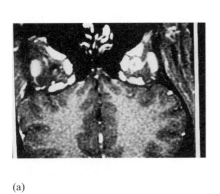
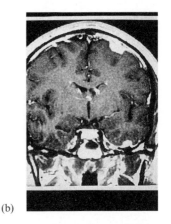

(a)   (b)

Figure 9.5 Magnetic resonance imaging (MRI) findings in a 54-year-old Caucasian housewife who presented with gradual painful visual loss in her left eye over the course of 9 months, associated with a rippling effect in her visual field. At the time there were no associated neurological abnormalities on examination outside the visual system. Temporal artery biopsy was normal and a course of intravenous methylprednisolone made no difference to her blindness. The pain became much worse 7 months after the onset and was exacerbated by adducting the left eye. At that stage there was no perception of light in the left eye and the fundus showed a swollen disc with peri-papillary haemorrhage. Routine blood and cerebrospinal fluid investigations were normal, with no oligoclonal bands detectable. MRI (shown above) demonstrated thickening of the left optic nerve extending from behind the globe to the chiasm (a) with abnormal contrast enhancement (T_1-weighted gadolinium-enhanced coronal MRI (b) showing a thickening and enhancement of the dural sheath of the right optic nerve with widespread dural enhancement with focal thickening of the meninges over the convexity and the left temporal region). Transection and biopsy of the optic nerve demonstrated non-caseating granulomata with multinucleate giant cells, confirming the diagnosis of optic nerve sarcoidosis. The patient was initially treated with intravenous methylprednisolone followed by oral prednisolone.

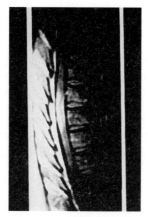

Figure 9.6 A previously well 49-year-old Caucasian company director started to experience band-like sensory phenomena around his waist which progressed over the course of 4 months to produce difficulty in walking with sphincter dysfunction. Examination revealed a spastic paraparesis with a sensory level at T_8. Magnetic resonance imaging of the spinal column (seen here) revealed an expanded spinal cord with pathological contrast enhancement at this site, which was felt to be an intramedullary tumour (T_1-weighted gadolinium-enhanced sagittal MRI of the thoracic spinal cord showing focal contrast enhancement and expansion of the cord at T_6–T_7 level). A laminectomy was performed and biopsy showed the typical appearances of sarcoidosis. The patient was treated with oral prednisolone and intravenous cyclophosphamide at 400 mg/day until his peripheral leukocyte count fell to below 4×10^6/ml. When last reviewed, over 2 years after the presentation of his illness, he was virtually asymptomatic and able to walk long distances unaided. He was maintained on 25 mg of prednisolone on alternate days together with amytriptyline for residual paraesthesiae.

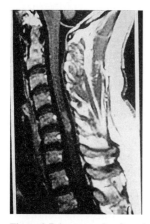
(a)   (b)
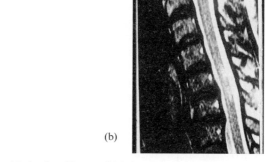

Figure 9.7 An example of a spinal cord lesion in a 37-year-old Asian man who presented with a progressive paraplegia with a positive Kveim test, normal cerebrospinal fluid and a positive ^{67}Ga scan (with uptake in the lacrimal and parotid glands and hilar region). (a) T_2-weighted sagittal magnetic resonance image showing focal area of abnormal high signal at C_5–C_6. (b) T_1-weighted gadolinium-enhanced image shows focal contrast enhancement at that level.

Figure 9.5 also shows optic nerve enhancement, which was seen in eight patients (28%). Examples of spinal cord involvement are shown in Figures 9.6 and 9.7. Computed tomography generally produced less information than MRI, particularly in the posterior fossa. Pathological meningeal contrast enhancement occurred on CT in four patients (20%), white matter lesions were detected in six (30%) and lesions of the optic nerve or chiasm were seen in two (10%).

All these abnormalities have been described in previous series of cases (Miller *et al.*, 1988; Seltzer *et al.*, 1991). The distinction of neurosarcoidosis from multiple sclerosis can sometimes be very difficult. Although none of the appearances is specific for neurosarcoidosis, meningeal enhancement or persistent enhancement (more than a few weeks) of parenchymal lesions are much more suggestive of a granulomatous process and are not expected in multiple sclerosis. Occasionally, white matter lesions are seen in sarcoidosis which are indistinguishable from multiple sclerosis.

It is recognized that the diagnostic criteria suggested here will inevitably exclude a number of patients with neurosarcoidosis. However, the further detailed prospective study of patients, so defined, may permit identification of diagnostic factors and patterns which will assist in the diagnosis of milder or atypical forms of the disease.

Treatment and clinical course

It is difficult to produce valid observations concerning the effectiveness of treatment for neurosarcoidosis unless patients have been followed up for long periods of time. In the British series this was at least 18 months. Forty-seven patients meeting this criterion were analysed according to treatment received and overall clinical course. The mainstay of medical treatment in neurosarcoidosis is corticosteroids and 34 patients received this therapy alone, usually as a combination of long-term oral prednisolone with or without intravenous methylprednisolone boluses. Ten out of 34 (29%) improved or stabilized, whereas 24 out of 34 (71%) deteriorated. Other therapies were tried only as steroid treatment was becoming ineffective or side effects were too severe; such treatments included methotrexate, azathioprine and hydroxychloroquine. The number of patients treated with any other single regime was too small to draw firm conclusions. Cyclosporin was used in three instances and was associated with improvement in one. Cranial irradiation was used in two instances, in one case after cyclosporin had failed and in one case after corticosteroids proved ineffective. Intravenous cyclophosphamide was used at high dosage (400 mg/day until the peripheral white cell count fell to below 4×10^6/ml) in three cases, who all improved.

Although the British series was the largest single series of cases with neurosarcoidosis yet reported, with the most extensive follow-up details, it remains impossible to identify those patients in whom early aggressive immunotherapy would be beneficial. As no prospective data are available in this condition, analysis of the available data would suggest that disease presenting in the spinal cord or optic nerve, together with epilepsy, carry a poorer prognosis than facial nerve palsies. Most patients are treated with systemic corticosteroids which often carry significant side effects as dosages tend to be high and prolonged. Although some patients improve on this treatment, many continue to have troublesome disease. It is often the case that symptoms tend to recur at doses of prednisolone less than 20–25 mg/day (or the equivalent in other corticosteroid type), making cessation of corticosteroids difficult. The incidence of steroid-related side effects is extremely high with such prolonged treatment. Concomitant anticonvulsant therapy, which induces hepatic microsomal enzymes, may reduce prednisolone concentration and efficacy, necessitating even higher oral doses. Bolus pulsed intravenous methylprednisolone gives a high initial loading dose of corticosteroid and may help to avoid side effects associated with long-term oral treatment.

Even fewer data exist concerning the efficacy of other forms of immunomodulatory therapy. The use of chlorambucil (Kataria, 1980), methotrexate (Lower and Baughman, 1990; Soriano et al., 1990), chloroquine (Morse et al., 1961), cyclosporin (Kavanaugh et al., 1987; Cunnah et al., 1988; Stern et al., 1992), radiotherapy (Grizzanti et al., 1982; Bejar et al., 1985; Gelwan et al., 1988) and in the British series cyclophosphamide, have all been reported. Recent experience suggests that methotrexate, usually used weekly in a dose of 10 mg, may be of value in maintaining optimal suppression together with intravenous/oral prednisolone, and this is often used as a first line steroid-sparing agent. Hydroxychloroquine has also proved to be a very useful adjunct to steroids (Sharma, 1998); at a dose of 200 mg/day the Ophthalmological Society has approved its use without recourse to examination with red light. This can be used daily for up to about 1 year and is worth considering as a first line agent together with methotrexate. Cyclosporin, cyclophosphamide and fractionated radiotherapy all need further assessment. One regime for the management of neurosarcoidosis consists of initiating treatment with 1 g intravenous methylprednisolone for 3 days together with at least 25 mg of oral prednisolone or equivalent per day. Intravenous methylprednisolone 1 g is then continued on a weekly basis for a number of weeks, allowing a reduction of oral prednisolone to 15–20 mg/day. During this period oral methotrexate and hydroxychloroquine may be added, especially with severe disease or a poor initial response to steroids. In severe cases, the intravenous methylprednisolone may be continued for some months, with a gradually increasing inter-dose interval. However, it must be emphasized that clear guidelines and indications for treatment together with the drugs which should be used in different clinical circumstances remain matters for further scientific enquiry.

In an uncommon illness, progress in management requires co-operation on a large scale, to establish a large prospective series in order to validate the diagnostic criteria and to enable more trials of treatment. Better data are needed concerning the prognosis of clinical presentations, the usefulness of particular investigations and in the early diagnosis of neurosarcoidosis. It is only with such information that a rational approach to treatment can be designed. At the present time neurosarcoidosis continues to carry one of the poorer prognoses of any of the protean manifestations of the disease.

References

Balbi, B., Moller, D. R., Kirby, M., et al. (1990) Increased numbers of T-lymphocytes with $\gamma\delta$ T antigen receptors in a subgroup of individuals with pulmonary sarcoidosis. J. Clin. Invest., **85**, 1353–1361.

Bejar, J. M., Kerby, G. R., Ziegler, D. K. and Festoff, B. W. (1985) Treatment of central nervous system sarcoidosis with radiotherapy. *Ann. Neurol.*, **18**, 258–260.

British Thoracic and Tuberculous Association (1973) Familial associations in sarcoidosis: a report to the research committee of the British Thoracic and Tuberculous Association. *Tubercle*, **54**, 87–97.

Chilosi, M., Mombello, A., Montagna, L., *et al.* (1990) Multimarkers immunohistochemical staining of calgranulins, chloracetate esterase, and S100 for simultaneous demonstration of inflammatory cells on paraffin sections. *J. Histochem. Cytochem.*, **38**, 1669–1675.

Cunnah, D., Chew, S. and Wass, J. (1988) Cyclosporin for central nervous system sarcoidosis. *Am. J. Med.*, **85**, 580–581.

DiAlberti, L., Piatelli, A., Artese, L., *et al.* (1997) Human herpesvirus 8 variants in sarcoid tissues. *Lancet*, **350**, 1655–1661.

Delaney, P. (1977) Neurologic manifestations of sarcoidosis review of the literature with a report of 23 cases. *Ann. Intern. Med.*, **87**, 336–345.

DuBois, R. M., Geddes, D. M, and Mitchell, D. N. (1993) Moratorium on Kveim test. *Lancet*, **342**, 173.

Epstein, W. L. (1991) Ultrastructural heterogeneity of epithelioid cells in cutaneous organised granulomata of diverse aetiology. *Arch. Dermatol.* 127, 821–826.

Gelwan, M. J., Kellen, R. I., Burde, R. M. and Kupersmith, M. J. (1988) Sarcoidosis of the anterior visual pathway: successes and failures. *J. Neurol. Neurosurg. Psychiat.*, **51**, 1473–1480.

Grizzanti, J. N., Knapp, A. B., Schecter, A. J. and Williams, M. H. (1982) Treatment of sarcoid meningitis with radiotherapy. *Am. J. Med.*, **73**, 605–608.

Hagerstrand, I. and Linel, F. (1964) The prevalence of sarcoidosis in the autopsy material from a Swedish town. In *Proc. IIIrd Int. Conf. on Sarcoidosis* (Lofgren, S., ed.), *Acta Med. Scand.* **(Suppl)** 425, 171.

Iwai, K., Tachibana, T., Takemura, T., Matsui, Y., Kitaichi, M. and Kawabata, Y. (1993) Pathological studies on sarcoidosis autopsy. 1. Epidemiological features of 320 cases in Japan. *Acta Path. Japon.*, **43**, 372–376.

James, D. G. and Hosoda, Y. (1994) Epidemiology of sarcoidosis. In *Sarcoidosis and other Granulomatous Diseases* (James, D. G., ed.), pp. 729–743. New York: Marcel Dekker.

James, D. G. and Sharma, O. P. (1967) Neurosarcoidosis. *Proc. R. Soc. Med.*, **60**, 1169–1170.

Kataria, Y. P. (1980) Chlorambucil in sarcoidosis. *Chest*, **78**, 36–43.

Kavanaugh, A. F., Andrew, S. L., Cooper, B., Lawrence, E. C. and Huston, D. P. (1987) Cyclosporin therapy of central nervous system sarcoidosis. *Am. J. Med.*, **82**, 387.

Keane, J. R. (1994) Bilateral seventh nerve palsy: and analysis of 43 cases and review of the literature. *Neurology*, **44**, 1198–1202.

Lower, E. E. and Baughman, R. P. (1990) The use of low dose methotrexate in refractory sarcoidosis. *Am. J. Med. Sci.*, **299**, 153–157.

Mangiapan, G. and Hance, A. J. (1995) Mycobacteria and sarcoidosis: an overview and summary of recent molecular biological data. *Sarcoidosis*, **12**, 20–37.

Maycock, R. L., Bertrand, P., Morrison, C. E. and Scott, J. H. (1963) Manifestations of sarcoidosis: analysis of 145 patients with a review of the literature. *Am. J. Med.*, **35**, 67–89.

Miller, D. H., Kendall, B. E., Barter, S., *et al.* (1988) Magnetic resonance imaging in central nervous system sarcoidosis. *Neurology*, **38**, 378–383.

Mitchell, D. N. (1997) Mycobacteria and sarcoidosis. *Lancet*, **348**, 768–769.

Modlin, R. L., Hofmann, F. M., Scharma, O. P., *et al.* (1984) Demonstration in situ of subsets of T-lymphocytes in sarcoidosis. *Am. J. Dermatopathol.*, **6**, 423–427.

Morse, S. I., Cohn, Z. A., Hirsch, J. G. and Schaedler, R. W. (1961) The treatment of sarcoidosis with chloroquine. *Am. J. Med.*, **30**, 779–784.

Newman, L. S., Rose, C. S. and Maier, L. A. (1997) Sarcoidosis. *N. Engl. J. Med.*, **336**, 1224–1234.

Ohara, K., Okubo, A., Kamata, K., Sasaki, H., Kobayashi, J. and Kitamura, S. (1993) Transbronchial lung biopsy in the diagnosis of suspected ocular sarcoidosis. *Arch. Ophthalmol.*, **111**, 642–644.

Oksanen, V. (1986) Neurosarcoidosis: clinical presentations and course in 50 patients. *Acta Neurol. Scand.*, **73**, 283–290.

Poulter, L. W. (1983) Antigen presenting cells *in situ*: their identification and involvement in immunopathology. *Clin. Exp. Immunol.*, **53**, 520–523.

Prescott, C. A. J. (1988) Idiopathic facial nerve palsy (the effect of treatment with steroids). *J. Laryng. Otol.*, **102**, 403–407.

Scadding, J. G. and Mitchell, D. N. (1985) The Kveim reaction. In *Sarcoidosis* (Scadding, J. G. and Mitchell, D. N., eds), pp. 444–481. London: Chapman & Hall.

Semenzato, G., Agostini, C., Chilosi, M. (1994) Immunology and immunohistology. In *Sarcoidosis and other Granulomatous Diseases* (James, D. G., ed.), New York: Marcel Dekker.

Seltzer, S., Mark, A. S. and Atlas, S. W. (1991) CNS sarcoidosis: evaluation with contrast-enhanced MR imaging. *Am. J. Neuroradiol.*, **12**, 1227–1233.

Sharma, O. P. (1998) Effectiveness of chloroquine and hydroxychloroquine in treating selected patients with sarcoidosis with neurological involvement. *Arch. Neurol.*, **55**, 1248–1254.

Soriano, F. G., Caramelli, P., Nitrini, R. and Rocha, A. S. (1990) Neurosarcoidosis: therapeutic success with methotrexate. *Postgrad. Med. J.*, **66**, 142–143.

Stern, B. J., Krumholz, A., Johns, C., Scott, P. and Nissim, J. (1985) Sarcoidosis and its neurological manifestations. *Arch. Neurol.*, **42**, 909–917.

Stern, B. J., Schonfeld, S. A., Sewell, C., Krumholz, A., Scott, P. and Belendiuk, G. (1992) The treatment of neurosarcoidosis with cyclosporin. *Arch. Neurol.*, **49**, 1065–1072.

Stilzbach, L. E. (1996) An international Kveim test study 1960–1966. In *La Sarcoidose Rapports de la IV Conference Internationale* (Turief, J. and Chabot, J., eds), pp. 200–213. Paris: Masson.

Stilzbach, L. E., James, D. G., Neville, E., Turiaf, J., Battesti, J. P., Sharma, O. P., Hosoda. Y., Mikami, R. and Odaka, M. (1974) Course and prognosis of sarcoidosis around the world. *Am. J. Med.*, **57**, 847–885.

van der Oord, J. J., de Wolf-Peeters, C., Facchetti, F. and Desmet, V. J. (1984) Cellular composition of hypersensitivity-type granuloma. Immunohistochemical analysis of tuberculous and sarcoidal lymphadenitis. *Hum. Pathol.*, **15**, 559–565.

Wallaert, B., Ramon, P., Fournier, E. C., Prin, L., Tonnel, A. B. and Voisin, C. (1986) Activated alveolar macrophage and lymphocyte alveolitis in extrathoracic sarcoidosis without radiological mediastinopulmonary involvement. *Ann. N. Y. Acad. Sci.*, **465**, 201–210.

Wilson, S. A. K. (1940) Uveoparotid paralysis. In *Neurology* (Wilson, S. A. K., ed.), pp. 599–601. London: Edward Arnold.

Zajicek, J. P. (1990) Sarcoidosis of the cauda equina: a report of three cases. *J. Neurol.*, **237**, 244–246.

Zajicek, J. P., *et al.* (1999) Central nervous system sarcoidosis diagnosis and management based on a large series. Submitted for publication.

Chapter 10

Cerebral vasculitis

Neil Scolding

Introduction	210
Classification	211
Histopathology	212
Mechanisms of tissue damage in vasculitis	213
The clinical features of central nervous system vasculitis	218
Investigation and diagnosis	219
The treatment of cerebral vasculitis	234
Giant cell arteritis and Takayasu's disease	237
Behçet's disease	240
Vogt–Koyanagi–Harada syndrome	243
References	244

Introduction

Cerebral vasculitis is a serious but uncommon condition. In a not atypical neurology unit, it accounts for a maximum of 0.5% admissions, with a very crudely estimated minimum annual incidence of perhaps 1–2 per million. This may be compared with a more accurately estimated incidence of systemic vasculitis of 39 per million (Watts and Scott, 1997). Cerebral vasculitis may be primary and idiopathic; alternatively, cerebral vasculitis may occur in the context of a number of systemic disorders – inflammatory and otherwise – or be precipitated by extraneous agents. An enormous range of clinical features, reflecting diffuse, focal or multifocal involvement of any part of the brain, is possible. The natural history is also widely variable, with acute, chronic, relapsing, fulminant or benign monophasic courses all well described. There is no perfect diagnostic test – angiography, widely perceived to be a powerful diagnostic tool, has significant false negative and positive rates, while biopsy is invasive and may not prove definitive. Furthermore, not a single one of the currently recommended therapeutic regimes has been subjected to the rigours of a randomized treatment trial.

In recent years there have been a number of important advances in the diagnostic approach to multisystem vasculitis, with new serological, imaging and clinical procedures rapidly finding their places in the routine management of patients with renal, pulmonary, dermatological or other organ involvement (Savage *et al.*, 1997; Watts and Scott, 1997). Significant progress in our understanding of the pathological processes underlying vasculitis has been accompanied by the development of novel and successful immunological therapies, and there has been a clear improvement in the prognosis of systemic vasculitic disorders (Lai *et al.*, 1990; Mathieson *et al.*, 1990; Jayne *et al.*, 1991; Jennette and Falk, 1991; Jennette *et al.*, 1994a, b). It therefore becomes timely to re-examine vasculitic disease of the nervous system, and to investigate whether these recent advances present new opportunities for improving the diagnosis, treatment and outlook of these difficult and challenging disorders.

Classification

The vasculitides are an heterogeneous group of disorders which share certain pathological features, in particular intramural inflammation and necrotic changes within the walls of blood vessels. Classification has proved difficult and a number of systems have been proposed which depend variably on additional histological characteristics, such as the size of vessel involved and the presence or otherwise of granulomata, or on to the clinical context and organ involved. Primary vasculitic disorders include Wegener's granulomatosis, microscopic polyangiitis and temporal arteritis, while vasculitis may alternatively be secondary to collagen vascular or rheumatologic disorders, malignancy (particularly myeloproliferative disease), drugs, or infections such as hepatitis B or C.

The most recent classification systems (e.g. Jennette *et al.*, 1994a; Scott and Watts, 1994; Watts and Scott, 1997) depend largely on vessel size – giant cell and Takayasu's arteritis mainly affecting large vessels (i.e. the aorta and large regional branches), classical polyarteritis nodosa and Kawasaki disease principally involving medium-sized vessels (the main visceral arteries), and (most) of the remaining vasculitides, e.g. Wegener's disease, Churg–Strauss syndrome, etc., predominantly affecting small vessels. Scott and Watts have modified this system, incorporating a useful 'primary' and 'secondary' subclassification (Table 10.1).

Table 10.1

Dominant vessel involved	Primary	Secondary
Large arteries	Giant cell arteritis	Aortitis with rheumatoid disease;
	Takayasu's arteritis	infection (e.g. syphilis)
Medium arteries	Classical polyarteritis nodosa	Infection (e.g. hepatitis B)
	Kawasaki disease	
Small vessels and medium arteries	Wegener's granulomatosis	Vasculitis with rheumatoid disease,
	Churg–Strauss syndrome	Systemic lupus erythematosus,
	Microscopic polyangiitis	Sjögren's syndrome, drugs, infection (e.g. HIV)
Small vessels	Henoch–Schönlein purpura	Drugs (e.g. sulphonamides, etc.)
	Essential cryoglobulinaemia	Infection (e.g. hepatitis C)
	Cutaneous leukocytoclastic vasculitis	

Reproduced with permission from Scott and Watts (1994).

Organ-specific vasculitis compounds the difficulties of classification. Certain tissues – in particular, kidney and lung – are especially susceptible to vasculitic diseases, and are commonly involved in many systemic vasculitides. Occasionally, however, vasculitic processes appear to confine themselves exclusively to single organs. Giant cell arteritis involving only the mesenteric vessels is described (Smith *et al.*, 1988), as is organ-restricted polyarteritis. In Eale's disease and Cogan's syndrome, the vasculitic process is found respectively only in the retina and in the eye and audiovestibular apparatus.

Involvement of the central nervous system (CNS) or peripheral nervous system (PNS) can occur in any of the systemic vasculitides (Sigal, 1987; Moore and Calabrese, 1994b). Additionally, primary isolated vasculitis of the CNS or of the PNS is recognized, where little or no inflammation is apparent outside the nervous system (Dyck *et al.*, 1987; Calabrese and Mallek, 1988; Moore, 1994a). Vasculitis restricted to the CNS was first described only in 1959 by Cravioto and Feigin, who used the term 'granulomatous angiitis' (Cravioto and Feigin, 1959). It was later suggested that the occurrence of granulomata was variable and non-specific (though others propose that the presence of granulomata is prognostically useful, indicating more aggressive disease (Hankey, 1991)) and that 'isolated vasculitis of the CNS' was a more useful term. However, disease apparently confined to the CNS may have systemic manifestations both clinically, on careful direct enquiry, and pathologically (Cravioto and Feigin, 1959; Sigal, 1987), so that the term 'primary angiitis of the CNS' (PACNS) may be preferable. In both primary and secondary CNS vasculitis, the neurological features arising from inflammation and necrosis of the vasculature – principally, the consequences of infarction – can be devastating and permanent, but CNS vasculitis remains under-recognized and notoriously difficult to diagnose, further accentuating the clinical problem.

Histopathology

The classical pathological change in vasculitis is that of an inflammatory infiltrate within the vascular wall associated with destructive changes, commonly described as fibrinoid necrosis (Figure 10.1). In many organs, this vascular injury results in occlusion and infarction, usually the principal cause of clinical manifestations. Onto this histopathological template, additional features are associated with specific vasculitic syndromes (Lie, 1995, 1997).

In *classical polyarteritis nodosa*, which is rather an uncommon disorder, erosion of the vascular wall commonly and characteristically results in aneurysm formation. Microscopically, necrotising changes are present with mixed cells, some authors suggesting that neutrophils are less prominent than CD4$^+$ lymphocytes and macrophages (Cid *et al.*, 1994). Granulomata are rare both in this disorder and in *microscopic polyangiitis* – from which histopathological distinction may be difficult. In *Churg–Strauss* syndrome, extravascular granulomata are prominent and diagnostically important, as is the presence of a prominent eosinophilic infiltrate. It may not surprise even the unwary that granulomata are similarly a key feature of *Wegener's granulomatosis*; a necrotising, leukocytoclastic picture is apparent. The latter is a characteristic feature of *hypersensitivity vasculitis*, usually with a neutrophilic infiltrate, though lymphocytic disease is well described.

A variety of pathological pictures are described in *isolated CNS angiitis*

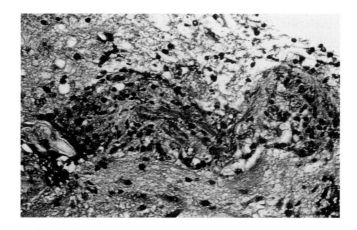

Figure 10.1 Cerebral biopsy, 28-year-old female with isolated cerebral vasculitis. Clear changes of necrotising leukocytoclastic vasculitis are present, with an intense cellular infiltrate predominantly comprising neutrophils.

(Lie, 1992a). Characteristically, small vessels – arteries much more frequently than veins – in the cerebral parenchyma and the leptomeninges are involved, but vessels of varying calibre may be affected (Younger *et al.*, 1988). Typically, the process is patchy and multifocal, with skip lesions, contributing to the significant false negative diagnostic rate of cerebral biopsy. Any part of the vessel wall may be involved. Granulomata may or may not be present; some authors have suggested that their presence indicates a poor prognosis (Hankey, 1991), but the presence of both granulomatous and non-granulomatous angiitis in adjacent vessels of the same patient (Lie, 1992a) undermines this proposal.

In granulomatous lesions, the cellular infiltrate is generally mixed, and includes lymphocytes, plasma cells and histiocytes. Langerhans and foreign body-type giant cells are present. In non-granulomatous angiitis, there is either an infiltrate predominantly of lymphocytes, or a polyarteritis-like picture, with marked necrotic change (Hankey, 1991; Lie, 1992a).

Notwithstanding the characteristic pathological pictures in classical instances of each of the many specific vasculitic syndromes, including the size of vessel involved, presence of granulomata, etc., the point may be made that in most cases, the principal function of biopsy is to confirm the presence of vasculitis. Quite often, it may only serve as a diagnostic guide for distinguishing the various subtypes and must be used in conjunction with the clinical picture; alone it can be a poor arbitrator (Lie, 1995).

Mechanisms of tissue damage in vasculitis

Whilst recent systems of classification of the vasculitides, such as those described above, represent a considerable improvement over previous methods, an aetiologically- or pathogenetically-based system would have a more rational biological basis and might be expected to be more useful in predicting therapies. Unfortunately, the current very limited understanding both of the initiating causes of vasculitis – in contrast to many autoimmune disorders, there does not even appear to be a Class II major histocompatibility complex (MHC) association upon which to build hypotheses of causation (Zhang *et al.*, 1995) – and of the mechanisms of tissue damage, does not yet permit such an approach to be applied to the whole spectrum of vasculitic syndromes.

The exception to this general rule of aetiological ignorance is that group of vasculitides occurring in the context of infectious diseases, where direct bacterial (e.g. Neisserial, spirochaetal), viral (e.g. herpes zoster), atypical bacterial (e.g. rickettsial) or fungal invasion of the vascular wall causes the vasculitic process. It should be stressed that the clinical picture produced by these microbial vasculitides may not differ from that in primary immunologically driven vasculitis, patients having come to grief when their (infectious) vasculitic syndrome was treated vigorously but inappropriately with immune suppressants, a vivid illustration of the therapeutic value of an aetiologically based approach to classifying vasculitis.

Antibody-dependent mechanisms of vascular injury

Of the two classical effector limbs of the immune system, cellular and humoral, the latter appears far more important in the development of the vasculitic process than cell-mediated events, although the constant qualification of this simplified approach to immune mechanisms – that humoral and cellular immunity are interdependent and cannot truly be divorced – again applies.

Three principal pathways of vascular injury are commonly invoked (e.g. (Jennette *et al.*, 1994b)): immune complex-mediated vasculitis, direct antibody attack of the vasculature, and anti-neutrophil cytoplasmic antibody (ANCA)-related vasculitis; all depend ultimately on antibodies. T cell-dependent mechanisms are rather less commonly implicated in vasculitis, but will also be discussed.

Immune complex-mediated vasculitis

Immune complex deposition in the wall of blood vessels triggers activation of the complement cascade and the consequent recruitment of polymorphs and macrophages, amplification of inflammation, and the generation of lytic and injurious membrane attack complexes. This sequence of events is widely quoted as a cause of the vasculitic process, although there are in fact rather few examples in which this has been demonstrated unequivocally.

Vasculitis associated with certain infections may, however, arise as a result of this process (although in others mentioned above, direct invasion of the vessel wall by the perpetrating contagion, rather than the immunological sequelae, is responsible). Hepatitis B associated vasculitis has long been considered an immune complex-mediated process, and more recently, hepatitis C infection and subsequent immune complex formation and deposition has been found to underlie many cases of cryoglobulinaemic vasculitis (Agnello *et al.*, 1992) – we and others have observed mononeuritis multiplex in this context (Scolding *et al.*, unpublished observations; Khella *et al.*, 1995; Apartis *et al.*, 1996).

Henoch–Schönlein purpura, serum sickness and the uncommon true vasculitis associated with lupus also share this mechanism. A common clinical correlate of vasculitis driven by immune complex formation is (type I membranoproliferative or mesangiocapillary) glomerulonephritis.

Direct antibody attack
Antibodies directed against the glomerular basement membrane (GBM) provide the most robust example of vascular injury directly caused by specific antibodies. In Goodpasture's syndrome, the vasculitic process induced by these antibodies (which are directed against type IV collagen antigens (Wieslander *et al.*, 1987)) is limited to capillaries in the lungs and the glomeruli. Systemic vasculitis associated with anti-GBM antibodies also occurs and here involves vessels larger than capillaries, but in these cases anti-GBM antibodies are usually accompanied by ANCA.

Antibodies directed against endothelial cells have been reported in a variety of disorders, including multiple sclerosis and experimental allergic encephalomyelitis (Tsukada *et al.*, 1987), where a pathological role has been suggested. Studies of patients with vasculitic syndromes have also revealed the presence of anti-endothelial cell antibodies. Such antibodies have been shown to activate or to injure endothelial cells (Carvalho *et al.*, 1996), though their lack of specificity, coupled with rather variable rates of detection, has left questions concerning their relevance (Chan *et al.*, 1993). Medium and large vessel vasculitis (and therefore less often cerebral disease) are more frequently associated with anti-endothelial cell antibodies than small vessel disease (Salojin *et al.*, 1996).

A slightly more complete – although still far from wholly compelling – story has emerged concerning a possible role for anti-endothelial cell antibodies in *Kawasaki disease* (Leung *et al.*, 1986; Tizard *et al.*, 1991; Jacobs, 1996). This disorder was originally described in 1967 in Japan (Kawasaki *et al.*, 1974) as an acute febrile childhood disease with conjunctival injection, dryness of the lips with a strawberry tongue, cervical lymphadenopathy, a polymorphic rash and a hand–foot syndrome. Acutely, a pan-carditis and a coronary arteritis may complicate the illness; coronary artery aneurysm represents a longer term complication. Neurologically there is commonly an aseptic meningitis; hemiplegic stroke, encephalopathy and facial palsy have also been recorded. Pathologically, an acute systemic inflammatory vasculitis, with little or no fibrinoid necrosis, underlies the disease. Circulating antibodies of IgG and IgM classes exert cytotoxic effects on cultured endothelial cells stimulated by tumour necrosis factor or interleukin (IL)-1 (Leung *et al.*, 1986); more recently, a toxic effect in the absence of cytokine stimulation has been demonstrated (Kaneko *et al.*, 1994), though clearly, this still falls well short of proving a role *in vivo*. An alternative suggested role for bacterial superantigen immune stimulation now appears unlikely following detailed studies of V_β and T cell activation markers in patients (Pietra *et al.*, 1994).

Anti-neutrophil cytoplasmic antibody-related vasculitis
The description of antibodies directed against cytoplasmic antigens in polymorphonuclear cells in patients with systemic vasculitis represented a major advance in serological diagnosis of these disorders (Niles, 1996).

Indirect immunofluorescence testing using ethanol-fixed neutrophils reveals two patterns of reactivity – cytoplasmic ('cANCA'), associated with Wegener's granulomatosis, and perinuclear, ('pANCA'), rather less specific, but commonly seen in microscopic polyangiitis and Churg–Strauss syndrome (and with glomerulonephritis). These fluorescence reactivities are associated with specificity for a neutrophil serine protease, proteinase (PR)-3, and myeloperoxidase (MPO), respectively. More recently, antibodies of a third specificity have been described, associated with cANCA or pANCA fluorescence patterns. These react with another component of neutrophil granules termed bactericidal/permeability-increasing protein (BPI), which has potent anti-bacterial activity against Gram-negative organisms (Zhao *et al.*, 1995). No specific disease association of this reactivity is apparent, positive results occurring with samples from patients with Wegener's granulomatosis, microscopic polyarteritis, Behçet's syndrome and organ-specific vasculitis. Other specificities continue to be described (Kain *et al.*, 1995), answers awaiting the correct question.

It should, however, be emphasized that disease specificity of ANCAs antibodies is far from absolute or perfect: positive results are seen occasionally in individuals with no clinically apparent vasculitic disorder and less rarely in patients with connective tissue disorders, particularly lupus (Spronk *et al.*, 1996; Merkel *et al.*, 1997), again with no discernible vasculitic component to their disease.

Despite the diagnostically useful specificity of these circulating antibodies, it has been observed that detailed histological studies of ANCA-related vasculitis often reveal little evidence of antibody-dependent tissue damage – neither immune complexes, complement components, nor immunoglobulins are readily identifiable – suggesting that the ANCAs may not play a direct role in tissue damage. One potential explanation for this apparent paradox offers an indirect role for these antibodies, i.e. the suggestion that ANCAs activate circulating mononuclear cells, stimulating an inflammatory cell attack on the vessel wall (Jennette, 1994; Jennette *et al.*, 1994b). Clearly, the cytoplasmic antigens within neutrophils (and monocytes) constituting the ANCA targets are ordinarily inaccessible to antibodies, but it has been shown that, upon stimulation of polymorphonucleocytes with the cytokines tumour necrosis factor (TNF)-α or IL-8, small amounts of PR-3 are translated to the surface of neutrophils (Csernok *et al.*, 1994). Once there, PR-3 becomes accessible to circulating ANCAs and it has been shown that the ensuing antibody–antigen binding triggers a neutrophil response, dependent on antigen-bound ANCAs interacting with Fc receptors (Porges *et al.*, 1994; Mulder *et al.*, 1995); changes in intracellular calcium regulation are seen (Lai *et al.*, 1994; Porges *et al.*, 1994); ultimately, degranulation with free radical production follows (Falk *et al.*, 1990). Cross-linking of ANCA antigens plays an important role in this process (Kettritz *et al.*, 1997).

Following movement from primary granules in the cytoplasm to the cell surface, enzymes are released, including PR-3 and MPO. These can be identified in the lesions of, for example, Wegener's granulomatosis (Brouwer *et al.*, 1994a), where they may play a role in tissue damage (Brouwer *et al.*, 1994a). PR-3 may lyse human endothelia, or indeed induce apoptosis of these cells (Yang *et al.*, 1996)

A potential further role for ANCAs later in this putative sequence of events is proposed. cANCA (specific to PR-3) inhibits inactivation of this enzyme, blocking the binding of the naturally occurring regulator α_1-antitrypsin (Dolman *et al.*, 1993). Paradoxically, some of the destructive effects of PR-3 can, however, also be directly inhibited by ANCA (Ballieux *et al.*, 1994); the overall effect of these antibodies on enzyme function *in vivo* therefore remains unknown.

Yet other mechanisms by which ANCA might induce tissue damage have been suggested, centred on involvement of vascular endothelial cells. ANCA binding to neutrophils precipitates adherence to endothelial cells (Keogan *et al.*, 1993), probably via β_2 integrin (Reumaux *et al.*, 1995), followed by endothelial cell damage (Ewert *et al.*, 1992; Savage *et al.*, 1992).

Cytokines (including TNF-α, interferon (IFN)-γ, and IL-1α and -1β) also induce endothelial cell PR-3 expression followed by its translocation to the cell surface (Mayet *et al.*, 1993), re-emphasizing the possibility of a direct effect of circulating ANCAs on blood vessels. Circulating MPO and PR-3 enzymes also bind to endothelial cells (Pall and Savage, 1994), where they might then bind ANCAs. The postulate of direct ANCA-mediated endothelial damage would, however, be difficult to reconcile with the suggestion that immunoglobulins are not detectable in pathological studies of ANCA-related vasculitis; furthermore, *in vivo*, PR-3 expression in affected endothelia cannot be demonstrated (Mrowka *et al.*, 1995).

Cell-mediated vasculitis

Interactions between adhesion molecules on endothelial cells and circulating lymphocytes and other inflammatory cells play a vital role in the development of inflammatory lesions (Springer, 1994). The *selectins* are important in leukocyte rolling along vessel walls, while the *integrin* and *immunoglobulin gene superfamily* adhesion molecule groups mediate adherence of leukocytes followed by penetration of the vascular endothelium. Various of these molecules are found in elevated serum concentrations, or to be expressed on monocytes at higher levels, in vasculitic syndromes (e.g. vascular cellular adhesion molecule (VCAM)-1, intracellular adhesion molecule (ICAM)-1, lymphocyte function-associated molecule (LFA)-3, and monocyte expression of ICAM-1 and LFA-3 in Wegener's granulomatosis (Wang *et al.*, 1993; Stegeman *et al.*, 1994)), reflecting vascular inflammation without illuminating the underlying reason. ICAM-1 and VCAM-1 are up-regulated in hypertrophic endothelial cells within vasculitic lesions (Bradley *et al.*, 1994).

Received wisdom has T lymphocytes forming a rather inconsequential component of the cellular infiltrate within the vessel wall in most systemic vasculitides, with the important exceptions of both giant cell and Takayasu's arteritis which will be discussed below. As mentioned above, neutrophils and monocytes are dominant. A relative paucity of lymphocytes applies in the main to acute lesions, and chronically affected vessels may contain substantial numbers of T cells, but it is commonly suggested that the majority of the systemic vasculitides are not T cell driven.

Recent studies have, however, more clearly identified activated T cells and (putatively) antigen-presenting MHC Class II[+] dendritic cells in the lesions of microscopic polyarteritis nodosa (Cid *et al.*, 1994) and Wegener's granulomatosis (Pall and Savage, 1994). Furthermore, in the latter disorder circulating T cells responsive to PR-3 have been demonstrated (Brouwer *et al.*, 1994b). MPO and PR-3-directed T cell responses are increasingly studied in systemic vasculitis (Griffith *et al.*, 1996), and significant involvement of T cells seems more than likely (Mathieson and Oliveira, 1995; Weyand and Goronzy, 1996).

In both primary CNS and peripheral nerve vasculitic lesions, the predominant infiltrate is in fact of $CD4^+$ and $CD8^+$ T lymphocytes and monocytes (Kissel, 1989; Cid *et al.*, 1994; Lie, 1997). Eosinophils rarely are found to be prominent. B cells and plasma cells are also present, with giant cells of both Langerhans and foreign body type.

The clinical features of central nervous system vasculitis

Published reviews of the manifestations of CNS vasculitis have rightly emphasized the protean manifestations, wide variation in disease activity, course and severity, and the absence of a pathognomic or even typical clinical picture (Moore and Cupps, 1983; Sigal, 1987; Kissel, 1989; Moore, 1989; Moore, 1994; Moore and Calabrese, 1994b) – all of which contribute to the notorious difficulties of recognition and diagnosis. Focal or multifocal infarction, or diffuse ischaemia, affecting any part of the brain, explain the occurrence of almost any neurological symptom, sign or syndrome. Thus, headache, focal and generalized seizures, stroke-like episodes causing hemispheric or brainstem deficits, acute and subacute encephalopathies, progressive cognitive changes, chorea, myoclonus and other movement disorders, optic and other cranial neuropathies are all seen, and this spectrum applies equally to primary intracranial vasculitis and to cerebral involvement by systemic vasculitis in the context of, for example, microscopic polyangiitis or rheumatoid disease (Moore and Cupps, 1983; Sigal, 1987; Kissel, 1989). Intracranial haemorrhage is less commonly encountered. Systemic features may be present (though often only revealed on direct enquiry) even in so-called isolated CNS vasculitis. These include fever and night sweats, livedo reticulares or oligoarthropathy, features which very rarely emerge unless directly and specifically sought. The course is commonly acute or subacute, but chronic progressive presentations are also well described, as are spontaneous relapses and remissions.

We studied a small number of patients with cerebral vasculitis (Scolding *et al.*, 1998) and, despite the typically disconcertingly wide range of clinical presentations, were able to delineate three broad clinical categories:

1. Atypical multiple sclerosis ('MS-plus') – with a spontaneously relapsing and remitting course, neurological features which may include optic neuropathy and brainstem episodes, but with additional neurological symptoms or signs which are less common in multiple sclerosis – seizures, severe and persisting headaches, encephalopathic episodes, or hemispheric stroke-like episodes.
2. Acute or subacute encephalopathy, commonly presenting as an acute confusional state, progressing to drowsiness and coma.
3. Intracranial mass lesion – with headache, drowsiness, focal signs and

(often) raised intracranial pressure, CT scanning usually revealing a single lesion (though in our cases, subsequent MRI – after biopsy – revealed multiple lesions invisible to CT).

On reviewing the literature, we found the great majority of cases detailed also conformed to these patterns. Clearly this grouping should not necessarily carry pathological or pathogenetic implications, or influence prognostication or therapy. However, that cerebral vasculitis should be suspected when these clinical pictures are encountered may help improve recognition of this condition (Scolding *et al.*, 1998).

Investigation and diagnosis

Suspicion having been entertained, the diagnosis of cerebral vasculitis is very far from straightforward. Three processes are involved – the exclusion of alternative possibilities, the confirmation of intracranial vasculitis, and pursuit of causes of vasculitis.

Differential diagnosis

A number of disorders may cause a pleomorphic combination of encephalopathy, strokes, seizures and focal deficits or acute or subacute onset, and must therefore be considered in the differential diagnosis of cerebral vasculitis (Hamuryudan *et al.*, 1997a). Infective endocarditis causing multiple cerebral emboli must vigorously be pursued, as must other causes of multiple emboli, both cardiac – such as atrial myxoma – and systemic coagulopathies, such as thrombotic thrombocytopenic purpura (Ruggenenti and Remuzzi, 1996); cerebral sinus thrombosis must also be considered. Multiple cholesterol emboli may cause a picture suggestive of cerebral vasculitis (Rosansky, 1982).

In the rare Köhlmeyer–Degos disease, an occlusive non-inflammatory vasculopathy involves (particularly) the skin, gastro-intestinal tract and the CNS, causing a combination of papular skin lesions, perforation of the gut and peritonitis, and haemorrhagic strokes (McFarland *et al.*, 1978; Dastur *et al.*, 1981; Subbiah *et al.*, 1996). Susac's syndrome is another unusual, non-inflammatory microvasculopathy, predominantly (but not exclusively) affecting females, and causing a recognizable triad of deafness, retinal microinfarction and encephalopathy (Susac *et al.*, 1979; Susac, 1994). The disorder is typically monophasic and self-limiting. It is of unknown cause; one case is reported in which the Factor VIII Leiden mutation was present (Barker *et al.*, submitted).

The list of other vasculopathies causing multiple strokes in a young person is long, and includes fibromuscular dysplasia, Moyamoya disease, amyloid angiopathy, CADASIL, Marfan's syndrome, pseudoxanthoma elasticum, Fabry's disease, homocysteinuria and Ehlers–Danlos syndrome. Mitochondrial disease, classically MELAS, may similarly account for stroke-like presentations, while strokes, seizures and encephalopathy also occur in Leigh's disease. Infections must intensively be sought, especially in those patients who appear to have cerebral vasculitis in the context of previously established systemic inflammatory disorders who have received immuno-suppressant treatments. Finally, non-vasculitic inflammatory diseases, including sarcoidosis, lupus and anti-phospholipid disease, must be considered.

In practice, a properly taken history and reasonably thorough examination may exclude much of this rather alarmingly long list. A full blood count, coagulation screen, blood cultures and echocardiography are mandatory, as are serology, microscopy and culture, where possible supplemented by molecular studies – (polymerase chain reaction (PCR)) on blood and spinal fluid to seek infections; CSF lactate and cytology should also be performed. Angiography and, where appropriate, skin (possibly with fibroblast culture) or muscle biopsy (for mitochondrial studies), and genetic studies will help exclude the majority of angiopathies and inherited collagen vascular and mitochondrial disorders.

Confirming cerebral vasculitis

No single simple investigation is universally useful in the diagnosis of cerebral vasculitis, a point repeatedly made in the literature (Calabrese and Mallek, 1988; Moore, 1994; Moore and Calabrese, 1994; Stone et al., 1994; Scolding et al., 1998). The erythrocyte sedimentation rate (ESR) and/or C-reactive protein (CRP) levels are often abnormal – in approximately two-thirds of cases of primary intracranial vasculitis (Calabrese and Mallek, 1988; Hankey, 1991) and more in cases secondary to systemic disease, but obviously lack specificity. (Interestingly, in the small number of cases reported, CRP levels have been normal in primary CNS disease (Calabrese and Mallek, 1988).)

Specific serological testing is important in excluding lupus as an alternative to suspected cerebral vasculitis and in seeking causes for an established intracranial vasculitic process (see below), but is of very limited value in confirming or refuting cerebral vasculitis. In primary angiitis of the CNS, serological markers are, by definition, negative (Calabrese and Mallek, 1988; Hankey, 1991; Moore, 1994). We studied the value of testing for ANCA in five cases of primary cerebral vasculitis and found a positive result in only one case, in whom there was no clinical evidence of conventional ANCA[+] systemic disease (Scolding et al., 1998); we have also performed ANCA testing on CSF samples (in patients with systemic and cerebral vasculitis, and positive serum tests), but found no detectable antibody (Scolding et al., 1998; Scolding and Lockwood, unpublished observations).

Spinal fluid examination is, like ESR testing, often abnormal, but lacks specificity. Pooled case reviews suggest changes in cell count (averages of 60–80 cells/high power field are quoted) and protein both occurring in 65–80% of cases (Sigal, 1987; Calabrese and Mallek, 1988; Hankey, 1991). More recent studies give slightly lower figures – Abu Shakra finding five out of 12 samples to be abnormal (Abu Shakra et al., 1994), Stone et al. found eight out of 15 samples to be abnormal (Stone et al., 1994) and Moore quoting a figure of 50% (Moore, 1994a). The criteria defining an abnormal result vary significantly between groups, however (in Calabrese and Mallek (1988), for example, more than one cell per high power field was described as abnormal; Sigal (1987) gives no information on definitions), making comparison

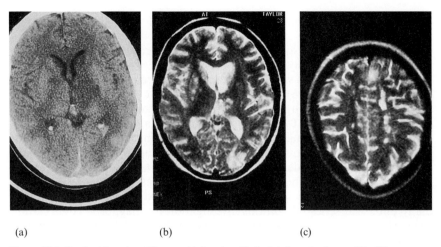

(a)   (b)   (c)

Figure 10.2 Cerebral imaging, 28-year-old female with isolated cerebral vasculitis (biopsy illustrated in Figure 10.1. (a) Computed tomography brain scan. A non-enhancing lesion is shown in the left thalamus, exhibiting slight mass effect. Magnetic resonance imaging (b and c) showed multiple T_2-weighted high signal intensity lesions in the periventricular areas, with larger areas in the left thalamus, the heads of both caudate nuclei, and the left occipital cortex.

difficult. We found a significantly elevated cell count (38 lymphocytes) in only one of eight cases, although two others had very marginally abnormal routine laboratory test results (a protein of 0.6 g/dl and a total cell count of six inflammatory cells) (Scolding *et al.*, 1998).

We also assessed the value of spinal fluid oligoclonal immunoglobulin band analysis in cerebral vasculitis, of which there have been no previous published systematic studies (although Hilt *et al.* (1983), describing four cases of Herpes zoster-related cerebral vasculitis, reports the presence of oligoclonal bands in two). Three out of seven of our cases showed abnormalities (Scolding *et al.*, 1998). Interestingly, we did not commonly observe the pattern perhaps most typical of multiple sclerosis, bands present in CSF but not serum. One of our patients had different immunoglobulin bands in CSF and in serum, one identical, and the third showed a fluctuating pattern on serial testing over a 2 year period, initial testing showing several spinal fluid bands and one serum band, while repeat analysis showed several bands in both serum and spinal fluid, all different, and a third test showed normal serum electrophoresis, but the continuing presence of oligoclonal bands in the spinal fluid. We suggested that oligoclonal band analysis is worthwhile in all cases of suspected cerebral vasculitis, an abnormal result (and perhaps particularly of variable pattern, or indicating intrathecal and systemic immunoglobulin synthesis) providing support, albeit without specificity, for an inflammatory process involving the CNS.

Magnetic resonance imaging (MRI) (Figure 10.2) has been suggested as a sensitive, but not specific screening test in cerebral vasculitis: ischaemic areas, periventricular white matter lesions, haemorrhagic lesions and parenchymal or meningeal enhancing areas may be shown (Harris *et al.*, 1994). The latter authors reported significant abnormalities in nine out of nine cases of proven disease, and no negative scans with subsequent positive angiography, and Vollmer *et al.* (1993), in a retrospective analysis including only pathologically proven cases, also suggested a diagnostic sensitivity approaching 100%.

However, in an interesting correlative study, Greenan et al. (1992) found that careful regional analysis of each of seven cases revealed that in 12 out of 33 vascular distributions with angiographic evidence of vasculitis, no lesions were present on MRI. Stone et al. reviewed 20 cases and confirmed the imperfect sensitivity, with five normal scans (Stone et al., 1994), while Alhalabi et al. recorded four cases with abnormal angiography, histopatho-logically confirmed vasculitis, but normal MRI (Alhalabi and Moore, 1994). Pathologically proven cases with normal MRI and normal angiography have also been reported (Vanderzant et al., 1988). MR angiography is not (yet) of sufficient resolution to show changes in cerebral vasculitis.

The value of contrast angiography is more difficult to assess, not least since many published series rely on this investigation for diagnostic confirmation (Abu Shakra et al., 1994; Stone et al., 1994). Segmental (often multifocal) narrowing and areas of localized dilatation or beading, often with areas of occlusion, rarely also with aneurysms (Koo and Massey, 1988) occur, though it has been pointed out that these changes are *not* specific to vasculitis (Hankey, 1991), and may be seen in infective or carcinomatous lepto-meningitis, vasospasm (e.g. in migraine), fibromuscular dysplasia, radiation, sickle cell disease, moyamoya and other disorders. Studies depending on pathological examination indicate a false negative rate for angiography of 30–45% (Calabrese and Mallek, 1988; Hankey, 1991), while Vollmer et al. (1993) and Koo and Massey (1988), respectively, found angiography to be diagnostically useful in only 27% and 20% of cases; we also found only one of four cases to have abnormal angiography. Perhaps this is not surprising, the affected vessels commonly being less than 0.5 mm in diameter (Hankey, 1991) – others suggest 100–200 μm (Kendall, 1984), again, significantly beyond the resolution of conventional contrast angiography. Hellmann et al. reported a 10% risk of transient neurological deficit in patients undergoing angiography for suspected vasculitis and permanent deficit in 1% (Hellmann et al., 1992). Although the value of this investigation may have been over-emphasized in the past, it clearly remains important to exclude atheromatous and other disease (see above).

Indium-labelled white cell nuclear scanning is of recognized value in the diagnosis of systemic vasculitides (Reuter et al., 1995), disclosing areas of inflammation often unsuspected clinically. We assessed its value in three cases of cerebral vasculitis (Scolding et al., 1998), but found abnormal cerebral accumulation of indium-labelled leukocytes in only one (Figure 10.3). However, in two cases, accumulation in the lungs (with no accompanying symptoms, signs, or X-ray abnormalities) provided indirect supportive evidence of an inflammatory multisystem process. Functional cerebral imaging, including single particle emission computed tomography (SPECT), was abnormal in eight out of 12 patients in one series (Vollmer et al., 1993); cerebral perfusion SPECT may well therefore be a useful, if non-specific test in cerebral vasculitis, demonstrating focal or multifocal ischaemia secondary to the vasculitic process (Figure 10.4). Positron emission tomography scanning may become a valuable diagnostic tool in the future (Hiraiwa et al., 1983).

The value of studying the ocular vasculature in the diagnosis of systemic

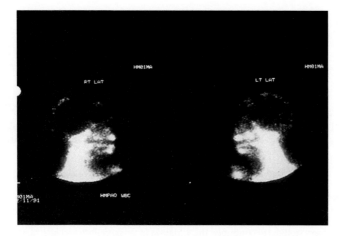

Figure 10.3 Indium-labelled white cell scan, 61-year-old female with clinically isolated cerebral vasculitis. Patchy uptake is apparent in both cerebral hemispheres, more marked in the left (A and B).

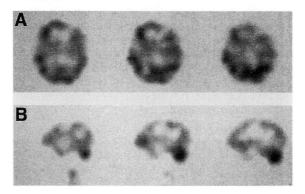

Figure 10.4 Perfusion HMPAO single particle emission computed tomography scanning, patient illustrated in Figure 10.3. Multiple focal ischaemic defects are demonstrated; these involved the left posterior parietal region, the left fronto-parietal and the right temporal areas.

vasculitic syndromes has recently been clearly established (Charles *et al.*, 1991). Conventional slit lamp microscopy and fundus fluorescein angiography can be used to study both anterior and posterior ocular circulations, but this may be supplemented by dynamic recording of erythrocyte flow using video slit lamp microscopic recording, coupled with low-dose anterior segment fluorescein angiography, to examine in greater detail the vasculature of the anterior ocular chamber (Meyer and Watson, 1987; Meyer, 1988). In vasculitis, the range of recorded abnormalities include marked slowing of flow, multifocal attenuation of arterioles and erythrocyte aggregates. Fluorescein studies may confirm these changes and also demonstrate areas of small vessel infarction, together with multifocal segments of intense leakage from post-capillary and collecting venules. We have found these techniques to make a substantial contribution to the diagnosis of cerebral

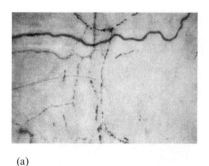

(a)

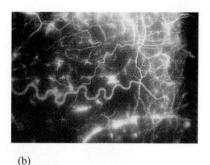

(b)

Figure 10.5 Anterior ocular vascular study, 66-year-old male with cerebral vasculitis in the context of rheumatoid disease. Still frames from slit-lamp video recording are shown. Abnormalities included multifocal attenuation of arterioles and erythrocyte aggregates (a). Low-dose fluorescein studies (b) confirmed the variation in vessel calibre and also demonstrated areas of small vessel infarction, together with multifocal segments of intense leakage from post-capillary and collecting venules.

vasculitis (Figure 10.5), changes occurring in four of six cases studied (Scolding *et al.*, 1998).

In a disease of such severity, where the diagnosis may carry with it the implication of long-term immunosuppressive treatment, histopathological confirmation is clearly highly desirable. Brain biopsy should therefore be undertaken in suspected cerebral vasculitis. Ideally, an abnormal area, preferably in the non-dominant hemisphere, should be biopsied; if this is not possible, a 'blind' biopsy, incorporating meninges, white and grey matter, usually from the non-dominant temporal tip – which is more likely to include longitudinally orientated surface vessel (Moore, 1989) – may be taken. Whether perfusion abnormalities illustrated by SPECT scanning may serve as better targets for biopsy when static imaging is normal has not been explored. Focal segmental intense inflammatory changes may be seen, more commonly in arterioles than veins. In primary angiitis of the CNS, the infiltrate usually comprises lymphocytes with some monocytes and plasma cells; there may be giant cells and necrosis may or may not be prominent. Surrounding changes of ischaemia and haemorrhage may be seen. Intracranial involvement secondary to multisystem vasculitis *may* show changes more specific to the systemic disease (Allen, 1993; see above). Alternatively and no less importantly, biopsy may reveal an underlying process not otherwise suspected with profound therapeutic implications, such as infective or neoplastic (principally lymphomatous) vasculopathies.

Not surprisingly, there are substantial differences in the clinical pattern of disease in pathologically proven cases of cerebral vasculitis and in those where the diagnosis has been reached on the basis of ancillary investigations, principally angiography, but without histology (e.g. Calabrese *et al.*, 1993; Calabrese and Duna, 1995). A more predictable course is suggested when pathological proof of vasculitis is available: stroke is less common (approximately 15% of cases), and a subacute encephalopathy with headache, obtundation and confusion is the rule (Vollmer *et al.*, 1993, Younger *et al.*, 1988). The spinal fluid tends to be more active (Calabrese *et al.*, 1993). A uniformly poor prognosis is described, with approximately 50% of patients dying within 6 weeks and overall a fatal outcome in 85–90% of cases.

By contrast, Calabrese *et al.* defined the subset of patients within the PACNS spectrum diagnosed without histology (Calabrese *et al.*, 1993). Among 108 cases of PACNS drawn from the English literature, these authors found 25 in whom the diagnosis was reached on the basis of angiography alone. These patients, as a group, were younger, with a greater preponderance of women; they often presented with an isolated focal stroke-like onset and had a considerably less aggressive course, commonly exhibiting a favourable outcome, often with monophasic, self-resolving disease. The authors suggested the term *benign angiopathy of the CNS*, emphasizing both the distinctive prognosis and that such cases, lacking histopathological data, were likely to be heterogeneous and include patients with a variety of the pathological entities known to generate similar angiographic appearances. Two years earlier, Hankey had also analysed cases according to the presence or absence of histological proof of diagnosis, and drawn attention to the female preponderance, younger age of onset and monophasic, benign course in those cases in whom the diagnosis rested upon angiography alone (Hankey, 1991; Vollmer *et al.*, 1993): again, noting and listing the disorders which angiographically mimic vasculitis, he suggested the term *isolated angiopathy of the CNS*. Recent suggestions confirm that this is unlikely to represent a true subset, and in fact may not have a benign outcome (Woolfenden *et al.*, 1988).

It is axiomatic but important that lack of pathological confirmation of cerebral vasculitis allows the unsatisfactory inclusion of a range of different pathological processes and that angiography alone represents insufficient grounds upon which to base the diagnosis. For precisely these reasons, it must also be emphasized that *benign angiopathy of the CNS* is a syndrome, not a 'disease that is distinctive', and has a long list of possible underlying causal disorders, each of which requires specific investigation and exclusion. The universally good outcome apparently associated with the syndrome may artefactually reflect the entirely retrospective nature of the data upon which the 'diagnosis' is reached – patients with a more severe clinical picture are far more likely to undergo cerebral biopsy than those with angiographic appearances of vasculitis but a relatively trivial syndrome. The observations are not practically helpful or indeed applicable to the management of patients with suspected CNS vasculitis.

The difficulties and complexities of the biopsy question are further emphasized by examination of the data concerning biopsy and mortality (Younger *et al.*, 1988). In only 10 out of 78 cases of pathologically proven disease was the diagnosis made ante-mortem on the basis of cerebral biopsy – in 50% of the (20) cases biopsied, a non-diagnostic result emerged, while in 68 out of 78 cases the vasculitic pathology was revealed only after post-mortem examination. It is self-evident that this group represents the more severe end of the spectrum of cerebral vasculitis; it cannot be argued from these data that histologically proven disease carries a more severe prognosis and non-pathologically proven disease is more benign.

The issue of biopsy is not, therefore, at all straightforward. Cerebral biopsy is not a trivial procedure, carrying a significant risk – that of serious morbidity estimated at 0.5–2% (Barza and Pauker, 1980). A significant false negative rate of 30–50% is described (Calabrese and Mallek, 1988; Younger *et al.*, 1988; Hankey, 1991). Often it is difficult to build a compelling case for biopsy – in one of our cases, for example, findings included strongly positive rheumatoid serology, positive ANCA serology, marked elevations of both ESR and CRP, and unequivocal evidence of small vessel vasculitis in the anterior ocular circulation, with no other explanation for a subacute encephalopathy after extensive investigation (Scolding *et al.*, 1998). In the light of the established false negative rate, a non-diagnostic biopsy might not have influenced the decision to treat with cyclophosphamide (to which there was a brisk response) – though the importance of excluding alternative processes also enters the equation, and must not be underestimated. Reviews indicate that ante-mortem biopsies had been performed in only 14 out of 48 (29%) and 37 out of 71 (52%) of published cases (Calabrese and Mallek, 1988; Hankey, 1991).

In this author's view, the case for biopsy can be much more compellingly built on the negative grounds of excluding alternative diagnoses, than positively to prove vasculitis. In the last 2 years, four patients seen by the author had a presumptive diagnosis of cerebral angiitis, with supportive and wholly consistent clinical and paraclinical evidence – upon cerebral biopsy, two had lymphoma, one had Susac's syndrome, while the fourth (non-insulin dependent but otherwise previously perfectly well), ANCA$^+$ when first tested and then commenced on steroids, had invasive mycotic vasculitis.

Cause of the vasculitic process; specific diseases and syndromes

Primary angiitis of the central nervous system
A diagnosis of *PACNS* (Calabrese and Mallek, 1988; Moore, 1989, 1994; Lie, 1992a) is established when clinical, serological and imaging findings all fail to disclose evidence of a specific systemic process, vasculitic or otherwise. Whether non-specific symptoms, signs or laboratory changes are permissible is not clear inasmuch as the literature is inconsistent. Thus, some authors note the presence of fever in 10–25% (Sigal, 1987; Calabrese and Mallek, 1988), while others indicate that there is no fever in isolated cerebral angiitis (Moore, 1994). The extent to which general malaise, weight loss or anorexia may occur also vary in published series (some suggest 20% for the latter (Hankey, 1991; Vollmer *et al.*, 1993)). Again, in some series a raised ESR was reported in 35–66% of cases, while Moore suggests a normal ESR is a prerequisite to the diagnosis (Moore, 1994). In practice, confidence in the complete restriction of the vasculitic process to the CNS – as implied by the absence of non-specific systemic symptoms and a normal ESR – is difficult to achieve: asymptomatic vasculitic changes in other organs – including lung, kidney, and prostate – are often apparent only at post-mortem examination (reviewed in Calabrese and Mallek, 1988; Younger *et al.*, 1988; Lie, 1992a).

Isolated cerebral angiitis is therefore essentially a diagnosis of exclusion, although (as mentioned above) some histological features may be specific to this disorder. A syndrome which may be clinically identical – although more commonly (and fascinatingly) only a single (ipsilateral) hemisphere is involved – may occur in the context of Herpes zoster ophthalmicus (Hilt *et al.*, 1983; Sigal, 1987), though most would put this disorder in the category of vasculitis secondary to infection. Occasionally, the isolated CNS disease is yet further confined, the vasculitic process affecting only the spinal cord (Feasby *et al.*, 1975; Caccamo *et al.*, 1992).

Whether *benign angiopathy of the CNS*, angiographically defined, non-pathologically proven but assumed primary angiitis, ultimately emerges as a separate entity remains to be established (see above discussion), but seems unlikely.

Two eponymous primary disorders may involve the CNS. *Cogan's syndrome* is an unusual disorder, mostly affecting young adults, character-ized by recurrent episodes of interstitial keratitis and/or scleritis with vestibulo-auditory symptoms (Haynes *et al.*, 1980; Vollertsen *et al.*, 1986; Rosenbaum *et al.*, 1997), which may be complicated by CNS, PNS or systemic vasculitis (Bicknell and Holland, 1978; Vollertsen, 1990). In *Eale's disease*, an isolated retinal vasculitis occurs, causing visual loss; again, neurological complications are well described (Dastur and Singhal, 1976; Renie *et al.*, 1983; Katz *et al.*, 1991; Weber and Conrad, 1993).

Primary systemic vasculitides with central nervous disease
Each of the systemic vasculitides may be complicated by cerebral involvement; each has a number of defining characteristics which must be sought (or may be obvious) in patients suspected or proving to have cerebral vasculitis. In most, constitutional disturbance – fever, night sweats, severe malaise, weight loss – is marked; a rash or arthropathy may be obvious.

Wegener's granulomatosis predominantly affects the upper and lower respiratory tracts – nose (often with destructive cartilaginous change causing saddle nose deformity), sinuses, larynx, trachea and lungs. Ocular involve-ment may occur; renal disease is usual. cANCA is positive, with PR-3 specificity, and the biopsy is characteristic, with granulomatous vasculitis. The diagnostic features are shown in Table 10.2.

Table 10.2 Wegener's granulomatosis: diagnostic criteria

At least two of the following:

- bloody or purulent nasal discharge
- nodules, cavities or infiltrates on chest X-ray
- microscopic haematuria or red cell casts
- granulomatous inflammation on biopsy

American College of Rheumatology criteria (Leavitt *et al.*, 1990).

Wegener's granulomatosis can rarely precipitate an intracerebral vascu-litis, causing neurological manifestations no different from those of other cerebral vasculitides; the diagnosis is suggested by the additional and specific clinical and serological findings (Yamashita *et al.*, 1986; Nishino *et al.*, 1993a,b). Overall, around 30% of patients with Wegener's disease experience neurological complications (Nishino *et al.*, 1993a); but in the majority of these, the peripheral nerve bears the brunt of the damage. Direct effects of the granulomatous process – either by contiguous invasive spread, or from remote metastatic granulomata – represent a mode of neurological involve-

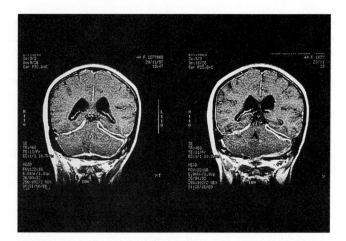

Figure 10.6 Gadolinium-enhanced T$_1$-weighted magnetic resonance imaging scan of a 38-year-old female with established Wegener's disease and biopsy-confirmed meningeal involvement. Meningeal thickening and enhancement are apparent in the posterior falx and in the tentorium cerebelli, in the dura overlying the cerebellum and the occiput (together with the antral, sphenoid and ethmoid sinuses).

ment unique to Wegener's disease and occur more commonly than cerebral vasculitis. Orbital pseudotumour was reported in 5% of 324 patients with Wegener's granulomatosis (Nishino *et al.*, 1993a); other cranial neuropathies were found in approximately 6% and were also thought to represent direct effects of granulomatous meningitis (Nishino *et al.*, 1993a). The latter may be clearly – and occasionally dramatically (Figure 10.6) – demonstrated by gadolinium-enhanced MRI scanning, and can cause headaches and reactive spinal fluid changes. The seventh and eighth nerves are particularly susceptible to involvement from middle ear disease.

Microscopic polyangiitis is a multisystem small vessel vasculitis which can involve almost any organ or may rarely be confined to a single organ. Renal involvement is almost invariable; the lungs are too commonly involved. PNS involvement, with mononeuritis multiplex, is more common than CNS disease. The diagnosis usually rests upon a combination of renal biopsy (indications for which might include loin pain, enlarged kidneys, impaired renal function or proteinuria with casts) and ANCA serology (commonly pANCA, directed against MPO).

Classical polyarteritis nodosa is now recognized as an unusual disorder which may have some overlap and co-exist with microscopic polyangiitis, but often occurs alone. The importance of distinguishing between microscopic polyangiitis (MPA) and (classical) polyarteritis nodosa (PAN), has been repeatedly stressed over the last decade or more and has recently been re-emphasized (Guillevin and Lhote, 1995), although it is still not universally accepted (for a critique of the Chapel Hill consensus proposals regarding MPA and PAN, see Lie, 1994). Medium sized vessels are affected in PAN and the kidneys are again commonly involved; renal angiography may help in diagnosis, often revealing microaneurysms. The gut and the CNS are also often affected, though mononeuritis multiplex is much the commoner neurological manifestation of classical PAN (up to 70% of cases (Guillevin *et al.*, 1992; Guillevin and Lhote, 1995)). In contrast to microscopic polyangiitis, hypertension is almost invariable and ANCA serology is usually negative (Guillevin *et al.*, 1993).

The great majority of published reports of neurological disease complicating polyarteritis antedate the (moderately) recently emphasized distinction between microscopic polyangiitis and classical PAN – early series also include cases which would now be classified as Wegener's granulomatosis (e.g. Moore and Fauci, 1981); in general, there appears agreement that in these disorders, the PNS is far more commonly involved than the CNS (up to 60% of patients developing involvement of the former, perhaps 20% the latter).

Churg–Strauss syndrome is a multisystem disease characterized pathologically by a granulomatous necrotising vasculitis and clinically by prominent asthma with an eosinophilia. ANCA testing is often positive, with MPO specificity. As with microscopic polyangiitis, peripheral nerve complications – usually mononeuritis multiplex – are commoner than CNS disease, but biopsy-proven choroid plexus disease, presenting with subarachnoid haemorrhage, is reported (Chang *et al.*, 1993).

Small vessel vasculitis commonly affects post-capillary venules, causing a leukocytoclastic change with predominant polymorphonucleocyte and mononuclear cell infiltrate. Complement and immune complex deposition is apparent. The skin is most commonly involved, usually with purpura or urticaria; the common presence of an allergic precipitant has led historically to the term *hypersensitivity vasculitis* often being used synonymously in this context; *cutaneous leukocytoclastic vasculitis* is the currently preferred epithet (Table 10.1). Peripheral neuropathy was reported in three out of 38 patients with cutaneous small vessel vasculitis (Winkleman *et al.*, 1964), with two patients exhibiting a stroke syndrome. Miller *et al.* reported two patients with CNS disease, one with frequent transient ischaemic attacks, one with an encephalopathy (Miller *et al.*, 1984).

Kawasaki disease
The characteristic clinical features of this largely childhood onset disorder, usually readily distinguished from other vasculitides, have been described above (p. 215).

Cerebral vasculitis complicating non-vasculitic systemic disorders
Systemic lupus erythematosus (SLE). The neurological complications of SLE have been described elsewhere (Chapter 7); the clinical picture of cerebral vasculitis may closely be mimicked by CNS lupus, but the underlying cause is very rarely vasculitis (though this is reported (Ellis and Verity, 1979; Bacon and Carruthers, 1995)). A non-inflammatory vasculopathy is far more commonly responsible for the various clinical pictures of cerebral lupus.

The diagnostic criteria for lupus have been described in Chapter 7; the usual emphasis is placed on serology and on specifically seeking systemic features – rash, arthropathy, etc. In the primary anti-phospholipid syndrome (APS), with its characteristic clinical picture of small vessel strokes and chorea, the underlying pathology is likewise not conventionally one of vasculitis (Hughson *et al.*, 1993; Lie, 1996b), although (again) isolated instances of vasculitis in the context of the primary APS are described (Goldberger *et al.*, 1992).

Connective tissue diseases. Cerebral vasculitis is an unusual complication of various of the connective tissue disorders, as described in Chapter 7. Seropositive rheumatoid disease is a well-recognized precipitant (Ramos and Mandybur, 1975; Sigal, 1987), though the association is uncommon; skin involvement accompanied by mononeuritis multiplex is a more typical manifestation of rheumatoid vasculitis (Bacon and Carruthers, 1995). Some doubt has recently been cast on the previously suggested poorer prognosis of rheumatoid disease when complicated by vasculitis (Voskuyl *et al.*, 1996). There are rare reports of CNS vasculitis in the context of systemic sclerosis, Sjögren's syndrome and mixed connective tissue disease (Bennett *et al.*, 1978; Estey *et al.*, 1979; Bennett and O'Connell, 1980; Graf *et al.*, 1993). The neurological manifestations are no different from other cerebral vasculitides; rarely, there is no preceding history of systemic symptoms, the patient presenting with a neurological syndrome. Thus, in all cases of suspected cerebral vasculitis, the specific systemic features of each disorder must be directly sought, and appropriate serology and, occasionally, biopsy (e.g. salivary gland in Sjögren's syndrome), performed.

Cryoglobulinaemia. Cryoglobulins are circulating immunoglobulins so named since they (reversibly) precipitate in the cold. In 25% of cases, a monoclonal IgG or IgM (or, rarely, IgA) is responsible – type 1 cryoglobulinaemia – and there is a predictable association with myeloproliferative disorders. A further 25% are due to a mixture of polyclonal IgG and monoclonal IgM, the latter exhibiting rheumatoid factor activity (type 2 cryoglobulins), while in the remaining 50% – type 3 cryoglobulinaemia – the circulating immunoglobulins comprise polyclonal IgM rheumatoid factor with polyclonal IgG.

In types 2 and 3 disease (collectively mixed cryoglobulinaemia), an underlying infectious, autoimmune or lymphoproliferative process is commonly associated. A significant proportion of the remaining cases of so-called essential mixed cryoglobulinaemia have recently been shown to be due to hepatitis C infection (Cacoub *et al.*, 1993, 1994; Ferri *et al.*, 1993a). In one study, PCR analysis showed hepatitis C viraemia in 86% of patients with mixed cryoglobulinaemia, and the identification of virus within peripheral monocytes was consistent with a direct lymphotrophic role of the hepatitis C virus in the development of lymphoproliferative disorders. (Fifty-four percent of patients with chronic hepatitis C infection had cryoglobulinaemia in a prospective study (Cacoub *et al.*, 1993).) Interferon-α has been shown to be of benefit both in the resolution of symptoms and clearance of virus, though discontinuation of treatment consistently precipitated recurrence of viraemia and disease (Ferri *et al.*, 1993b).

The clinical features represent the consequences of hyperviscosity – causing peripheral thrombotic and ischaemic phenomena, which predominate in type 1 disease – and of immune complex deposition-triggered vasculitis in mixed cryoglobulinaemia, particularly when associated with hepatitis C infection. Skin disease, with purpura progressing to necrotic ulceration, and renal and joint involvement are common. Leukocytoclastic vasculitis is apparent on skin biopsy, with prominent deposits of immune complexes and complement. The diagnosis, however, will only be made if blood is collected into a plain tube, immediately placed in water in a thermos at 37°C, taken to the laboratory and tested forthwith.

Large series or literature-based reviews indicate that peripheral neuropathy occurs in 22–32% of patients with essential cryoglobulinaemia (Abel et al., 1993; Monti et al., 1995). Mononeuritis multiplex is the commonest phenotype and leukocytoclastic vasculitis is found on biopsy. Central nervous system involvement is rare; occasional patients with compatible clinical syndromes – seizures, stroke, or mixed pictures with recurrent encephalomyelopathy and/or strokes – are reported (Abramsky and Slavin, 1974; Gorevic et al., 1980) but no histological confirmation of an intracranial vasculitic process was apparent in the one case examined.

Sarcoidosis. The neurology of sarcoidosis is dealt with in Chapter 9. In the interests of completeness it may here be reiterated that, usually in the context of granulomatous meningitis (with accompanying signs of meningism and cranial neuropathy), histologically and angiographically evident vasculitis of the CNS may occur (Lawrence et al., 1974; Caplan et al., 1983).

Drug-induced vasculitis. The issue of vasculitis and drugs is complex (reviewed in Giang, 1994; Calabrese and Duna, 1996). The most compelling evidence of a direct association relates to amphetamines. In 1970, Citron et al. described 14 patients, all of whom had abused amphetamines, with clinical and histological evidence of multisystem necrotising vasculitis (Citron et al., 1970). Other cases with histopathological confirmation of intracranial vasculitis have also been reported (Weiss et al., 1970), while studies of experimental animals revealed that the angiographic appearances of vasculitis could be induced by intravenous amphetamines (Rumbaugh et al., 1971; Wang et al., 1990).

Intracerebral or subarachnoid haemorrhage, or stroke, have been reported in the context of a variety of other sympatheticomimetic agents, occasionally with angiography showing changes consistent with vasculitis. In only a few cases, however, has CNS histopathology confirmed that vasculitis, rather than spasm, was the underlying cause (Glick et al., 1987), although cases with both clinical and pathological pictures indistinguishable from isolated CNS angiitis have been reported (Lie, 1992c).

A similar picture emerges regarding cocaine or 'crack'. Histologically proven cerebral vasculitis does occur (Krendel et al., 1990), occasionally with normal angiography, but studies specifically addressing the issue have indicated that the majority of strokes occurring with cocaine abuse were *not* associated with vasculitis. In pathological series studying patients dying from intracerebral haemorrhages in the context of cocaine abuse, not a single case of intracranial vasculitis was found (Aggarwal et al., 1996; Nolte et al., 1996). Arterial spasm, platelet aggregation, severe abrupt hypertension or migraine-related phenomena have been invoked as alternative mechanisms. It is also possible that in a significant proportion of cases associated with intravenous recreational drug abuse, the vasculitic process is driven not directly by the toxin, but rather by associated hepatitis C infection – certainly the picture of small vessel non-granulomatous vasculitis described in cocaine-associated disease is compatible.

Infections. There is a recent resurgence in interest in vasculitis associated with infections (Somer and Finegold, 1995; Lie, 1996a). It has even been suggested that chronic viral infection – specifically, with parvovirus B19 – might be the (or at least a) cause of polyarteritis nodosa, Kawasaki disease and Wegener's granulomatosis, although most would consider the case far from proven as yet (Lie, 1996a).

At least three mechanisms may underlie microbe-related vascular damage – direct invasion, immune complex formation and deposition, and (in part related to the second), secondary cryoglobulinaemia. Although the association of hepatitis C infection with cryoglobulinaemia and small vessel vasculitis has been stressed above, other infections, including hepatitis B, Epstein–Barr virus and cytomegalovirus (CMV), Lyme disease and syphilis, malaria and coccidiomycosis all have also been linked to mixed cryoglobulinaemia.

Primary invasion of the vascular wall by the infectious agent is, however, the commonest precipitant of infection-associated vasculitis. Histoplasma, coccidioides and aspergillus are among the fungal causes of this picture. The disorder usually occurs only in immune suppressed patients, though it may be emphasized that diabetes represents an extremely prevalent and often overlooked cause of compromised immunity. We have seen mucomycosis-induced cerebral vasculitis in a female non-insulin dependent diabetic. Toxoplasma-related vasculitis is also caused by direct invasion (Huang and Chou, 1988), but is more or less confined to patients with more explicit and severe immune suppression, usually HIV-related (Navia et al., 1986), as is the much less common CMV vasculitis (Golden et al., 1994). Cerebral vasculitis directly triggered by HIV itself, and not apparently by associated secondary infections or lymphoma, has been reported (Gray et al., 1992). HIV has also been responsible for a re-emergence of syphilitic cerebral vasculitis (reviewed in Calabrese, 1991).

A more extensive historical literature has accumulated concerning the relationship between herpes zoster and cerebral vasculitis. The association of zoster ophthalmicus with cerebral vasculitis (usually) localized to the ipsilateral hemisphere has been mentioned above, and occurs in approximately 0.5% of cases of the former (Marsh and Cooper, 1993). A monophasic illness, with hemiparesis contralateral to the eye disease, is the conventional picture (Hilt et al., 1983). However, more generalized necrotising and granulomatous vasculitis can also occur with either ophthalmic or more remote herpes (Rosenblum and Hadfield, 1972).

More general causes of meningeal or cerebral infection – mycobacteria, pneumococci and *Haemophilus influenzae* – may also trigger intracranial vasculitis. Tuberculosis-associated vasculitis may be driven by tuberculo-protein immune complexes (Chan and Pang, 1990; Lie, 1996a).

The obvious and vital importance of exhaustively seeking and excluding infection in patients with suspected or proven cerebral vasculitis has already been emphasized.

Malignancy, lymphomatoid granulomatosis and malignant angioendothelioma. Vasculitis may occur in association with a variety of malignancies (Kurzrock and Cohen, 1993; Fortin, 1996) as what might best be described as a paraneoplastic phenomenon. Greer et al. described 13 such patients, in whom the principal clinical vasculitic manifestation was dermatological, biopsy showing a leukocytoclastic vasculitic picture without complement or immunoglobulin deposition (Greer et al., 1988). Interestingly (and in common with other paraneoplastic disorders; see Chapter 5), in 10 out of 13 patients, vasculitic symptoms antedated diagnosis of the malignancy by a mean of 10 months. Lympho- or myeloproliferative disorders predominate – granulomatous vasculitis of the CNS in the context of Hodgkin's disease is well described (Greco et al., 1976; Yuen and Johnson, 1996), including isolated CNS disease with a pathological picture indistinguishable from conventional isolated CNS angiitis (Lie, 1992c). A particularly compelling case for polyarteritis nodosa occurring as a paraneoplastic consequence of hairy cell leukaemia has also been presented (Carpenter and West, 1994; Fortin, 1996) – but other tumours, e.g. renal (Lacour et al., 1993) – may also be associated with vasculitis (Kurzrock and Cohen, 1993).

A more direct effect is seen in *lymphomatoid granulomatosis*, a rare disease, first described only in 1972 (Liebow et al., 1972). This was originally described as a multisystem granulomatous vasculitic disorder characterized pathologically by destructive infiltrates of lymphoreticular cells with plasmacytoid features centred upon the walls of small arteries; an accompanying inflammatory infiltrate in the vascular wall and sparse formation of granulomata were also found. Others have since asserted that there is an absence of both multinucleate giant cells and of true granulomata (Kleinschmidt et al., 1992). Cutaneous and pulmonary involvement are common, with nodular cavitating lung infiltrates, and neurological manifestations occur in 25–30% of cases (Katzenstein et al., 1979; Hogan et al., 1981; Kleinschmidt et al., 1992); they are the presenting feature in approximately 20%, and disease confined to the brain has been described (Kokmen et al., 1977; Schmidt et al., 1984). The primary aetiology is unknown, but it was early recognized that the disease not uncommonly transforms to malignant lymphoma (Katzenstein et al., 1979). Later it became clear that lymphomatoid granulomatosis is itself primarily a pre-malignant or frankly lymphomatous disorder centred on the vascular wall, with destructive change and secondary inflammatory infiltration lending the appearance of true vasculitis; the infiltrating neoplastic cell is of T lymphocyte derivation (Jaffe, 1984), contrasting with the great majority of primary CNS lymphomas, which are of B cell origin.

Neoplastic or *malignant angioendotheliosis* is also a rare disorder (Wick et al., 1982; LeWitt et al., 1983). Although described by some as synonymous with *lymphomatoid granulomatosis* (Berlit, 1994), it is a nosologically separate and more overtly malignant condition. The neurological features of each disorder are similar, largely representing those of cerebral vasculitic disease; the additional systemic features of lymphomatoid granulomatosis are mentioned above, while in malignant angioendotheliomatosis lung involvement is not the rule; skin manifestations are characteristic, but here, fixed subcutaneous haemorrhagic or non-haemorrhagic nodules are seen with overlying telangiectasia and/or ulceration, largely found over the trunk or extremities. Descriptions of the histopathology indicate that some features are held in common – like lymphomatoid granulomatosis, malignant angioendotheliomatosis is characterized by the proliferation, centred upon blood vessels, of abnormal mononuclear cells which show numerous features of malignancy; granulomata are not apparent.

Both disorders therefore appear to fall within that spectrum of lymphomatous disease wherein the malignant process is largely centred upon the vasculature. However, there end the pathological similarities. For while it has now been clearly established by immunohistochemical, ultrastructural and molecular techniques that the neoplastic cells in both malignant angioendotheliomatosis (Wick *et al.*, 1982; Bhawan, 1987; Petroff *et al.*, 1989) and in lymphomatoid granulomatosis (Jaffe, 1984; Donner *et al.*, 1990) are of lymphoid origin, there remain two crucial differences. Lymphomatoid granulomatosis belongs to the post-thymic T cell proliferative disorders (Lipford *et al.*, 1988), specifically among those centred upon blood vessels – angiocentric, angiodestructive lymphoma. Importantly, the neoplastic process occurs *within* the vascular wall. Contrariwise, in malignant angioendotheliomatosis, the process is intravascular, i.e. within the lumen, and the lymphomatous cells characteristically do not invade the vascular wall. Furthermore, this is a B cell malignancy – intravascular B cell immunoblastic lymphoma.

The treatment of cerebral vasculitis

Increasingly successful therapies for other inflammatory neurological diseases – most conspicuously, plasmapheresis and intravenous immunoglobulin for inflammatory neuropathies and myopathies, but also the prospect of emerging useful treatments for multiple sclerosis (Hohlfeld, 1997; Rudick *et al.*, 1997), together with reports of successful new therapies for multisystem vasculitis (Mathieson *et al.*, 1990; Jayne *et al.*, 1991) – provide new hope for the treatment of cerebral vasculitis.

However, the low incidence of vasculitic cerebral disease, together with the absence of any unifying or commonly accepted diagnostic criteria, renders formal prospective therapeutic trials extremely difficult: none has so far been reported. There are also few lessons to be drawn from multisystem vasculitis, where again treatment is empirical, and very few randomized therapeutic trials have been performed. An informed approach to treatment therefore depends on the cumulative experience described in published retrospective and pooled series.

It was on just such a basis that a recommendation for therapy with cyclophosphamide plus steroids was made and largely accepted in 1973 (Fauci and Wolff, 1973). Prospective controlled randomized trials remain conspicuous by their absence, but retrospective analyses support the use of these drugs. In Wegener's disease, a remission rate of 75% is quoted (Hoffman *et al.*, 1990, 1992).

Quite how best to use these agents remains debated. In proven non-infectious cerebral vasculitis, a reasonable induction regime might comprise high-dose steroids (perhaps best started with intravenous methylprednisolone, 1 g daily for 3 days, followed by prednisolone 60 mg/day, decreasing at weekly intervals by 10 mg increments to 10 mg/day if possible), together with oral cyclophosphamide 2.5 mg/kg (in practice usually rounded *down*, not up, to the nearest 50 mg). In older patients, a starting dose of 2.0 mg/kg might more commonly be employed – some authorities suggest this dose for all patients (Scott and Bacon, 1984; Cupps, 1990; Haubitz *et al.*, 1991; Adu *et al.*, 1997). Lower doses are required if there is renal failure.

The steroid/cyclophosphamide combination should be continued for an induction phase of 9–12 weeks – though some suggest 4–6 months (Savage *et al.*, 1997); the dose of cyclophosphamide must be reduced if there occurs a leukopenia (total white blood cell count falling to below 4.0×10^9) or neutropenia (below 2.0×10^9). All being well, conversion to a maintenance regime of alternate day steroids (10–20 mg prednisolone), and substituting azathioprine (2 mg/kg/day) for cyclophosphamide, may occur at this stage; this should be continued for a further 10 months, then gradually withdrawn. Cyclophosphamide has also been advocated in systemic rheumatoid vasculitis (Luqmani *et al.*, 1994) and should, it may be presumed, also be used in cerebral disease.

Pulsed weekly intravenous cyclophosphamide (three intravenous pulses of 15 mg/kg at 0, 2 and 4 weeks, given with MESNA, then three oral pulses at weeks 7, 10 and 13 (same total dose, 15 mg/kg, on each occasion but taken in three aliquots of 5 mg/kg), then three similar doses at 4 week intervals, three at 5 week intervals, then six at 6 week intervals is a representative recommendation) appears to differ insignificantly in efficacy and side effects from daily oral treatment (Scott and Bacon, 1984; Cupps, 1990; Haubitz *et al.*, 1991; Adu *et al.*, 1997), despite a total dose of cyclophosphamide far in excess of that used in oral regimes. Others, however, have suggested (based on retrospective analyses) that, despite an initial advantage, relapse may be substantially commoner than with oral therapy – 79% of patients representing treatment failures (Hoffman *et al.*, 1990). In a larger study of 43 patients with Wegener's disease treated with pulse cyclophosphamide, patients with severe disease were found to respond poorly to this mode of administration and the authors concluded that pulse cyclophosphamide should not be used for rapidly progressive or severe disease (Reinhold *et al.*, 1994).

However, a recent study suggested lower dose pulsed cyclophosphamide – 500 mg weekly intravenously – may be equally efficacious but less toxic (Martin *et al.*, 1997). Whilst comparable data are not available for specifically intracranial vasculitis, it would certainly be true that cerebral involvement in systemic vasculitis represents an indication of quite considerable severity; the current author at present uses oral, not pulsed, cyclophosphamide.

Cyclophosphamide carries a number of serious risks, not only of bone marrow suppression, but also of haemorrhagic cystitis and bladder cancer – risk of the latter is increased some 33-fold over the background age- and sex-matched prevalence. Other malignancies, infertility in females, and, more rarely, cardiotoxicity and pulmonary fibrosis, constitute the other major side effects (Hoffman *et al.*, 1990; Fraiser *et al.*, 1991). Haemorrhagic cystitis is probably caused by the toxic metabolite acrolein; MESNA, which binds to acrolein, can help prevent this complication, but whether it has a beneficial effect over and above that of adequate hydration has not been determined.

Azathioprine is less toxic. The suggested increased risk of cancers has been questioned (Singh *et al.*, 1989); hepatotoxicity is rare, but reversible marrow suppression can occur. Teratogenicity is said not to have been reported in humans (Anonymous, 1994).

As mentioned above, Hankey and Calabrese have drawn attention to a subset of patients with angiographically-diagnosed, histologically-challenged disease: 'benign (or isolated) cerebral vasculopathy' (Hankey, 1991). Some authors suggest that, depending on the clinical context and before embarking upon potentially hazardous treatments, patients considered to have this disorder should be treated simply with a trial of high-dose steroids alone – or that even this may not be necessary, since self-limiting, monophasic disease with complete spontaneous resolution is reported (Calabrese and Duna, 1995). However, the difficulties of prospectively applying this retrospective diagnosis – which amount to deciding when not to pursue biopsy – have been mentioned above. Relapses when steroids alone are used are well described (Koo and Massey, 1988) and most authors would firmly advocate early recourse to cyclophosphamide in patients not responding very rapidly to steroids, and its immediate use in those with life-threatening illness. Adopting an expectant approach in patients without histological verification, rather than seeking tissue biopsy and thence more aggressive therapy, is hard to justify in a disorder of not uncommonly fatal outcome, except in the most trivially affected. Recent evidence confirms that angiographically defined vasculitis is not at all necessarily benign or induced monophasic (Woolfenden et al. 1998).

Monitoring the therapeutic response is (yet another) substantial and unresolved problem in the management of patients with systemic vasculitis (Exley and Bacon, 1996; Luqmani et al., 1997), and is arguably an even greater challenge in patients with cerebral disease. It is clear that when much of the clinical picture may be the consequence of (established) cerebral infarction, the most successful treatment is unlikely to be mirrored by a brisk improvement in clinical signs or in disability. In systemic disease, monitoring the ESR and CRP, together with systemic symptoms (fever, malaise, etc.) have conventionally proved helpful – although of course are non-specific, and might mislead through intercurrent infection, irrelevant or severe. More recently (in systemic vasculitis) ANCA levels have been reported to be useful in predicting relapse (Jayne et al., 1995), though the temporal relationship, often weak, may not be useful in therapeutic decision making and there is little unanimity concerning the value of serial ANCA testing (reviewed in Exley and Bacon, 1996). White cell scanning is also reported to be useful in systemic vasculitis (Reuter et al., 1995).

Neither ANCA testing nor labelled leukocyte imaging provide data which are useful in following isolated intracranial vasculitis. Serial video recording of ocular vasculitic change offers one possibility in that group of patients with initially abnormal findings (Scolding et al., 1998). Spinal fluid analysis and angiography are a little invasive for routine monitoring – though the latter has been used (Alhalabi and Moore, 1994), and may be considered justified by the potential severity of both disease and treatment. For the future, serum cytokines and/or adhesion molecules are currently under assessment for monitoring disease activity in systemic vasculitis, with promising preliminary results (Nassonov et al., 1995; reviewed in Exley and Bacon, 1996); these molecules can naturally also be measured in spinal fluid and one may speculate that, notwithstanding their diagnostic non-specificity (thus far), such assays may fulfil a role in monitoring disease activity.

In disease which deteriorates or otherwise fails to respond to cyclophosphamide plus steroids, or in patients unable to tolerate this treatment, other agents may be (more or less) speculatively assayed. Furthermore, the severity of side effects of conventional treatment has properly stimulated interest in other potentially first-line therapeutic approaches (Lockwood, 1994;

Langford, 1997; Luqmani *et al.*, 1997).

Methotrexate, given at 10–25 mg doses on a once weekly basis, is occasionally used as a second-line agent (again, with steroids), either during induction or maintenance phases; preliminary evidence of its value (in combination with steroids) as first-line treatment for Wegener's disease has been presented (Hoffman *et al.*, 1992). It may cause bone marrow suppression, pneumonitis and hepatotoxicity, all of which are dose related (the last rarely occurring before the cumulative dose has reached 1.5 g (Anonymous, 1995)). Folinic acid helps prevent marrow suppression; patients should be warned that penicillin, trimethoprim (alone or in sulphonamide combinations), aspirin and other non-steroidal anti-inflammatory drugs all can increase the harmful effects of methotrexate (by interfering with renal excretion). *Cyclosporin* is neurotoxic (and nephrotoxic) and appears of little value in vasculitis; we have experience of a single patient with cerebral vasculitis whose disease was entirely unresponsive to cyclosporin (though patients unresponsive to cyclophosphamide are also, of course, well described (e.g. Abu Shakra M. *et al.*, 1994).

Intravenous immunoglobulin (0.4 mg/kg/day), of established value in some large vessel vasculitides, has been found useful in open studies of patients with systemic vasculitis (Tuso *et al.*, 1992; Jayne and Lockwood, 1993, 1996; Lockwood, 1996a), though in another series of 14 patients, 60% of cases achieved partial remission but none reached complete remission (Richter *et al.*, 1993). Its very good safety record is clearly of considerable attraction, and further studies are underway. In *Kawasaki disease* the current treatment recommendation is for intravenous immunoglobulin, used as four to five doses of 400 mg/kg/day or a single dose of 2 g/kg, with aspirin.

Plasmapheresis has been the subject of one of the few randomized controlled studies in vasculitis; no benefit over and above that of steroids alone was found in patients with small vessel systemic vasculitis (Guillevin *et al.*, 1992). It is, however, valuable in cryoglobulinaemia (Campion, 1992; Taylor and Samanta, 1993). *Campath-1H* is a humanized monoclonal antibody directed against the CD52 antigen, present on most lymphocytes (excluding natural killer cells). Though still experimental, treatment with Campath-1H, particularly in combination with a second humanized monoclonal antibody, against CD4, has exhibited demonstrable long-term benefit in systemic vasculitis (Mathieson *et al.*, 1990; Lockwood *et al.*, 1996b). We have not as yet treated patients with cerebral vasculitis with Campath-1H. *Interferon-α* is effective in controlling hepatitis C-associated hepatitis, cryoglobulinaemia and vasculitis (Shindo *et al.*, 1992; Misiani *et al.*, 1994), but disease recurs reasonably reliably within months of treatment withdrawal. *Oxpentifylline (pentoxifylline)* is increasingly studied in a variety of inflammatory disorders, vasculitis included, as are *dapsone* and *thalidomide*.

Giant cell arteritis and Takayasu's disease

These disorders represent the two principal large vessel vasculitides.

Giant cell arteritis rarely affects individuals less than 55 years of age. It affects women twice as commonly as men, and has an overall prevalence of

100–150 per 100 000 (Huston *et al.*, 1978). Generally it presents with uni- or bilateral scalp pain, often severe, with exquisite tenderness. Additional symptoms, often only offered on direct enquiry, include those of jaw claudication, and of polymyalgia rheumatica, with stiffness and aching of the shoulder girdle, worse in the mornings, and occasionally general malaise. The affected temporal artery(-ies) may be thickened and cord-like, often non-pulsatile and tender. A raised ESR, often accompanied by a normochromic normocytic anaemia, is the usual pointer to the diagnosis, which must be confirmed by temporal artery biopsy – a specimen of several centimetres' length is recommended (Fernandez, 1988; Kent and Thomas, 1990) to help avoid false negative results, which may occur because of the focal or multifocal nature of the disorder.

Histopathological examination of the vessel reveals changes of vasculitis, with an inflammatory infiltrate comprising mononuclear and giant cells; the latter phagocytose the elastic laminae (Parker *et al.*, 1975), accounting for the characteristic fragmentation. The latter is an important diagnostic feature which persists after inflammatory changes have subsided and may therefore be a useful finding in patients biopsied after treatment has been started. This said, it may be mentioned that recent evidence indicates that vasculitic changes may still be apparent in biopsies taken 14 days or more after the commencement of steroids, a useful practical aid to managing patients (Achkar *et al.*, 1994). Acutely, granulomata may be present.

Immunological aspects

Immunoglobulin and complement deposits are apparent in lesions (Liang *et al.*, 1974), but activated T cells predominate in the inflammatory infiltrate, suggesting cell-mediated immune damage (Martinez *et al.*, 1996a). An association with human leukocyte antigen (HLA)-DR (Weyand *et al.*, 1994b; Weyand and Goronzy, 1995a) supports this possibility. Molecular analysis of T cells expanded from separate lesions indicates that a very small fraction of the infiltrating T lymphocytes has undergone clonal proliferation and that identical proliferating T cells are present in non-contiguous lesions, providing powerful evidence that these cells are recognizing local antigen and are responsible for initiating immune attack (Weyand *et al.*, 1994c, 1996; Martinez *et al.*, 1996a,b; Weyand and Bartley, 1997). Cytokine analysis of lesions suggests a pattern typical of activated macrophages interacting with $CD4^+$ helper T lymphocytes (Weyand *et al.*, 1994a, 1997).

Neurological complications

Blindness is a serious hazard, occurring in approximately one-sixth of *treated* patients with temporal arteritis (Caselli *et al.*, 1988; Caselli and Hunder, 1994), as a consequence of anterior ischaemic optic neuropathy following vasculitic involvement of the posterior ciliary arteries and/or the ophthalmic artery, from which they are derived; central retinal artery occlusion is much less common (Mehler and Rabinowich, 1988). A typical picture comprises (locally) painless loss of acuity, commonly severe, often with an altitudinal field defect. The fundal appearances may be normal, although swelling (usually mild) may be seen. Intracranial involvement is much less common

(Caselli *et al.*, 1988), but can occur with a clinical picture more or less typical of cerebral vasculitis with perhaps two exceptions. First, vertebral artery involvement and brainstem ischaemia is more common (Wilkinson and Russell, 1972; Caselli and Hunder, 1994), perhaps because the posterior cerebellar artery retains an internal elastic lamina. Second, stroke is possibly a more common manifestation, perhaps reflecting the size of vessel involved, although it has also been suggested that embolus more usually accounts for stroke than arteritic narrowing (Wilkinson and Russell, 1972).

Treatment

There is little or no dissent from the view that oral steroids remain the treatment of choice, used immediately there is serious suspicion of the disease (in the happy knowledge that biopsy may be deferred by at least a few days without losing diagnostic value) and in high doses in view of the risk of permanent blindness. Between 60 and 80 mg daily are generally recommended. It has been suggested on the basis of prospective studies that lower doses (20 mg daily) may be equally efficacious (Mason and Walport, 1992; Myles *et al.*, 1992); a further recent study suggests that a starting dose of 30–40 mg daily, decreasing to 10 mg daily within 6 months and to 5–7.5 mg within 12 months, is equivalent in efficacy to higher dose regimes (Nesher *et al.*, 1997). Caution, however, has fed an understandable inertia in adopting such changes. Oral steroids are generally reduced slowly – perhaps 5 mg increments weekly – after 1 week (some would say 4 days, particularly if a higher starting dose is used), to a maintenance dose of perhaps 10 mg daily; thereafter, some would suggest continuing for periods of 12–24 months before complete (closely monitored and phased) withdrawal, others a slow (1 mg increments/month) continued reduction (Mason and Walport, 1992). Cessation of steroids after 6 months' symptom-free treatment on only 2.5 mg daily has been suggested (Nordborg *et al.*, 1995). Some patients appear still to require steroids 25 years on (Kyle and Hazelman, 1990). The ESR, whilst not perfect, is the most commonly used guide to treatment efficacy (Kyle *et al.*, 1989; Kyle and Hazleman, 1993); serum IL-6 levels are a promising alternative (Roche *et al.*, 1993). This duration of steroid therapy, particularly in a necessarily elderly population, should properly direct attention to the treatable or preventable long-term consequences of corticosteroids (Nesher *et al.*, 1994), particularly osteoporosis (appropriate supplementation should clearly be considered early, if not before), diabetes, cataract and peptic ulceration.

Steroid-resistant disease is almost unheard of; the role of azathioprine, which is of established value, is more therefore one of steroid sparing. Dapsone has been shown to be of value (Liozon *et al.*, 1993), but the significant side effects – two out of 24 patients in this series developed agranulocytosis – limit its more general use. Acute visual loss may in some cases be reversible, and high-dose intravenous methylprednisolone (e.g. 1 g daily for 3 days) should be exhibited (Model, 1978).

Takayasu's disease is a rare chronic giant cell panarteritis involving the great vessels – mainly the aortic arch and its principal branches. Patients present with acute limb ischaemia – the white, cold, pulseless picture of arterial occlusion, often with visual disturbance and strokes – and intracranial arteries also represent a major target in Takayasu's arteritis. Pronounced systemic symptoms are common (Hall *et al.*, 1985; Kerr, 1995). An HLA association is described, though with little consensus (reviewed in Kerr, 1995; Weyand and Goronzy, 1995b; Kimura *et al.*, 1996).

The histopathological abnormalities are similar to those of giant cell arteritis, though marked involvement of the vasa vasora is typical of Takayasu's arteritis, and the cellular infiltrates are more often in the adventitia and outer media; in giant cell arteritis, the infiltrate is more closely centred upon the elastic lamina (Weyand and Goronzy, 1995b). $\gamma\delta$ T cells are present; these and cytotoxic lymphocytes produce perforin in lesions, a pore-forming complex similar and related to the complement membrane attack complex. Perforin is also demonstrable on the surface of arterial vascular cells (Seko *et al.*, 1994) and it has been postulated that its targeted release is triggered by $\gamma\delta$ T cell recognition of heat shock protein (HSP).

Not surprisingly, angiography forms the mainstay of diagnosis (Kerr, 1995). As with giant cell arteritis, steroids are the first line treatment, but the more chronic nature of Takayasu's disease render steroid-sparing strategies more important still. Steroid-resistant disease is also more common (Kerr, 1995). Methotrexate has been shown to be of value in this context (Kerr *et al.*, 1994); cyclophosphamide is also used. The ESR has been reported to be of little value in monitoring progress (Kerr *et al.*, 1994).

Behçet's disease

Behçet's disease is a chronic relapsing multisystem inflammatory disorder whose clinical manifestations vary. The classical triad of recurrent uveitis with oral and genital aphthous ulceration remains clinically useful, though formal diagnostic criteria have now been proposed and generally adopted (Anonymous 1990; Rigby *et al.*, 1995). Recurrent oral ulceration (at least three times in one 12 month period) is an absolute criterion; any two of (i) recurrent genital ulceration, (ii) uveitis (anterior or posterior) or retinal vasculitis, (iii) skin lesions, including erythema nodosum, or acneiform nodules, pseudofolliculitis or papulopustular lesions, or (iv) a positive pathergy test (read at 24–48 h) are also required to confirm the diagnosis. (The latter is performed by injecting a small volume of sterile normal saline subcutaneously – some authorities suggest no inoculation, simply a sub-cutaneous puncture; a local pustular reaction when read constitutes a positive result. The test appears more useful in patients of Eastern extraction.)

The aetiology is unknown. Classically thought to be much commoner in the Middle and Far East, with a prevalence in Japan of around 1 per 10 000, a figure of the same order, 1 per 15 000, has recently been quoted for Olmsted County, Minnesota (O'Duffy, 1994) – though a prevalence 10- to 20-fold lower is more commonly quoted for the UK or the US (e.g. Jankowski *et al.*, 1992). An association with HLA-B51 occurs in patients of non-European extraction, with recent studies raising the possibility that the susceptibility gene may be more closely linked with the MHC Class 1-associated (M1CA) transmembrane protein (Mizuki *et al.*, 1997a; Mizuki *et al.*, 1997b).

The predominance of activated T cells in lesions (Charteris *et al.*, 1992) has emphasized the possible pathogenetic role of lymphocytes. Circulating $\gamma\delta$ T cells and NK cells are increased in number (Suzuki *et al.*, 1992); the former are also active at sites of inflammation (Hamzaoui *et al.*, 1994). $\gamma\delta$ T cells have a predilection for HSP reactivity (Kaneko *et al.*, 1997), and many infectious organisms bear antigens exhibiting marked human HSP cross-reactivity. Behçet's disease has a tendency to relapse in the face of a variety of intercurrent bacterial or viral infections. It has been suggested that autoimmune HSP-directed $\gamma\delta$ T cell reactivity might therefore be important in the development of tissue damage in Behçet's disease (Pervin *et al.*, 1993; Yamashita *et al.*, 1997). Lymphocytes from patients with Behçet's disease are reactive with HSP peptides and the latter may precipitate uveitis when inoculated into rodents (Stanford *et al.*, 1994). Recent work indicates that 76% of patients with Behçet's disease exhibit $\gamma\delta$ T cell responses to mycobacterial HSP peptides, suggesting not only important insights into the pathogenesis of the disorder, but also a potential diagnostic role (Hasan *et al.*, 1996).

Other suggestions have also been made: anti-endothelial cell antibodies are reported in patients with Behçet's disease (Direskeneli *et al.*, 1995; reviewed in Navarro *et al.*, 1997). Direct involvement of infectious organisms has been suggested, but never proven; parvoviruses were implicated at one stage, though more recent studies have failed to provide evidence of a firm link (Kiraz *et al.*, 1996).

The histopathological change is of epithelial lymphocytic infiltration also seen around small blood vessels, which may also exhibit endothelial cell proliferation and occlusion. Polymorphonuclear cell infiltration and fibrinoid necrosis within the vascular wall, i.e. frank vasculitic change, also may be seen. Vascular involvement – usually subcutaneous thrombophlebitis and/or venous occlusion in the extremities – occurs in 28% of patients (Koc *et al.*, 1992); Lie has emphasized small vessel vasculitis as the pathological basis underlying the vascular and more general clinical manifestations (Lie, 1992b).

Neurological features

In total, approximately one-third of patients with Behçet's disease develop some form of neurological involvement (O'Duffy, 1994), although some studies have suggested a rate of 5% may be more accurate (Serdaroglu *et al.*, 1989). Part of this discrepancy may be due to the variable inclusion of headache as a specific complication, a symptom which, when isolated, has been shown in a 7-year follow-up study not to carry serious long-term implications – two-thirds of such patients remaining free of neurological involvement (Akman *et al.*, 1996).

Cerebral venous sinus thrombosis is one of the principal neurological complications of Behçet's disease, some studies suggesting an incidence of approximately 10% (Wechsler *et al.*, 1992). It is more common in patients who have experienced subcutaneous thrombophlebitis (Koc *et al.*, 1992) and clearly represents a CNS complication particularly prevalent in Behçet's disease compared with other inflammatory disorders.

Sinus thrombosis apart, the commonly quoted manifestations – sterile meningoencephalitis, encephalopathy, brain stem syndromes, cranial neuropathies, cortical sensory and motor symptoms and signs, often of stroke-like onset – have the familiar echo of cerebral vasculitis. A picture resembling multiple sclerosis has also been described. Investigation may reveal an active CSF, with modest elevations in cell count or protein levels. Oligoclonal IgA and IgM bands – and not IgG – may be present (Sharief *et al.*, 1991); other studies indicate that electrophoretic evidence of blood–brain barrier breakdown may be more common (five out of 12 patients) than intrathecal immunoglobulin synthesis (McLean *et al.*, 1995). Evoked potentials may be diagnostically useful (Stigsby *et al.*, 1994).

An abnormal MRI is the rule – though, again in parallel with cerebral vasculitis, there are no specific or diagnostic changes. A prospective study of 31 patients with neurological Behçet's disease showed that multiple, small high signal intensity lesions (on T_2-weighted scans) in the hemispheric white matter, brain stem, basal ganglia or thalamus, or cortex occurred in 13 patients (Wechsler *et al.*, 1993). In cases where there is clinical diagnostic confusion, this distribution, i.e. white and grey matter lesions, may help distinguish Behçet's from multiple sclerosis. Optic nerve and spinal cord lesions are also found (Morrissey *et al.*, 1993). Changes of venous sinus thrombosis were present in over one-third of Wechsler's 31 patients (Wechsler *et al.*, 1993). Isolated hemispheric lesions were also described.

Treatment of Behçet's disease

Treatment, needless to say, can be difficult. Topical steroids are usually effective for ulceration (lozenges for the oral mucosa) and for uveitis. Colchicine and dapsone are also commonly used. Systemic and/or neurological disease most commonly respond to oral steroids; azathioprine may be used as an adjunct. Recent retrospective studies have indicated an improved survival in patients with CNS Behçet's treated with steroids and immunosuppressants (Hatzinikolaou *et al.*, 1993). Monitoring treatment is also difficult – neither the ESR nor CRP levels are useful (Rigby *et al.*, 1995); MRI might have such a role (Morrissey *et al.*, 1993; Wechsler *et al.*, 1993). Serum levels of TNF-α and soluble IL-2 receptor, while elevated in Behçet's disease, are not useful in monitoring disease activity (Sayinalp *et al.*, 1996).

The place of thalidomide in steroid-unresponsive Behçet's is currently under review; there is a slightly greater consensus regarding the use of cyclosporin (2.5–5.0 mg/kg) in such patients (Atmaca and Batioglu, 1994; Whitcup *et al.*, 1994), though again, proper trial data are lacking. In a single masked trial, cyclosporin was compared with cyclophosphamide and, despite an apparent initial benefit, long-term follow-up showed no clear difference (Ozyazgan *et al.*, 1992). Others much experienced in Behçet's disease advocate 6–12 months' treatment with the relatively less toxic chlorambucil for neurological disease (O'Duffy, 1994). The newer cyclosporin-like immunosuppressant FK-801 may be useful; there is some evidence of the value of IFN-α (Hamuryudan *et al.*, 1994). Azathioprine has been suggested to be of long-term value (Hamuryudan *et al.*, 1997b). Immunotherapy for Behçet's disease has recently been reviewed (Mochizuki, 1997).

The management of cerebral sinus thrombosis in Behçet's disease is also

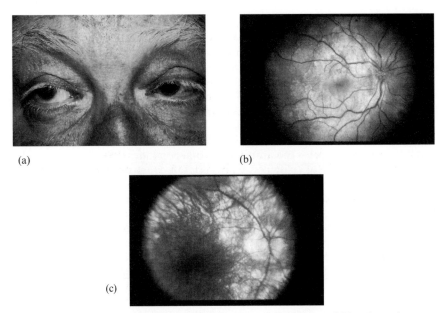

Figure 10.7 Vogt–Koyanagi–Harada syndrome. (a) Acute Vogt–Koyanagi–Harada syndrome, showing multiple retinal detachments and a swollen hyperaemic disc. (b) Convalescent phase Vogt–Koyanagi–Harada – the so-called 'sunset-glow' appearance, with orange-red discolouration of the optic fundus, and a pale atrophic disc. (c) Convalescent phase Vogt–Koyanagi–Harada: vitiligo and poliosis are obvious at this stage. (Illustrations courtesy Dr Ramana Moorthy, Elsevier.)

controversial (as is the treatment of sinus thrombosis outwith this context). The French experience suggests steroids with heparin and then warfarin are beneficial (Wechsler *et al.*, 1992); others consider formal anticoagulation hazardous (O'Duffy, 1994).

Vogt–Koyanagi–Harada syndrome

This is a rare disorder, inflammatory in nature but not truly vasculitic, and which might therefore count itself lucky to be included in this chapter, though not the book. The principal features are ocular (Figure 10.7b and c), with uveitis and retinal haemorrhages, and dermatological, with patches of depigmentation in the eyebrows, eyelashes and scalp hair (poliosis), as well as vitiligo (Moorthy *et al.*, 1995).

Sensorineural deafness is common, but the principal neurological manifestation is that of an aseptic meningitis. Other cranial nerves, particularly ocular motor, may become embroiled in the inflammatory process and headache is usually prominent. Neuropsychiatric changes may occur, as may signs of parenchymal involvement, including hemiplegia and transverse myelitis, though more often the disorder is relatively benign.

Spinal fluid analysis usually reveals a lymphocytic pleocytosis with a variably raised protein. Computed tomography and MRI may reveal characteristic choroidal changes and in some patients MRI shows high signal density periventricular lesions (Ibanez *et al.*, 1994). Both MRI and contrast angiography have shown vasculopathic changes suggestive of vasculitis, but without correlative histopathological confirmation (Ryan and Pettigrew, 1995). Cases with documentation of neuropathology are very rare; inflammatory changes, with perivascular cuffing and a brisk microglial reaction are recorded, without true vasculitis (Alema *et al.*, 1981).

A close Class II MHC association has been reported (DR4 and DQ4) (Islam *et al.*, 1994). The aqueous fluid contains a predominance of activated T lymphocytes, and peripheral cellular and humoral immune responses to uveal and retinal antigens have been described. Melanocytes represent the most obvious target – melanin-laden macrophages are found in the cerebrospinal fluid of patients with Vogt–Koyanagi–Harada syndrome (Nakamura *et al.*, 1996) – and considerable evidence of cytotoxic T cell activity against these cells has been presented (Norose and Yano, 1996; Sugita *et al.*, 1996).

Conventional treatment comprises high-dose intravenous steroids (Ikeda *et al.*, 1997); cyclosporin has been advocated in refractory cases. Intravenous immunoglobulin has also been suggested (Helveston and Gilmore, 1996). Sixty percent of patients retain moderate to good vision (Rubsamen and Gass, 1991).

References

Anonymous (1990) Criteria for diagnosis of Behçet's disease. International Study Group for Behçet's Disease. *Lancet*, **335**, 1078–1080.

Anonymous (1994) Immunosuppressive drugs and their complications. *Drug Therap. Bull.*, **32**, 66–70.

Anonymous (1995) Immunosuppression is mainstay of therapy for vasculitides. *Drugs Ther. Perspect.*, **6**, 9–11.

Abel, G., Zhang, Q. X. and Agnello, V. (1993) Hepatitis C virus infection in type II mixed cryoglobulinemia. *Arthritis Rheum.*, **36**, 1341–1349.

Abramsky, O. and Slavin, S. (1974) Neurologic manifestations in patients with mixed cryoglobulinemia. *Neurology*, **24**, 245–249.

Abu Shakra, M., Khraishi, M., Grosman, H., Lewtas, J., Cividino, A. and Keystone, E. C. (1994) Primary angiitis of the CNS diagnosed by angiography. *Quart. J. Med.*, **87**, 351–358.

Achkar, A. A., Lie, J. T., Hunder, G. G., Ofallon, W. M. and Gabriel, S. E. (1994) How does previous corticosteroid treatment affect the biopsy findings in giant cell (temporal) arteritis? *Ann. Intern. Med.*, **120**, 987–992.

Adu, D., Pall, A., Luqmani, R. A., Richards, N. T., Howie, A. J., Emery, P., *et al.* (1997) Controlled trial of pulse versus continuous prednisolone and cyclophosphamide in the treatment of systemic vasculitis. *Quart. J. Med.*, **90**, 401–409.

Aggarwal, S. K., Williams, V., Levine, S. R., Cassin, B. J. and Garcia, J. H. (1996) Cocaine-associated intracranial haemorrhage: absence of vasculitis in 14 cases. *Neurology*, **46**, 1741–1743.

Agnello, V., Chung, R. T. and Kaplan, L. M. (1992) A role for hepatitis C virus infection in type II cryoglobulinemia (see comments). *N. Engl. J. Med.*, **327**, 1490–1495.

Akman, D. G., Baykan, K. B., Serdaroglu, P., Gurvit, H., Yurdakul, S., Yazici, H., *et al.* (1996) Seven-year follow-up of neurologic involvement in Behçet syndrome. *Arch. Neurol.*, **53**, 691–694.

Alema, G., Appicciutoli, L., Corsi, F. M., Galgani, S., Piazza, G. and Sollazzo, D. (1981) Vogt–Koyanagi–Harada syndrome. Clinical and neuropathological report of a case. *Acta Neurol. Napoli.*, **3**, 680–686.

Alhalabi, M. and Moore, P. M. (1994) Serial angiography in isolated angiitis of the central nervous system. *Neurology*, **44**, 1221–1226.

Allen, N. B. (1993) Miscellaneous vasculitic syndromes including Behcet's disease and central nervous system vasculitis. *Curr. Opin. Rheumatol.*, **5**, 51–56.

Apartis, E., Leger, J. M., Musset, L., Gugenheim, M., Cacoub, P., Lyon, C. O., *et al.* (1996) Peripheral neuropathy associated with essential mixed cryoglobulinaemia: a role for hepatitis C virus infection? *J. Neurol. Neurosurg. Psychiat.*, **60**, 661–666.

Atmaca, L. S. and Batioglu, F. (1994) The efficacy of cyclosporin-a in the treatment of Behcet's disease. *Ophthalmic Surg.*, **25**, 321–327.

Bacon, P. A. and Carruthers, D. M. (1995) Vasculitis associated with connective tissue disorders. *Rheum. Dis. Clin. North Am.*, **21**, 1077–1096.

Ballieux, B. E., Zondervan, K. T., Kievit, P., Hagen, E. C., VanEs, L. A., van-de Woude, F., *et al.* (1994) Binding of proteinase 3 and myeloperoxidase to endothelial cells: ANCA-mediated endothelial damage through ADCC? *Clin. Exp. Immunol.*, **97**, 52–60.

Barza, M. and Pauker, S. G. (1980) The decision to biopsy, treat, or wait in suspected herpes encephalitis. *Ann. Intern. Med.*, **92**, 641–649.

Bennett, R. M., Bong, D. M. and Spargo, B. H. (1978) Neuropsychiatric problems in mixed connective tissue disease. *Am. J. Med.*, **65**, 955–962.

Bennett, R. M. and O'Connell, D. J. (1980) Mixed connective tisssue disease: a clinicopathologic study of 20 cases. *Semin. Arthritis Rheum.*, **10**, 25–51.

Berlit, P. (1994) The spectrum of vasculopathies in the differential diagnosis of vasculitis. *Semin. Neurol.*, **14**, 370–379.

Bhawan, J. (1987) Angioendotheliomatosis proliferans systemisata: an angiotropic neoplasm of lymphoid origin. *Semin. Diagn. Pathol.*, **4**, 18–27.

Bicknell, J. M. and Holland, J. V. (1978) Neurologic manifestations of Cogan syndrome. *Neurology*, **28**, 278–281.

Bradley, J. R., Lockwood, C. M. and Thiru, S. (1994) Endothelial cell activation in patients with systemic vasculitis. *Quart. J. Med.*, **87**, 741–745.

Brouwer, E., Huitema, M. G., Mulder, A. H., Heeringa, P., Van, G. H., Tervaert, J. W., *et al.* (1994a) Neutrophil activation *in vitro* and *in vivo* in Wegener's granulomatosis. *Kidney Int.*, **45**, 1120–1131.

Brouwer, E., Stegeman, C. A., Huitema, M. G., Limburg, P. C. and Kallenberg, C. G. (1994b) T cell reactivity to proteinase 3 and myeloperoxidase in patients with Wegener's granulomatosis (WG). *Clin. Exp. Immunol.*, **98**, 448–453.

Caccamo, D. V., Garcia, J. H. and Ho, K. L. (1992) Isolated granulomatous angiitis of the spinal cord. *Ann. Neurol.*, **32**, 580–582.

Cacoub, P., Lunel, F., Musset, L., Opolon, P. and Piette, J. C. (1993) Hepatitis C virus and cryoglobulinemia (letter; comment). *N. Engl. J. Med.*, **328**, 1121–1122.

Cacoub, P., Fabiani, F. L., Musset, L., Perrin, M., Frangeul, L., Leger, J. M., *et al.* (1994) Mixed cryoglobulinemia and hepatitis C virus. *Am. J. Med.*, **96**, 124–132.

Calabrese, L. H. (1991) Vasculitis and infection with the human immunodeficiency virus. *Rheum. Dis. Clin. North Am.*, **17**, 131–147.

Calabrese, L. H. and Duna, G. F. (1995) Evaluation and treatment of central nervous system vasculitis. *Curr. Opin. Rheumatol.*, **7**, 37–44.

Calabrese, L. H. and Duna, G. F. (1996) Drug-induced vasculitis. *Curr. Opin. Rheumatol.*, **8**, 34–40.

Calabrese, L. H. and Mallek, J. A. (1988) Primary angiitis of the central nervous system. Report of 8 new cases, review of the literature, and proposal for diagnostic criteria. *Medicine*, **67**, 20–39.

Calabrese, L. H., Gragg, L. A. and Furlan, A. J. (1993) Benign angiopathy: a subset of angiographically defined primary angiitis of the central nervous system. *J. Rheumatol.*, **20**, 2046–2050.

Campion, E. W. (1992) Desperate diseases and plasmapheresis (editorial; comment) (see comments). *N. Engl. J. Med.*, **326**, 1425–1427.

Caplan, L., Corbett, J., Goodwin, J., Thomas, C., Shenker, D. and Schatz, N. (1983) Neuro-ophthalmologic signs in the angiitic form of neurosarcoidosis. *Neurology*, **33**, 1130–1135.

Carpenter, M. T. and West, S. G. (1994) Polyarteritis nodosa in hairy cell leukemia: treatment with interferon-alpha. *J. Rheumatol.*, **21**, 1150–1152.

Carvalho, D., Savage, C. O., Black, C. M. and Pearson, J. D. (1996) IgG antiendothelial cell autoantibodies from scleroderma patients induce leukocyte adhesion to human vascular endothelial cells *in vitro*. Induction of adhesion molecule expression and involvement of endothelium-derived cytokines. *J. Clin. Invest.*, **97**, 111–119.

Caselli, R. J. and Hunder, G. G. (1994) Neurologic complications of giant cell (temporal) arteritis. *Semin. Neurol.*, **14**, 349–353.

Caselli, R. J., Hunder, G. G. and Whisnant, J. P. (1988) Neurologic disease in biopsy-proven giant cell (temporal) arteritis. *Neurology*, **38**, 352–359.

Chan, H. S. and Pang, J. (1990) Vasculitis in tuberculous infection (letter; comment) (see comments). *Chest*, **98**, 511.

Chan, T. M., Frampton, G., Jayne, D. R., Perry, G. J., Lockwood, C. M. and Cameron, J. S. (1993) Clinical significance of anti-endothelial cell antibodies in systemic vasculitis: a longitudinal study comparing anti-endothelial cell antibodies and anti-neutrophil cytoplasm antibodies. *Am. J. Kidney Dis.*, **22**, 387–392.

Chang, Y., Kargas, S. A., Goates, J. J. and Horoupian, D. S. (1993) Intraventricular and subarachnoid hemorrhage resulting from necrotizing vasculitis of the choroid plexus in a patient with Churg–Strauss syndrome. *Clin. Neuropathol.*, **12**, 84–87.

Charles, S. J., Meyer, P. A. R. and Watson, P. G. (1991) Diagnosis and management of systemic Wegener's granulomatosis presenting with anterior ocular inflammatory disease. *Br. J. Ophthalmol.*, **75**, 201–207.

Charteris, D. G., Barton, K., McCartney, A. C. and Lightman, S. L. (1992) CD4$^+$ lymphocyte involvement in ocular Behcet's disease. *Autoimmunity*, **12**, 201–206.

Cid, M. C., Grau, J. M., Casademont, J., Campo, E., Coll, V. B., Lopez, S. A., *et al.* (1994) Immunohistochemical characterization of inflammatory cells and immunologic activation markers in muscle and nerve biopsy specimens from patients with systemic polyarteritis nodosa. *Arthritis Rheum.*, **37**, 1055–1061.

Citron, B. P., Halpern, M., McCarron, M., Lundberg, G. D., McCormick, R., Pincus, I. J., *et al.* (1970) Necrotizing angiitis associated with drug abuse. *N. Engl. J. Med.*, **283**, 1003–1011.

Cravioto, F. and Feigin, I. (1959) Non-infectious granulomatous angiitis with a predilection for the nervous system. *Neurology*, **9**, 599–609.

Csernok, E., Ernst, M., Schmitt, W., Bainton, D. F. and Gross, W. L. (1994) Activated neutrophils express proteinase 3 on their plasma membrane *in vitro* and *in vivo*. *Clin. Exp. Immunol.*, **95**, 244–250.

Cupps, T. R. (1990) Cyclophosphamide: to pulse or not to pulse? (editorial; comment). *Am. J. Med.*, **89**, 399–402.

Dastur, D. K. and Singhal, B. S. (1976) Eales' disease with neurological involvement. Part 2. Pathology and pathogenesis. *J. Neurol. Sci.*, **27**, 323–345.

Dastur, D. K., Singhal, B. S. and Shroff, H. J. (1981) CNS involvement in malignant atrophic papulosis (Kohlmeier–Degos disease): vasculopathy and coagulopathy. *J. Neurol. Neurosurg. Psychiat.*, **44**, 156–160.

Direskeneli, H., Keser, G., D'Cruz, D., Khamashta, M. A., Akoglu, T., Yazici, H., *et al.* (1995) Anti-endothelial cell antibodies, endothelial proliferation and von Willebrand factor antigen in Behcet's disease. *Clin. Rheumatol.*, **14**, 55–61.

Dolman, K. M., Stegeman, C. A., van de Wiel, B. A., Hack, C. E., von dem Borne, A. E., Kallenberg, C. G., *et al.* (1993) Relevance of classic anti-neutrophil cytoplasmic autoantibody (C-ANCA)-mediated inhibition of proteinase 3-alpha 1-antitrypsin complexation to disease activity in Wegener's granulomatosis. *Clin. Exp. Immunol.*, **93**, 405–410.

Donner, L. R., Dobin, S., Harrington, D., Bassion, S., Rappaport, E. S. and Peterson, R. F. (1990) Angiocentric immunoproliferative lesion (lymphomatoid granulomatosis). A cytogenetic, immunophenotypic, and genotypic study. *Cancer*, **65**, 249–254.

Dyck, P. J., Benstead, T. J., Conn, D. L., *et al.* (1987) Nonsystemic vasculitic neuropathy. *Brain*, **110**, 843–854.

Ellis, S. G. and Verity, M. A. (1979) Central nervous system involvement in systemic lupus erythematosus: a review of neuropathologic findings in 57 cases, 1955–1977. *Semin. Arthritis Rheum.*, **8**, 212–221.

Estey, E., Lieberman, A., Pinto, R., Meltzer, M. and Ransohoff, J. (1979) Cerebral arteritis in scleroderma. *Stroke*, **10**, 595–597.

Ewert, B. H., Jennette, J. C. and Falk, R. J. (1992) Anti-myeloperoxidase antibodies stimulate neutrophils to damage human endothelial cells. *Kidney Int.*, **41**, 375–383.

Exley, A. R. and Bacon, P. A. (1996) Clinical disease activity in systemic vasculitis. *Curr. Opin. Rheumatol.*, **8**, 12–18.

Falk, R. J., Terrell, R. S., Charles, L. A. and Jennette, J. C. (1990) Anti-neutrophil cytoplasmic autoantibodies induce neutrophils to degranulate and produce oxygen radicals *in vitro*. *Proc. Natl Acad. Sci. USA*, **87**, 4115–4119.

Fauci, A. S. and Wolff, S. M. (1973) Wegener's granulomatosis: studies in eighteen patients and a review of the literature. *Med. Baltimore*, **52**, 535–561.

Feasby, T. E., Ferguson, G. G. and Kaufmann, J. C. (1975) Isolated spinal cord arteritis. *Can. J. Neurol. Sci.*, **2**, 143–146.

Fernandez, H. L. (1988) Temporal arteritis: clinical aids to diagnosis (published erratum appears in *J. Rheumatol.*, **16**, 260). *J. Rheumatol.*, **15**, 1797–1801.

Ferri, C., La, C. L., Longombardo, G., Greco, F. and Bombardieri, S. (1993a) Hepatitis C virus and mixed cryoglobulinaemia. *Eur. J. Clin. Invest.*, **23**, 399–405.

Ferri, C., Zignego, A. L., Longombardo, G., Monti, M., La, C. L., Lombardini, F., *et al.* (1993b) Effect of alpha-interferon on hepatitis C virus chronic infection in mixed cryoglobulinemia patients. *Infection*, **21**, 93–97.

Fortin, P. R. (1996) Vasculitides associated with malignancy. *Curr. Opin. Rheumatol.*, **8**, 30–33.

Fraiser, L. H., Kanekal, S. and Kehrer, J. P. (1991) Cyclophosphamide toxicity. Characterising and avoiding the problem. *Drugs*, **42**, 781–795.

Giang, D. W. (1994) Central nervous system vasculitis secondary to infections, toxins, and neoplasms. *Semin. Neurol.*, **14**, 313–319.

Glick, R., Hoying, J., Cerullo, L. and Perlman, S. (1987) Phenylpropanolamine: an over-the-counter drug causing central nervous system vasculitis and intracerebral hemorrhage. Case report and review. *Neurosurgery*, **20**, 969–974.

Goldberger, E., Elder, R. C., Schwartz, R. A. and Phillips, P. E. (1992) Vasculitis in the antiphospholipid syndrome. A cause of ischemia responding to corticosteroids (see comments). *Arthritis Rheum.*, **35**, 569–572.

Golden, M. P., Hammer, S. M., Wanke, C. A. and Albrecht, M. A. (1994) Cytomegalovirus vasculitis. Case reports and review of the literature. *Med. Baltimore*, **73**, 246–255.

Gorevic, P. D., Kassab, H. J., Levo, Y., Kohn, R., Meltzer, M., Prose, P., *et al.* (1980) Mixed cryoglobulinemia: clinical aspects and long-term follow-up of 40 patients. *Am. J. Med.*, **69**, 287–308.

Graf, W. D., Milstein, J. M. and Sherry, D. D. (1993) Stroke and mixed connective tissue disease. *J. Child Neurol.*, **8**, 256–259.

Gray, F., Lescs, M. C., Keohane, C., Paraire, F., Marc, B., Durigon, M., *et al.* (1992) Early brain changes in HIV infection: neuropathological study of 11 HIV seropositive, non-AIDS cases. *J. Neuropathol. Exp. Neurol.*, **51**, 177–185.

Greco, F. A., Kolins, J., Rajjoub, R. K. and Brereton, H. D. (1976) Hodgkin's disease and granulomatous angiitis of the central nervous system. *Cancer*, **38**, 2027–2032.

Greenan, T. J., Grossman, R. I. and Goldberg, H. I. (1992) Cerebral vasculitis: MR imaging and angiographic correlation. *Radiology*, **182**, 65–72.

Greer, J. M., Longley, S., Edwards, N. L., Elfenbein, G. J. and Panush, R. S. (1988) Vasculitis associated with malignancy. Experience with 13 patients and literature review. *Med. Baltimore*, **67**, 220–230.

Griffith, M. E., Coulthart, A. and Pusey, C. D. (1996) T cell responses to myeloperoxidase (MPO) and proteinase 3 (PR-3) in patients with systemic vasculitis. *Clin. Exp. Immunol.*, **103**, 253–258.

Guillevin, L., Fain, O., Lhote, F., Jarrousse, B., Le-Thi, H. D., Bussel, A., *et al.* (1992) Lack of superiority of steroids plus plasma exchange to steroids alone in the treatment of polyarteritis nodosa and Churg–Strauss syndrome. A prospective, randomized trial in 78 patients. *Arthritis Rheum.*, **35**, 208–215.

Guillevin, L. and Lhote, F. (1995) Distinguishing polyarteritis nodosa from microscopic polyangiitis and implications for treatment. *Curr. Opin. Rheumatol.*, **7**, 20–24.

Guillevin, L., Lhote, F., Jarrousse, B., Bironne, P., Barrier, J., Deny P., *et al.* (1992) Polyarteritis nodosa related to hepatitis B virus. A retrospective study of 66 patients. *Ann. Med. Interne. Paris.*, **143 (Suppl 1)**, 63–74.

Guillevin, L., Visser, H., Noel, L. H., Pourrat, J., Vernier, I., Gayraud, M., *et al.* (1993) Antineutrophil cytoplasm antibodies in systemic polyarteritis nodosa with and without hepatitis B virus infection and Churg–Strauss syndrome – 62 patients (see comments). *J. Rheumatol.*, **20**, 1345–1349.

Hall, S., Barr, W., Lie, J. T., Stanson, A. W., Kazmier, F. J. and Hunder, G. G. (1985) Takayasu arteritis. A study of 32 North American patients. *Med. Baltimore*, **64**, 89–99.

Hamuryudan, V., Moral, F., Yurdakul, S., Mat, C., Tuzun, Y., Ozyazgan, Y., *et al.* (1994) Systemic interferon alpha 2b treatment in Behcet's syndrome. *J. Rheumatol.*, **21**, 1098–1100.

Hamuryudan, V., Ozdogan, H. and Yazici, H. (1997a) Other forms of vasculitis and pseudovasculitis. *Baillière's Clin. Rheumatol.*, **11**, 335–355.

Hamuryudan, V., Ozyazgan, Y., Hizli, N., Mat, C., Yurdakul, S., Tuzun, Y., *et al.* (1997b) Azathioprine in Behcet's syndrome: effects on long-term prognosis. *Arthritis Rheum.*, **40**, 769–774.

Hamzaoui, K., Hamzaoui, A., Hentati, F., Kahan, A., Ayed, K., Chabbou, A., *et al.* (1994) Phenotype and functional profile of T cells expressing gamma delta receptor from patients with active Behcet's disease. *J. Rheumatol.*, **21**, 2301–2306.

Hankey, G. (1991) Isolated angiitis/angiopathy of the CNS. Prospective diagnostic and therapeutic experience. *Cerebrovasc. Dis.*, **1**, 2–15.

Harris, K. G., Tran, D. D., Sickels, W. J., Cornell, S. H. and Yuh, W. T. C. (1994) Diagnosing intracranial vasculitis: the roles of MR and angiography. *Am. J. Neuroradiol.*, **15**, 317–330.

Hasan, A., Fortune, F., Wilson, A., Warr, K., Shinnick, T., Mizushima, Y., *et al.* (1996) Role of gamma delta T cells in pathogenesis and diagnosis of Behcet's disease (see comments). *Lancet*, **347**, 789–794.

Hatzinikolaou, P., Vaiopoulos, G., Mavropoulos, S., Avdelidis, D., Stamatelos, G. and Kaklamanis, P. (1993) Adamantiadis–Behcet's syndrome: central nervous system involvement. *Acta Neurol. Scand.*, **87**, 290–293.

Haubitz, M., Frei, U., Rother, U., Brunkhorst, R. and Koch, K. M. (1991) Cyclophosphamide pulse therapy in Wegener's granulomatosis. *Nephrol. Dial. Transplant.*, **6**, 531–535.

Haynes, B. F., Kaiser, K. M., Mason, P. and Fauci, A. S. (1980) Cogan syndrome: studies in thirteen patients, long-term follow-up, and a review of the literature. *Med. Baltimore*, **59**, 426–441.

Hellmann, D. B., Roubenoff, R., Healy, R. A. and Wang, H. (1992) Central nervous system angiography: safety and predictors of a positive result in 125 consecutive patients evaluated for possible vasculitis. *J. Rheumatol.*, **19**, 568–572.

Helveston, W. R. and Gilmore, R. (1996) Treatment of Vogt–Koyanagi–Harada syndrome with intravenous immunoglobulin. *Neurology*, **46**, 584–585.

Hilt, D. C., Buchholz, D., Krumholz, A., Weiss, H. and Wolinsky, J. S. (1983) Herpes zoster ophthalmicus and delayed contralateral hemiparesis caused by cerebral angiitis: diagnosis and management approaches. *Ann. Neurol.*, **14**, 543–553.

Hiraiwa, M., Nonaka, C., Abe, T. and Iio, M. (1983) Positron emission tomography in systemic lupus erythematosus: relation of cerebral vasculitis to PET findings. *Am. J. Neuroradiol.*, **4**, 541–543.

Hoffman, G. S., Kerr, G. S., Leavitt, R. Y., Hallahan, C. W., Lebovics, R. S., Travis, W. D., *et al.* (1992) Wegener granulomatosis: an analysis of 158 patients (see comments). *Ann. Intern. Med.*, **116**, 488–498.

Hoffman, G. S., Leavitt, R. Y., Fleisher, T. A., Minor, J. R., Fauci, A. S. (1990) Treatment of Wegener's granulomatosis with intermittent high-dose intravenous cyclophosphamide (see comments). *Am. J. Med.*, **89**, 403–410.

Hogan, P. J., Greenberg, M. K. and McCarty, G. E. (1981) Neurologic complications of lymphomatoid granulomatosis. *Neurology*, **31**, 619–620.

Hohlfeld, R. (1997) Biotechnological agents for the immunotherapy of multiple sclerosis. Principles, problems and perspectives. *Brain*, **120**, 865–916.

Huang, T. E. and Chou, S. M. (1988) Occlusive hypertrophic arteritis as the cause of discrete necrosis in CNS toxoplasmosis in the acquired immunodeficiency syndrome. *Hum. Pathol.*, **19**, 1210–1214.

Hughson, M. D., McCarty, G. A., Sholer, C. M. and Brumback, R. A. (1993) Thrombotic cerebral arteriopathy in patients with the antiphospholipid syndrome. *Mod. Pathol.*, **6**, 644–653.

Huston, K. A., Hunder, G. G., Lie, J. T., Kennedy, R. H. and Elveback, L. R. (1978) Temporal arteritis: a 25-year epidemiologic, clinical, and pathologic study. *Ann. Intern. Med.*, **88**, 162–167.

Ibanez, H. E., Grand, M. G., Meredith, T. A. and Wippold, F. J. (1994) Magnetic resonance imaging findings in Vogt–Koyanagi–Harada syndrome. *Retina*, **14**, 164–168.

Ikeda, K., Suzuki, S., Ichijo, M., Matsuoka, Y. and Irimajiri, S. (1997) How high is high in steroid treatment of Vogt–Koyanagi–Harada syndrome? *Neurology*, **48**, 537.

Islam, S. M., Numaga, J., Fujino, Y., Hirata, R., Matsuki, K., Maeda, H., *et al.* (1994) HLA class II genes in Vogt–Koyanagi–Harada disease. *Invest. Ophthalmol. Vis. Sci.*, **35**, 3890–3896.

Jacobs, J. C. (1996) Kawasaki disease. *Curr. Opin. Rheumatol.*, **8**, 41–43.

Jaffe, E. S. (1984) Pathologic and clinical spectrum of post-thymic T cell malignancies. *Cancer Invest.*, **2**, 413–426.

Jankowski, J., Crombie, I. and Jankowski, R. (1992) Behcet's syndrome in Scotland. *Postgrad. Med. J.*, **68**, 566–570.

Jayne, D. R. and Lockwood, C. M. (1993) Pooled intravenous immunoglobulin in the management of systemic vasculitis. *Adv. Exp. Med. Biol.*, **336**, 469–472.

Jayne, D. R. and Lockwood, C. M. (1996) Intravenous immunoglobulin as sole therapy for systemic vasculitis. *Br. J. Rheumatol.*, **35**, 1150–1153.

Jayne, D. R., Gaskin, G., Pusey, C. D. and Lockwood, C. M. (1995) ANCA and predicting relapse in systemic vasculitis. *Quart J. Med.*, **88**, 127–133.

Jayne, D. R. W., Davies, M. J., Fox, C. J. V., Black, C. M. and Lockwood, C. M. (1991) Treatment of systemic vasculitis with pooled intravenous immunoglobulin. *Lancet*, **337**, 1137–1139.

Jennette J. C. (1994) Pathogenic potential of anti-neutrophil cytoplasmic autoantibodies (editorial; comment). *Lab. Invest.*, **70**, 135–137.

Jennette J. C. and Falk, R. J. (1991) Diagnostic classification of antineutrophil cytoplasmic autoantibody-associated vasculitides. *Am. J. Kidney Dis.*, **18**, 184–187.

Jennette J. C., Falk, R. J., Andrassy, K., Bacon, P. A., Churg, J., Gross, W. L., *et al.* (1994a) Nomenclature of systemic vasculitides: proposal of an international consensus conference. *Arthritis Rheum.*, **37**, 187–192.

Jennette J. C., Falk, R. J.and Milling, D. M. (1994b) Pathogenesis of vasculitis. *Semin. Neurol.*, **14**, 291–299.

Kain, R., Matsui, K., Exner, M., Binder, S, Schaffner, G., Sommer, E. M., *et al.* (1995) A novel class of autoantigens of anti-neutrophil cytoplasmic antibodies in necrotizing and crescentic glomerulonephritis: the lysosomal membrane glycoprotein h-lamp-2 in neutrophil granulocytes and a related membrane protein in glomerular endothelial cells. *J. Exp. Med.*, **181**, 585–597.

Kaneko, K., Savage, C. O., Pottinger, B. E., Shah, V., Pearson, J. D. and Dillon, M. J. (1994) Antiendothelial cell antibodies can be cytotoxic to endothelial cells without cytokine pre-stimulation and correlate with ELISA antibody measurement in Kawasaki disease. *Clin. Exp. Immunol.*, **98**, 264–269.

Kaneko, S., Suzuki, N., Yamashita, N., Nagafuchi, H., Nakajima, T., Wakisaka, S., *et al.* (1997) Characterization of T cells specific for an epitope of human 60-kD heat shock protein (hsp) in patients with Behcet's disease (BD) in Japan. *Clin. Exp. Immunol.*, **108**, 204–212.

Katz, B., Wheeler, D., Weinreb, R. N. and Swenson, M. R. (1991) Eales' disease with central nervous system infarction. *Ann. Ophthalmol.*, **23**, 460–463.

Katzenstein, A. L., Carrington, C. B. and Liebow, A. A. (1979) Lymphomatoid granulomatosis: a clinicopathologic study of 152 cases. *Cancer*, **43**, 360–373.

Kawasaki, T., Kosaki, F., Okawa, S., Shigematsu, I. and Yanagawa, H. (1974) A new infantile acute febrile mucocutaneous lymph node syndrome (MLNS) prevailing in Japan. *Pediatrics*, **54**, 271–276.

Kendall, B. (1984) Vasculitis in the central nervous system – contribution of angiography. *Eur. Neurol.*, **23**, 472–473.

Kent, R. B. and Thomas, L. (1990) Temporal artery biopsy. *Am. Surg.*, **56**, 16–21.

Keogan, M. T., Rifkin, I., Ronda, N., Lockwood, C. M. and Brown, D. L. (1993) Anti-neutrophil cytoplasm antibodies (ANCA) increase neutrophil adhesion to cultured human endothelium. *Adv. Exp. Med. Biol.*, **336**, 115–119.

Kerr, G. S. (1995) Takayasu's arteritis. *Rheum. Dis. Clin. North Am.*, **21**, 1041–1058.

Kerr, G. S., Hallahan, C. W., Giordano, J., Leavitt, R. Y., Fauci, A. S., Rottem, M., *et al.* (1994) Takayasu arteritis. *Ann. Intern. Med.*, **120**, 919–929.

Kettritz, R., Jennette, J. C. and Falk, R. J. (1997) Crosslinking of ANCA-antigens stimulates superoxide release by human neutrophils. *J. Am. Soc. Nephrol.*, **8**, 386–394.

Khella, S. L., Frost, S., Hermann, G. A., Leventhal, L., Whyatt, S., Sajid, M. A., *et al.* (1995) Hepatitis C infection, cryoglobulinemia, and vasculitic neuropathy. Treatment with interferon alfa: case report and literature review. *Neurology*, **45**, 407–411.

Kimura, A., Kitamura, H., Date, Y. and Numano, F. (1996) Comprehensive analysis of HLA genes in Takayasu arteritis in Japan. *Int. J. Cardiol.*, **54 (Suppl)**, S61–S69

Kiraz, S., Ertenli, I., Benekli, M. and Calguneri, M. (1996) Parvovirus B19 infection in Behcet's disease. *Clin. Exp. Rheumatol.*, **14**, 71–73.

Kissel, J. T. (1989) Neurologic manifestations of vasculitis. *Neurol. Clin.*, **7**, 655–673.

Kleinschmidt, D. B., Filley, C. M. and Bitter, M. A. (1992) Central nervous system angiocentric, angiodestructive T cell lymphoma (lymphomatoid granulomatosis). *Surg. Neurol.*, **37**, 130–137.

Koc, Y., Gullu, I., Akpek, G., Akpolat, T., Kansu, E., Kiraz, S., *et al.* (1992) Vascular involvement in Behcet's disease (see comments). *J. Rheumatol.*, **19**, 402–410.

Kokmen, E., Billman, J. K. J. and Abell, M. R. (1977) Lymphomatoid granulomatosis clinically confined to the CNS. A case report. *Arch. Neurol.*, **34**, 782–784.

Koo, E. H. and Massey, E. W. (1988) Granulomatous angiitis of the central nervous system: Protean manifestations and response to treatment. *J. Neurol. Neurosurg. Psychiat.*, **51**, 1126–1133.

Krendel, D. A., Ditter, S. M., Frankel, M. R. and Ross, W. K. (1990) Biopsy-proven cerebral vasculitis associated with cocaine abuse. *Neurology*, **40**, 1092–1094.

Kurzrock, R., Cohen, P. R. (1993) Vasculitis and cancer. *Clin. Dermatol.*, **11**, 175–187.

Kyle, V., Cawston, T. E. and Hazleman, B. L. (1989) Erythrocyte sedimentation rate and C reactive protein in the assessment of polymyalgia rheumatica/giant cell arteritis on presentation and during follow up. *Ann. Rheum. Dis.*, **48**, 667–671.

Kyle, V. and Hazleman, B. L. (1990) Stopping steroids in polymyalgia rheumatica and giant cell arteritis. *Br. Med. J.*, **300**, 344–345.

Kyle, V. and Hazleman, B. L. (1993) The clinical and laboratory course of polymyalgia rheumatica/giant cell arteritis after the first two months of treatment. *Ann. Rheum. Dis.*, **52**, 847–850.

Lacour, J. P., Castanet, J., Perrin, C., Vitetta, A. and Ortonne, J. P. (1993) Cutaneous leukocytoclastic vasculitis and renal cancer: two cases. *Am. J. Med.*, **94**, 104–108.

Lai, K. N., Jayne, D. R. W., Brownlee, A. and Lockwood, C. M. (1990) The specificity of anti-neutrophil cytoplasm autoantibodies in systemic vasculitis. *Clin. Exp. Immunol.*, **82**, 233–237.

Lai, K. N., Leung, J. C., Rifkin, I. and Lockwood, C. M. (1994) Effect of anti-neutrophil cytoplasm autoantibodies on the intracellular calcium concentration of human neutrophils (see comments). *Lab. Invest.*, **70**, 152–162.

Langford, C. A. (1997) Chronic immunosuppressive therapy for systemic vasculitis. *Curr. Opin.*

Rheumatol., **9**, 41–47.

Lawrence, W. P., el Gammal, T., Pool, W. H. J. and Apter, L. (1974) Radiological manifestations of neurosarcoidosis: report of three cases and review of literature. *Clin. Radiol.*, **25**, 343–348.

Leavitt, R. Y., Fauci, A. S., Bloch, D. A., Michel, B. A., Hunder, G. G., Arend, W. P., *et al.* (1990) The American College of Rheumatology 1990 criteria for the classification of Wegener's granulomatosis. *Arthritis Rheum.*, **33**, 1101–1107.

Leung, D. Y., Geha, R. S., Newburger, J. W., Burns, J. C., Fiers, W., Lapierre, L. A., *et al.* (1986) Two monokines, interleukin 1 and tumor necrosis factor, render cultured vascular endothelial cells susceptible to lysis by antibodies circulating during Kawasaki syndrome. *J. Exp. Med.*, **164**, 1958–1972.

Lewitt, P. A., Forno, L. S. and Brant, Z. M. (1983) Neoplastic angioendotheliosis: a case with spontaneous regression and radiographic appearance of cerebral arteritis. *Neurology*, **33**, 39–44.

Liang, G. C., Simkin, P. A. and Mannik, M. (1974) Immunoglobulins in temporal arteries. An immunofluorescent study. *Ann. Intern. Med.*, **81**, 19–24.

Lie, J. T. (1992a) Primary (granulomatous) angiitis of the central nervous system: a clinicopathologic analysis of 15 new cases and a review of the literature. *Hum. Pathol.*, **23**, 164–171.

Lie, J. T. (1992b) Vascular involvement in Behcet's disease: arterial and venous and vessels of all sizes (editorial; comment). *J. Rheumatol.*, **19**, 341–343.

Lie, J. T. (1992c) Vasculitis simulators and vasculitis look-alikes. *Curr. Opin. Rheumatol.*, **4**, 47–55.

Lie, J. T. (1994) Nomenclature and classification of vasculitis: plus ca change, plus c'est la meme chose (editorial). *Arthritis Rheum.*, **37**, 181–186.

Lie, J. T. (1995) Histopathologic specificity of systemic vasculitis. *Rheum. Dis. Clin. North Am.*, **21**, 883–909.

Lie, J. T. (1996a) Vasculitis associated with infectious agents. *Curr. Opin. Rheumatol.*, **8**, 26–29.

Lie, J. T. (1996b) Vasculopathy of the antiphospholipid syndromes revisited: thrombosis is the culprit and vasculitis the consort. *Lupus*, **5**, 368–371.

Lie, J. T. (1997) Biopsy diagnosis of systemic vasculitis. *Baillière's Clin. Rheumatol.*, **11**, 219–236.

Liebow, A. A., Carrington, C. R. and Friedman, P. J. (1972) Lymphomatoid granulomatosis. *Hum. Pathol.*, **3**, 457–458.

Liozon, F., Vidal, E. and Barrier, J. H. (1993) Dapsone in giant cell arteritis treatment. *Eur. J. Intern. Med.*, **4**, 207–214.

Lipford, E. H., Margolick, J. B., Longo, D. L., Fauci, A. S. and Jaffe, E. S. (1988) Angiocentric immunoproliferative lesions: a clinicopathologic spectrum of post-thymic T cell proliferations. *Blood*, **72**, 1674–1681.

Lockwood, C. M. (1994) Approaches to specific immunotherapy for systemic vasculitis. *Semin. Neurol.*, **14**, 387–392.

Lockwood, C. M. (1996a) New treatment strategies for systemic vasculitis: the role of intravenous immune globulin therapy. *Clin. Exp. Immunol.*, **104 (Suppl 1)**, 77–82.

Lockwood, C. M., Thiru, S., Stewart, S., Hale, G., Isaacs, J., Wraight, P., *et al.* (1996b) Treatment of refractory Wegener's granulomatosis with humanized monoclonal antibodies. *Quart. J. Med.*, **89**, 903–912.

Luqmani, R. A., Exley, A. R., Kitas, G. D. and Bacon, P. A. (1997) Disease assessment and management of the vasculitides. *Baillière's Clin. Rheumatol.*, **11**, 423–446.

Luqmani, R. A., Watts, R. A., Scott, D. G. and Bacon, P. A. (1994) Treatment of vasculitis in rheumatoid arthritis. *Ann. Med. Interne. Paris.*, **145**, 566–576.

McFarland, H. R., Wood, W. G., Drowns, B. V. and Meneses, A. C. (1978) Papulosis atrophicans maligna (Kohlmeier–Degos disease): a disseminated occlusive vasculopathy. *Ann. Neurol.*, **3**, 388–392.

McLean, B. N., Miller, D. and Thompson, E. J. (1995) Oligoclonal banding of IgG in CSF, blood–brain barrier function, and MRI findings in patients with sarcoidosis, systemic lupus erythematosus, and Behcet's disease involving the nervous system. *J. Neurol. Neurosurg.*

Psychiat., **58**, 548–554.

Marsh, R. J. and Cooper, M. (1993) Ophthalmic herpes zoster. *Eye*, **7**, 350–370.

Martin, S. I., D'Cruz, D., Mansoor, M., Fernandes, A. P., Khamashta, M. A. and Hughes, G. R. (1997) Immunosuppressive treatment in severe connective tissue diseases: effects of low dose intravenous cyclophosphamide. *Ann. Rheum. Dis.*, **56**, 481–487.

Martinez, T. V., Brack, A., Hunder, G. G., Goronzy, J. J. and Weyand, C. M. (1996a) The inflammatory infiltrate in giant cell arteritis selects against B lymphocytes. *J. Rheumatol.*, **23**, 1011–1014.

Martinez, T. V., Hunder, N. N., Hunder, G. G., Weyand, C. M. and Goronzy, J. J. (1996b) Recognition of tissue residing antigen by T cells in vasculitic lesions of giant cell arteritis. *J. Mol. Med.*, **74**, 695–703.

Mason, J. C. and Walport, M. J. (1992) Giant cell arteritis (editorial) (see comments). *Br. Med. J.*, **305**, 68–69.

Mathieson, P. W., Cobbold, S. P., Hale, G., Clark, M. R., Oliveira, D. B. G., Lockwood, C. M., *et al.* (1990) Monoclonal-antibody therapy in systemic vasculitis. *N. Engl. J. Med.*, **323**, 250–254.

Mathieson, P. W. and Oliveira, D. B. (1995) The role of cellular immunity in systemic vasculitis (editorial; comment). *Clin. Exp. Immunol.*, **100**, 183–185.

Mayet, W. J., Csernok, E., Szymkowiak, C., Gross, W. L., Meyer-Zum, B. K. (1993) Human endothelial cells express proteinase 3, the target antigen of anticytoplasmic antibodies in Wegener's granulomatosis. *Blood*, **82**, 1221–1229.

Mehler, M. F. and Rabinowich, L. (1988) The clinical neuro-ophthalmologic spectrum of temporal arteritis. *Am. J. Med.*, **85**, 839–844.

Merkel, P. A., Polisson, R. P., Chang, Y., Skates, S. J. and Niles, J. L. (1997) Prevalence of antineutrophil cytoplasmic antibodies in a large inception cohort of patients with connective tissue disease. *Ann. Intern. Med.*, **126**, 866–873.

Meyer, P. A. R. (1988) Patterns of blood flow in episcleral vessels studied by low dose fluorescein videoangiography. *Eye*, **2**, 533–546.

Meyer, P. A. R. and Watson, P. G. (1987) Low dose fluorescein angiography of the conjunctiva and episclera. *Br. J. Ophthalmol.*, **71**, 2–10.

Miller, D. H., Haas, L. F., Teague, C. and Neale, T. J. (1984) Small vessel vasculitis presenting as neurological disorder. *J. Neurol. Neurosurg. Psychiat.*, **47**, 791–794.

Misiani, R., Bellavita, P., Fenili, D., Vicari, O., Marchesi, D., Sironi, P. L., *et al.* (1994) Interferon alfa-2a therapy in cryoglobulinemia associated with hepatitis C virus (see comments). *N. Engl. J. Med.*, **330**, 751–756.

Mizuki, N., Inoko, H. and Ohno, S. (1997a) Pathogenic gene responsible for the predisposition of Behcet's disease. *Int. Rev. Immunol.*, **14**, 33–48.

Mizuki, N., Ota, M., Kimura, M., Ohno, S., Ando, H., Katsuyama, Y., *et al.* (1997b) Triplet repeat polymorphism in the transmembrane region of the MICA gene: A strong association of six GCT repetitions with Behcet disease. *Proc. Natl Acad. Sci. USA*, **94**, 1298–1303.

Mochizuki, M. (1997) Immunotherapy for Behcet's disease. *Int. Rev. Immunol.*, **14**, 49–66.

Model, D. G. (1978) Reversal of blindness in temporal arteritis with methylprednisolone (letter). *Lancet*, **i**, 340.

Monti, G., Galli, M., Invernizzi, F., Pioltelli, P., Saccardo, F., Monteverde, A., *et al.* (1995) Cryoglobulinaemias: a multicentre study of the early clinical and laboratory manifestations of primary and secondary disease. GISC. Italian Group for the Study of Cryoglobulinaemias. *Quart. J. Med.*, **88**, 115–126.

Moore, P. M. (1989) Diagnosis and management of isolated angiitis of the central nervous system (see comments). *Neurology*, **39**, 167–173.

Moore, P. M. (1994) Vasculitis of the central nervous system. *Semin. Neurol.*, **14**, 307–312.

Moore, P. M. and Calabrese, L. H. (1994) Neurologic manifestations of systemic vasculitides. *Semin. Neurol.*, **14**, 300–306.

Moore, P. M. and Cupps, T. R. (1983) Neurological complications of vasculitis. *Ann. Neurol.*, **14**, 155–167.

Moore, P. M. and Fauci, A. S. (1981) Neurologic manifestations of systemic vasculitis. A retrospective and prospective study of the clinicopathologic features and responses to therapy in 25 patients. *Am. J. Med.*, **71**, 517–524.

Moorthy, R. S., Inomata, H. and Rao, N. A. (1995) Vogt–Koyanagi–Harada syndrome. *Surv. Ophthalmol.*, **39**, 265–292.

Morrissey, S. P., Miller, D. H., Hermaszewski, R., Rudge, P., MacManus, D. G., Kendall, B., *et al.* (1993) Magnetic resonance imaging of the central nervous system in Behcet's disease. *Eur. Neurol.*, **33**, 287–293.

Mrowka, C., Csernok, E., Gross, W. L., Feucht, H. E., Bechtel, U. and Thoenes, G. H. (1995) Distribution of the granulocyte serine proteinases proteinase 3 and elastase in human glomerulonephritis. *Am. J. Kidney Dis.*, **25**, 253–261.

Mulder, A. H., Stegeman, C. A. and Kallenberg, C. G. (1995) Activation of granulocytes by anti-neutrophil cytoplasmic antibodies (ANCA) in Wegener's granulomatosis: a predominant role for the IgG3 subclass of ANCA. *Clin. Exp. Immunol.*, **101**, 227–232.

Myles, A. B., Perera, T. and Ridley, M. G. (1992) Prevention of blindness in giant cell arteritis by corticosteroid treatment (see comments). *Br. J. Rheumatol.*, **31**, 103–105.

Nakamura, S., Nakazawa, M., Yoshioka, M., Nagano, I., Nakamura, H., Onodera, J., *et al.* (1996) Melanin-laden macrophages in cerebrospinal fluid in Vogt–Koyanagi–Harada syndrome. *Arch. Ophthalmol.*, **114**, 1184–1188.

Nassonov, E., Samsonov, M., Beketova, T., Semenkova, L., Wachter, H. and Fuchs, D. (1995) Serum neopterin concentrations in Wegener's granulomatosis correlate with vasculitis activity. *Clin. Exp. Rheumatol.*, **13**, 353–356.

Navarro, M., Cervera, R., Font, J., Reverter, J. C., Monteagudo, J., Escolar, G., *et al.* (1997) Anti-endothelial cell antibodies in systemic autoimmune diseases: prevalence and clinical significance. *Lupus*, **6**, 521–526.

Navia, B. A., Cho, E. S., Petito, C. K. and Price, R. W. (1986) The AIDS dementia complex: II. Neuropathology. *Ann. Neurol.*, **19**, 525–535.

Nesher, G., Sonnenblick, M. and Friedlander, Y. (1994) Analysis of steroid related complications and mortality in temporal arteritis: a 15-year survey of 43 patients. *J. Rheumatol.*, **21**, 1283–1286.

Nesher, G., Rubinow, A. and Sonnenblick, M. (1997) Efficacy and adverse effects of different corticosteroid dose regimens in temporal arteritis: a retrospective study. *Clin. Exp. Rheumatol.*, **15**, 303–306.

Niles, J. L. (1996) Antineutrophil cytoplasmic antibodies in the classification of vasculitis. *Annu. Rev. Med.*, **47**, 303–313.

Nishino, H., Rubino, F. A., Deremee, R. A., Swanson, J. W. and Parisi, J. E. (1993a) Neurological involvement in Wegener's granulomatosis: an analysis of 324 consecutive patients at the Mayo Clinic. *Ann. Neurol.*, **33**, 4–9.

Nishino, H., Rubino, F. A. and Parisi, J. E. (1993b) The spectrum of neurologic involvement in Wegener's granulomatosis. *Neurology*, **43**, 1334–1337.

Nolte, K. B., Brass, L. M. and Fletterick, C. F. (1996) Intracranial hemorrhage associated with cocaine abuse: a prospective autopsy study. *Neurology*, **46**, 1291–1296.

Nordborg, E., Nordborg, C., Malmvall, B. E., Andersson, R. and Bengtsson, B. A. (1995) Giant cell arteritis. *Rheumatic Dis. Clin. N. Am.*, **21**, 1013–1026.

Norose, K. and Yano, A. (1996) Melanoma specific T_h1 cytotoxic T lymphocyte lines in Vogt–Koyanagi–Harada disease (see comments). *Br. J. Ophthalmol.*, **80**, 1002–1008.

O'Duffy, J. D. (1994) Behcet's disease. *Curr. Opin. Rheumatol.*, **6**, 39–43.

Ozyazgan, Y., Yurdakul, S., Yazici, H., Tuzun, B., Iscimen, A., Tuzun, Y., *et al.* (1992) Low dose cyclosporin A versus pulsed cyclophosphamide in Behcet's syndrome: a single masked trial. *Br. J. Ophthalmol.*, **76**, 241–243.

Pall, A. A. and Savage, C. O. (1994) Mechanisms of endothelial cell injury in vasculitis. *Springer Semin. Immunopathol.*, **16**, 23–37.

Parker, F., Healey, L. A., Wilske, K. R. and Odland, G. F. (1975) Light and electron microscopic studies on human temporal arteries with special reference to alterations related to senescence, atherosclerosis and giant cell arteritis. *Am. J. Pathol.*, **79**, 57–80.

Pervin, K., Childerstone, A., Shinnick, T., Mizushima, Y., van der, Zee, R., Hasan, A., *et al.*

(1993) T cell epitope expression of mycobacterial and homologous human 65–kilodalton heat shock protein peptides in short term cell lines from patients with Behcet's disease. *J. Immunol.*, **151**, 2273–2282.

Petroff, N., Koger, O. W., Fleming, M. G., Fishleder, A., Bergfeld, W. F., Tuthill, R., *et al.* (1989) Malignant angioendotheliomatosis: an angiotropic lymphoma. *J. Am. Acad. Dermatol.*, **21**, 727–733.

Pietra, B. A., De, I. J., Giannini, E. H. and Hirsch, R. (1994) TCR V beta family repertoire and T cell activation markers in Kawasaki disease. *J. Immunol.*, **153**, 1881–1888.

Porges, A. J., Redecha, P. B., Kimberly, W. T., Csernok, E., Gross, W. L. and Kimberly, R. P. (1994) Anti-neutrophil cytoplasmic antibodies engage and activate human neutrophils via Fc gamma RIIa. *J. Immunol.*, **153**, 1271–1280.

Ramos, M. and Mandybur, T. I. (1975) Cerebral vasculitis in rheumatoid arthritis. *Arch. Neurol.*, **32**, 271–275.

Reinhold, K. E., Kekow, J., Schnabel, A., Schmitt, W. H., Heller, M., Beigel, A., *et al.* (1994) Influence of disease manifestation and antineutrophil cytoplasmic antibody titer on the response to pulse cyclophosphamide therapy in patients with Wegener's granulomatosis. *Arthritis Rheum.*, **37**, 919–924.

Renie, W. A., Murphy, R. P., Anderson, K. C., Lippman, S. M., McKusick, V. A., Proctor, L. R., *et al.* (1983) The evaluation of patients with Eales' disease. *Retina.*, **3**, 243–248.

Reumaux, D., Vossebeld, P. J., Roos, D., Verhoeven, A. J. (1995) Effect of tumor necrosis factor-induced integrin activation on Fc gamma receptor II-mediated signal transduction: relevance for activation of neutrophils by anti-proteinase 3 or anti-myeloperoxidase antibodies. *Blood*, **86**, 3189–3195.

Reuter, H., Wraight, E. P., Qasim, F. J. and Lockwood, C. M. (1995) Management of systemic vasculitis: Contribution of scintigraphic imaging to evaluation of disease activity and classification. *Quart. J. Med.*, **88**, 509–516.

Richter, C., Schnabel, A., Csernok, E., Reinhold, K. E. and Gross, W. L. (1993) Treatment of Wegener's granulomatosis with intravenous immunoglobulin. *Adv. Exp. Med. Biol.*, **336**, 487–489.

Rigby, A. S., Chamberlain, M. A. and Bhakta, B. (1995) Behcet's disease. *Baillière's Clin. Rheumatol.*, **9**, 375–395.

Roche, N. E., Fulbright, J. W., Wagner, A. D., Hunder, G. G., Goronzy, J. J. and Weyand, C. M. (1993) Correlation of interleukin-6 production and disease activity in polymyalgia rheumatica and giant cell arteritis (see comments). *Arthritis Rheum.*, **36**, 1286–1294.

Rosansky, S. J. (1982) Multiple cholesterol emboli syndrome. *South. Med. J.*, **75**, 677–680.

Rosenbaum, J. T., Simpson, J. and Neuwelt, C. M. (1997) Successful treatment of optic neuropathy in association with systemic lupus erythematosus using intravenous cyclophosphamide. *Br. J. Ophthalmol.*, **81**, 130–132.

Rosenblum, W. I. and Hadfield, M. G. (1972) Granulomatous angiitis of the nervous system in cases of herpes zoster and lymphosarcoma. *Neurology*, **22**, 348–354.

Rubsamen, P. E. and Gass, J. D. (1991) Vogt–Koyanagi–Harada syndrome. Clinical course, therapy, and long-term visual outcome. *Arch. Ophthalmol.*, **109**, 682–687.

Rudick, R. A., Cohen, J. A., Weinstockguttman, B., Kinkel, R. P. and Ransohoff, R. M. (1997) Management of multiple sclerosis. *N. Engl. J. Med.*, **337**, 1604–1611.

Ruggenenti, P. and Remuzzi, G. (1996) The pathophysiology and management of thrombotic thrombocytopenic purpura. *Eur. J. Haematol.*, **56**, 191–207.

Rumbaugh, C. L., Bergeron, R. T., Scanlan, R. L., Teal, J. S., Segall, H. D., Fang, H. C., *et al.* (1971) Cerebral vascular changes secondary to amphetamine abuse in the experimental animal. *Radiology*, **101**, 345–351.

Ryan, S. J. and Pettigrew, L. C. (1995) Cranial arteriopathy in familial Vogt–Koyanagi–Harada syndrome. *J. Neuroimaging.*, **5**, 244–245.

Salojin, K. V., Le, T. M., Nassovov, E. L., Blough, M. T., Baranov, A. A., Saraux, A., *et al.* (1996) Anti-endothelial cell antibodies in patients with various forms of vasculitis. *Clin. Exp. Rheumatol.*, **14**, 163–169.

Savage, C. O., Pottinger, B. E., Gaskin, G., Pusey, C. D. and Pearson, J. D. (1992)

Autoantibodies developing to myeloperoxidase and proteinase 3 in systemic vasculitis stimulate neutrophil cytotoxicity toward cultured endothelial cells. *Am. J. Pathol.*, **141**, 335–342.

Savage, C. O., Harper, L. and Adu, D. (1997) Primary systemic vasculitis. *Lancet*, **349**, 553–558.

Sayinalp, N., Ozcebe, O. I., Ozdemir, O., Haznedaroglu, I. C., Dundar, S. and Kirazli, S. (1996) Cytokines in Behcet's disease. *J. Rheumatol.*, **23**, 321–322.

Schmidt, B. J., Meagher, V. K. and Del, C. J. (1984) Lymphomatoid granulomatosis with isolated involvement of the brain. *Ann. Neurol.*, **15**, 478–481.

Scolding, N. J., Jayne D. R., Zajicek, J. P., Meyer, P. A. R., Wraight, E. P. and Lockwood, C. M. (1997) The syndrome of cerebral vasculitis: recognition, diagnosis and management. *Quart. J. Med.*, **90**, 61–73.

Scott, D. G. and Bacon, P. A. (1984) Intravenous cyclophosphamide plus methylprednisolone in treatment of systemic rheumatoid vasculitis. *Am. J. Med.*, **76**, 377–384.

Scott, D. G. and Watts, R. A. (1994) Classification and epidemiology of systemic vasculitis (editorial) (see comments). *Br. J. Rheumatol.*, **33**, 897–899.

Seko, Y., Minota, S., Kawasaki, A., Shinkai, Y., Maeda, K., Yagita, H., *et al.* (1994) Perforin-secreting killer cell infiltration and expression of a 65-kD heat-shock protein in aortic tissue of patients with Takayasu's arteritis. *J. Clin. Invest.*, **93**, 750–758.

Serdaroglu, P., Yazici, H., Ozdemir, C., Yurdakul, S., Bahar, S. and Aktin, E. (1989) Neurologic involvement in Behcet's syndrome. A prospective study. *Arch. Neurol.*, **46**, 265–269.

Sharief, M. K., Hentges, R. and Thomas, E. (1991) Significance of CSF immunoglobulins in monitoring neurologic disease activity in Behcet's disease. *Neurology*, **41**, 1398–1401.

Shindo, M., Di, B. A. and Hoofnagle, J. H. (1992) Long-term follow-up of patients with chronic hepatitis C treated with alpha-interferon. *Hepatology*, **15**, 1013–1016.

Sigal, L. H. (1987) The neurologic presentation of vasculitic and rheumatologic syndromes. A review. *Med. Baltimore*, **66**, 157–180.

Singh, G., Fries, J. F., Spitz, P. and Williams, C. A. (1989) Toxic effects of azathioprine in rheumatoid arthritis. A national post-marketing perspective (see comments). *Arthritis Rheum.*, **32**, 837–843.

Smith, J. A., O'Sullivan, M., Gough, J. and Williams, B. D. (1988) Small-intestinal perforation secondary to localized giant-cell arteritis of the mesenteric vessels. *Br. J. Rheumatol.*, **27**, 236–238.

Somer, T. and Finegold, S. M. (1995) Vasculitides associated with infections, immunization, and antimicrobial drugs. *Clin. Infect. Dis.*, **20**, 1010–1036.

Springer, T. A. (1994) Traffic signals for lymphocyte recirculation and leukocyte emigration: the multistep paradigm. *Cell*, **76**, 301–314.

Spronk, P. E., Bootsma, H., Horst, G., Huitema, M. G., Limburg, P. C., Cohen, T. J., *et al.* (1996) Antineutrophil cytoplasmic antibodies in systemic lupus erythematosus. *Br. J. Rheumatol.*, **35**, 625–631.

Stanford, M. R., Kasp, E., Whiston, R., Hasan, A., Todryk, S., Shinnick, T., *et al.* (1994) Heat shock protein peptides reactive in patients with Behcet's disease are uveitogenic in Lewis rats. *Clin. Exp. Immunol.*, **97**, 226–231.

Stegeman, C. A., Tervaert, J. W., Huitema, M. G., De, J. P. and Kallenberg, C. G. (1994) Serum levels of soluble adhesion molecules intercellular adhesion molecule 1, vascular cell adhesion molecule 1, and E-selectin in patients with Wegener's granulomatosis. Relationship to disease activity and relevance during followup. *Arthritis Rheum.*, **37**, 1228–1235.

Stigsby, B., Bohlega, S., al Kauri, M. Z., al Dalaan, A. and el Ramahi, K. (1994) Evoked potential findings in Behcet's disease. Brain-stem auditory, visual, and somatosensory evoked potentials in 44 patients. *Electroencephalogr. Clin. Neurophysiol.*, **92**, 273–281.

Stone, J. H., Pomper, M. G., Roubenoff, R., Miller, T. J. and Hellmann, D. B. (1994) Sensitivities of noninvasive tests for central nervous system vasculitis: a comparison of lumbar puncture, computed tomography, and magnetic resonance imaging. *J. Rheumatol.*, **21**, 1277–1282.

Subbiah, P., Wijdicks, E., Muenter, M., Carter, J. and Connolly, S. (1996) Skin lesion with a fatal neurologic outcome (Degos' disease). *Neurology*, **46**, 636–640.

Sugita, S., Sagawa, K., Mochizuki, M., Shichijo, S. and Itoh, K. (1996) Melanocyte lysis by cytotoxic T lymphocytes recognizing the MART-1 melanoma antigen in HLA-A2 patients with Vogt–Koyanagi–Harada disease. *Int. Immunol.*, **8**, 799–803.

Susac, J. O. (1994) Susac's syndrome: the triad of microangiopathy of the brain and retina with hearing loss in young women. *Neurology*, **44**, 591–593.

Susac, J. O., Hardman, J. M. and Selhorst, J. B. (1979) Microangiopathy of the brain and retina. *Neurology*, **29**, 313–316.

Sizuki, Y., Hoshi, K., Matsuda, T. and Mizushima, Y. (1992) Increased peripheral blood gamma delta + T cells and natural killer cells in Behcet's disease. *J. Rheumatol.*, **19**, 588–592.

Taylor, H. G. and Samanta, A. (1993) Treatment of vasculitis. *Br. J. Clin. Pharmacol.*, **35**, 93–104.

Tizard, E. J., Baguley, E., Hughes, G. R. and Dillon, M. J. (1991) Antiendothelial cell antibodies detected by a cellular based ELISA in Kawasaki disease. *Arch. Dis. Child*, **66**, 189–192.

Tsukada, N., Koh, C. S., Yanagisawa, N., Okano, A., Behan, W. M. and Behan, P. O. (1987) A new model for multiple sclerosis: chronic experimental allergic encephalomyelitis induced by immunization with cerebral endothelial cell membrane. *Acta Neuropathol. Berl.*, **73**, 259–266.

Tuso, P., Moudgil, A., Hay, J., Goodman, D., Kamil, E., Koyyana, R., *et al.* (1992) Treatment of antineutrophil cytoplasmic autoantibody-positive systemic vasculitis and glomerulonephritis with pooled intravenous gammaglobulin. *Am. J. Kidney Dis.*, **20**, 504–508.

Vanderzant, C., Bromberg, M., MacGuire, A. and McCune, J. (1988) Isolated small-vessel angiitis of the central nervous system. *Arch. Neurol.*, **45**, 683–687.

Vollertsen, R. S. (1990) Vasculitis and Cogan's syndrome. *Rheum. Dis. Clin. North Am.*, **16**, 433–439.

Vollertsen, R. S., McDonald, T. J., Younge, B. R., Banks, P. M., Stanson, A. W. and Ilstrup, D. M. (1986) Cogan's syndrome: 18 cases and a review of the literature. *Mayo Clin. Proc.*, **61**, 344–361.

Vollmer, T. L., Guarnaccia, J., Harrington, W., Pacia, S. V. and Petroff, O. A. C. (1993) Idiopathic granulomatous angiitis of the central nervous system: diagnostic challenges. *Arch. Neurol.*, **50**, 925–930.

Voskuyl, A. E., Zwinderman, A. H., Westedt, M. L., Vandenbroucke, J. P., Breedveld, F. C. and Hazes, J. M. (1996) The mortality of rheumatoid vasculitis compared with rheumatoid arthritis. *Arthritis Rheum.*, **39**, 266–271.

Wang, A. M., Suojanen, J. N., Colucci, V. M., Rumbaugh, C. L. and Hollenberg, N. K. (1990) Cocaine- and methamphetamine-induced acute cerebral vasospasm: an angiographic study in rabbits. *Am. J. Neuroradiol.*, **11**, 1141–1146.

Wang, C. R., Liu, M. F., Tsai, R. T., Chuang, C. Y. and Chen, C. Y. (1993) Circulating intercellular adhesion molecules-1 and autoantibodies including anti-endothelial cell, anti-cardiolipin, and anti-neutrophil cytoplasma antibodies in patients with vasculitis. *Clin. Rheumatol.*, **12**, 375–380.

Watts, R. A. and Scott, D. G. (1997) Classification and epidemiology of the vasculitides. *Baillière's Clin. Rheumatol.*, **11**, 191–217.

Weber, F. and Conrad, B. (1993) Chronic encephalitis and Eales disease. *J. Neurol.*, **240**, 299–301.

Wechsler, B., Dell'lsola, B., Vidailhet, M., Dormont, D., Piette, J. C., Bletry, O., *et al.* (1993) MRI in 31 patients with Behcet's disease and neurological involvement: prospective study with clinical correlation. *J. Neurol. Neurosurg. Psychiat.*, **56**, 793–798.

Wechsler, B., Vidailhet, M., Piette, J. C., Bousser, M. G., Dell, I. B., Bletry, O., *et al.* (1992) Cerebral venous thrombosis in Behcet's disease: clinical study and long-term follow-up of 25 cases. *Neurology*, **42**, 614–618.

Weiss, S. R., Raskind, R., Morganstern, N. L., Pytlyk, P. J. and Baiz, T. C. (1970) Intracerebral and subarachnoid hemorrhage following use of methamphetamine ('speed'). *Int. Surg.*, **53**, 123–127.

Weyand, C. M. and Bartley, G. B. (1997) Giant cell arteritis: new concepts in pathogenesis and implications for management (editorial; comment). *Am. J. Ophthalmol.*, **123**, 392–395.

Weyand, C. M. and Goronzy, J. J. (1995a) Giant cell arteritis as an antigen-driven disease.

Rheum. Dis. Clin. North Am., **21**, 1027–1039.

Weyand, C. M. and Goronzy, J. J. (1995b) Molecular approaches toward pathologic mechanisms in giant cell arteritis and Takayasu's arteritis. *Curr. Opin. Rheumatol.*, **7**, 30–36.

Weyand, C. M. and Goronzy, J. J. (1996) The pathogenic role of T lymphocytes in vasculitis. *Sarcoidosis Vasc. Diffuse. Lung Dis.*, **13**, 217–220.

Weyand, C. M., Hicok, K. C., Hunder, G. G. and Goronzy, J. J. (1994a) Tissue cytokine patterns in patients with polymyalgia rheumatica and giant cell arteritis (see comments). *Ann. Intern. Med.*, **121**, 484–491.

Weyand, C. M., Hunder, N. N., Hicok, K. C., Hunder, G. G. and Goronzy, J. J. (1994b) HLA-DRB1 alleles in polymyalgia rheumatica, giant cell arteritis, and rheumatoid arthritis. *Arthritis Rheum.*, **37**, 514–520.

Weyand, C. M., Schonberger, J., Oppitz, U., Hunder, N. N., Hicok, K. C. and Goronzy, J. J. (1994c) Distinct vascular lesions in giant cell arteritis share identical T cell clonotypes. *J. Exp. Med.*, **179**, 951–960.

Weyand, C. M., Wagner, A. D., Bjornsson, J. and Goronzy, J. J. (1996) Correlation of the topographical arrangement and the functional pattern of tissue-infiltrating macrophages in giant cell arteritis. *J. Clin. Invest.*, **98**, 1642–1649.

Weyand, C. M., Tetzlaff, N., Bjornsson, J., Brack, A., Younge, B. and Goronzy, J. J. (1997) Disease patterns and tissue cytokine profiles in giant cell arteritis. *Arthritis Rheum.*, **40**, 19–26.

Whitcup, S. M., Salvo, E. C. J. and Nussenblatt, R. B. (1994) Combined cyclosporine and corticosteroid therapy for sight-threatening uveitis in Behcet's disease. *Am. J. Ophthalmol.*, **118**, 39–45.

Wick, M. R., Scheithauer, B. W., Okazaki, H. and Thomas, J. E. (1982) Cerebral angioendotheliomatosis. *Arch. Pathol. Lab. Med.*, **106**, 342–346.

Wieslander, J., Kataja, M. and Hudson, B. G. (1987) Characterization of the human Goodpasture antigen. *Clin. Exp. Immunol.*, **69**, 332–340.

Winkleman, R. K. and Ditto, W. B. (1964) Cutaneous and visceral syndromes of necrotizing or 'allergic' vasculitis. *Medicine*, 43, 59–89.

Wilkinson, I. M. and Russell, R. W. (1972) Arteries of the head and neck in giant cell arteritis. A pathological study to show the pattern of arterial involvement. *Arch. Neurol.*, **27**, 378–391.

Woolfenden, A. R., Tong, D. C., Marks, M. P., Ali, A. O. and Albers, G. W. (1988) Angiographically defined primary angiitis of the CNS: is it really benign? *Neurology*, **51**, 183–188.

Yamashita, N., Kaneoka, H., Kaneko, S., Takeno, M., Oneda, K., Koizumi, H., *et al.* (1997) Role of gammadelta T lymphocytes in the development of Behcet's disease. *Clin. Exp. Immunol.*, **107**, 241–247.

Yamashita, Y., Takahashi, M., Bussaka, H., Miyawaki, M. and Tosaka, K. (1986) Cerebral vasculitis secondary to Wegener's granulomatosis: computed tomography and angiographic findings. *J. Comput. Tomogr.*, **10**, 115–120.

Yang, J. J., Kettritz, R., Falk, R. J., Jennette, J. C. and Gaido, M. L. (1996) Apoptosis of endothelial cells induced by the neutrophil serine proteases proteinase 3 and elastase. *Am. J. Pathol.*, **149**, 1617–1626.

Younger, D. S., Hays, A. P., Brust, J. C. and Rowland, L. P. (1988) Granulomatous angiitis of the brain. An inflammatory reaction of diverse etiology. *Arch. Neurol.*, **45**, 514–518.

Yuen, R. W., Johnson, P. C. (1996) Primary angiitis of the central nervous system associated with Hodgkin's disease. *Arch. Pathol. Lab. Med.*, **120**, 573–576.

Zhang, L., Jayne, D. R., Zhao, M. H., Lockwood, C. M. and Oliveira, D. B. (1995) Distribution of MHC class II alleles in primary systemic vasculitis. *Kidney Int.*, **47**, 294–298.

Zhao, M. H., Jones, S. J. and Lockwood, C. M. (1995) Bactericidal/permeability-increasing protein (BPI) is an important antigen for anti-neutrophil cytoplasmic autoantibodies (ANCA) in vasculitis. *Clin. Exp. Immunol.*, **99**, 49–56.

Index

ACA (anti-cardiolipin antobodies) in SLE, 154, 158
  risk factor for stroke, 160, 165
Acute disseminated encephalomyelitis, see ADEM
Acute haemorrhagic leukoencephalomyelitis, 85
Acute necrotising myelitis, 81
Addressin MECA-325, 46
ADEM (acute disseminated encephalomyelitis), 82
  akin to transverse myelitis, 80
  close similarities with EAE, 84
  pathology, 84
  similarities with multiple sclerosis, 84
Adhesion molecules, see ICAM, VCAM
  in multiple sclerosis, 106
AHLE (acute haemorrhagic leukoencephalomyelitis), 85
Amphetamines, vasculitis, 231
Amphiphysin, 145
ANA (antinuclear antibody), 160
ANCA (anti-neutrophil cytoplasmic antibodies), 215
Anergy, 4
Angioendotheliosis, malignant, 233
Angiography in cerebral vasculitis, 222
Angiopathy of the CNS, benign or isolated, 225
Ankylosing spondylitis, neurological complications, 170
ANNA-1, 128
ANNA-2, (anti-Ri antibodies/type 2 anti-neuronal nuclear antibodies), 129
Antibodies, onconeural, 126
Anti-cardiolipin antibodies see ACA
  in SLE, 155
Anti-cardiolipin syndrome, 156
Antigen, oral administration, 108
Antigen-presenting cells in brain, 8
Antigen-specific immunotherapy of multiple sclerosis, 108
Anti-Hu antibodies/type I anti-neuronal nuclear antibodies (ANNA-1), 128
Anti-idiotypic network, 12
Anti-neutrophil cytoplasmic antibodies (ANCA), 215
Antinuclear antibody in SLE, 160
Anti-Ri antibodies/type 2 anti-neuronal nuclear antibodies (ANNA-2), 129
Anti-Yo antibodies/anti-Purkinje cell cytoplasmic antibodies (APCA), 127
APCA, see Anti-Yo antibodies
Apoptosis, lymphocytes, 8
Armadillo syndrome, 140

Arteritis, see also Vasculitis
  giant cell, 237
Aspergillus vasculitis, 232
Astrocytes:
  and blood–brain barrier, 44
  form scar tissue, 28
  type 1 and blood–brain barrier, 6
  type 2, 55
Ataxia in multiple sclerosis, 22
Australia, multiple sclerosis rare in, 34
Autoimmune disease, initiation, 12
  maintenance, 13
  therapeutic strategies, 13
  thyroid diseases, 8
Avonex, see, IFN-β
Axon damage in multiple sclerosis, 27, 52
  described by Charcot and Dawson, 37
Azathioprine for multiple sclerosis, 31, 97

B cell surface antigen B220, 11
  CD5$^+$, produce natural antibodies, 11
B7 family of receptors, 4
Bactericidal/permeability-increasing protein (BPI), 216
Balò's concentric sclerosis, 87
Barrier, blood–brain 1
  damage, 44
  immune privilege, 43
  incompetent in places, 7
  structure of, 6
Behçet's disease, 240
  neurological complications, 241
  treatment, 242
Benign angiopathy of the CNS, 225
Betaferon, see IFN-β
Bladder symptoms in multiple sclerosis, treatment, 31
BPI (bactericidal/permeability-increasing protein), 216
Brain biopsy:
  in cerebral vasculitis, 224–226
  in Whipple's disease, 185

Calcium flux by complement and perforin, 47
Calgranulin Mac 387, calcium binding protein, 195
Campath-1H, 26
  for cerebral vasculitis, 237
  for multiple sclerosis, 102
Cancer causing vasculitis, 232
CD28, 4
CD4$^+$ T cells:
  recognize HLA class II, 3

secrete cytokines that act on B cells, 3
in MS, 36, 41, 95, 109
CD8$^+$ T cells:
are cytotoxic, 3
recognize HLA class I, 3
in MS, 36, 41, 95, 109
Cerebellar degeneration, subacute, 119
in coeliac disease, 188
Cerebral:
emboli, multiple, 219
lupus, 154, 164
vasculitis, see Vasculitis
venous sinus thrombosis in Behçet's disease,
242
Chest radiograph in sarcoidosis, 201
Chorea in SLE, 161
Choroid plexus blood–brain barrier, 7
Churg–Strauss syndrome:
ANCA in, 216
histology, 212
neurological complications, 219
Clathrin-coated pits on endothelial cells, 45
Clonal deletion, 4, 10
Clonal ignorance, 10
Coccidioidosis vasculitis, 232
Coeliac disease:
cerebellar degeneration, 188
neurological complications, 187
Cogan's syndrome, 212, 227
Colitis, ulcerative, see Inflammatory bowel
disease
Complement:
activation, 6
causes calcium flux, 47
in MS, 47–50
in vasculitis, 217
Conduction, saltatory, disrupted, 24
Connective tissue diseases, autoantibodies in,
150
Copolymer-1 $\alpha_4\beta_1$, in multiple sclerosis treat-
ment, 54
see Glatirimer acetate
Corticosteroids:
for multiple sclerosis treatment, 30
side effects, 207
Co-stimulatory molecules, 4
Crohn's disease, see Inflammatory bowel
disease
Cryoglobinaemia and hepatitis C, 230
CTLA-4 (cytotoxic T lymphocyte antigen-4),
4
Cuprizone-induced demyelination, 44
Cyclophosphamide
in MS, 96–97
in vasculitis, 235
Cytokines, suppression of pro-inflammatory,
14
MS 41–43, 50, 109
vasculitis, 218
Cytotoxic T lymphocyte antigen-4 (CTLA-4),
4

Dawson's histopathology of multiple sclerosis, 35
Dementia in SLE, 158
Demyelination, 21
combined central and peripheral, 88
cuprizone-induced, 44
inflammatory, other than multiple sclerosis,
74
primary, in multiple sclerosis, 35
repair by systemic immunoglobulins, 56
repair by transplant of glial cells, 55
Denny–Brown, histology of paraneoplastic
disorders, 125
Dermatomyositis linked with cancer, 125
Devic's disease, 80

EAE (experimental allergic encephalomyelitis), 1
and multiple sclerosis, 39, 54, 95
is suppressed by anti-IFN-γ antibodies and
IL-4, 5
similarities with ADEM, 84
Eale's disease, 212, 227
Electrophoretic examination of CFS, 29
Encephalitis:
brainstem, 121
limbic, 121
periaxalis concentrica, 87
periaxalis diffusa, 87
periaxalis scleroticans, 87
Encephalomyelitis, post-infectious and post-
vaccinal, 82
Encephalopathy:
acute ischaemic in SLE, 160
Hashimoto's, 189
in SLE, 158
of myxoedema, 189
vasculitis, 218
Endocarditis, Libman Sacks, 166
Endothelial cell clathrin-coated pits, 45
Epithelioid cells in sarcoid lesions, 197
Epitope spread results in secondary immuni-
zation, 52
ESR, SLE, 163,
vasculitis, 220, 226
Experimental allergic encephalomyelitis, see
EAE
Facial nerve paralysis in sarcoidosis, 198
Fas, 40
Foix Alajuanine syndrome, 81
Fundus examination in cerebral vasculitis, 223

GABA (γ-amino butyric acid), 141
GAD (glutamic acid decarboxylase), 142
Gadolinium enhanced MRI, 29, 44
Galactocerebroside, 53
Gallium scan in sarcoidosis, 202
Gamma-amino butyric acid (GABA), 141

GBS (Guillain Barré syndrome), 80
Giant cell arteritis, 237
    treatment, 239
Gitter cells, 51
Glatirimer acetate, treatment of multiple
    sclerosis, 54, 102
Glia limitans, 44
Glial cells to repair demyelinated lesions, 55
Glutamate, 50
Glutamic acid decarboxylase (GAD) antibo-
    dies in stiff man syndrome, 142
Goodpasture's syndrome, 215
Granulomatous reactions, causes, 194
Guillain Barré syndrome, see GBS

Hashimoto's disease, 8
    encephalopathy, 189
Heparan sulphate endoglycosidase, 45
Hepatitis C and cryoglobinaemia, 230
Herpes zoster and cerebral vasculitis, 232
HHV-6 (human herpes virus-6), 96
Histoplasma vasculitis, 232
HLA (human leukocyte antigen) classes 1 and
    2, 3
    in multiple sclerosis, 95
Hodgkin's disease and vasculitis, 232
Human herpes virus-6, 96
Human leukocyte antigen, see HLA

ICAM-1 (intercellular adhesion molecule-1), 4, 45
    in Wegener's granuloma, 216
    in MS, 44–46, 106–107
IFN-β 100, 101
IFN-γ (interferon-γ), 5
IL-10 treatment of multiple sclerosis, 105
IL-12 antibody treatment of multiple sclerosis,
    105
Immune:
    deviation, 11
    privilege in CNS, 43
    response, 2
        antigen non-specific, 6
        antigen-specific, 3
    suppressants for multiple sclerosis treat-
        ment, 31
    tolerance, 4
Immunization, secondary, in demyelination,
    52
Immunoglobulin, intravenous for treatment
    of:
    cerebral vasculitis, 237
    multiple sclerosis, 99
    SLE, 170
Impotence in multiple sclerosis, sildenafil for,
    31
Indium-labelled white cell scanning in cerebral
    vasculitis, 222
Inflammatory bowel disease:
    and multiple sclerosis, possible association, 181

epilepsy in, 183
    neurological complications, 183
    vasculitis in, 183
Integrin $\alpha_1\beta_1$, 46, 54, 217
    and emigration of lymphocytes, 7
Intercellular adhesion molecule-1, see ICAM-1
Interferonγ, see IFN-γ
Interferon β, see IFN-β
Interleukin, see IL
Isaac's syndrome, 140
Isolated angiopathy of the CNS, 225

Kawasaki disease, 215
Kohlmeyer Degos disease, 219
Kveim test, 201

Lambert–Eaton myasthenic syndrome, 119
Leber's hereditary optic neuropathy, 75
LEMS (Lambert–Eaton myasthenic syn-
    drome), 119.
Leprosy, tuberculoid, 9
LFA-1 (lymphocyte function associated anti-
    gen-1), 4
LFA-3, 45
    in Wegener's granuloma, 217
Lhermitte's sign, 27
Libman–Sacks endocarditis, 166
Lung cancer, small cell:
    association with paraneoplastic disorders,
        118
    express Anti-Hu/ANNA-1 antigen, 128
Lupoid sclerosis, 162
Lupus:
    anticoagulants, 158
    cerebral, 154, 164
    encephalopathy, 158
Lymphocyte function associated antigen, see
    LFA
Lymphocytes:
    in sarcoid lesions, 195
    in MS, 36, 40–43, 44–47
    traffic into the brain, 45
Lymphocytic choriomeningitis viral glycopro-
    tein, 11
Lymphomatoid granulomatosis, 233
Lymphotoxin, see TNF-β

MAG (myelin-associated glycoprotein), 42
    antibodies cause oligodendrocytemyelin da-
        mage, 49
Magnetic resonance:
    Imaging, see MRI
    Spectroscopy (MRS), 27
Major histocompatibility complex (MHC), 7,
    see also HLA
Marburg disease, 86
Marcus Gunn pupil, 75
MBP (myelin basic protein)-reactive T cells, 11

Measles, ADEM, 85
Membrane attack complex, 49
Memory cells, 3
Meningitis in rheumatoid arthritis, 149
Metalloproteinase inhibitors, treatment of multiple sclerosis, 106
MHC (major histocompatibility complex), 7, *see also* HLA
Microglia:
  activated, may present antigen to T cells, 3, 46
  are macrophages and secrete cytokines, 6
  may express class II MHC molecules. 7
Micrographia in multiple sclerosis, 23
Mixed connective tissue disease, 153
MMP, *see* Metalloproteinase
Moersch and Woltman, 141
MOG (myelin-oligodendrocyte glycoprotein), 15
  antibodies cause oligodendrocytemyelin damage, 49
Molecular mimics, 12
MRI (magnetic resonance imaging), gadolinium-enhanced, 24, 29
  in Behçet's disease, 242
  in cerebral vasculitis, 221
  in sarcoidosis, 203
  in SLE encephalopathy, 168
MRS (magnetic resonance spectroscopy), 27
Multiple sclerosis:
  acute, 86
  antigen, 42
  axon damage, 27
  clinical features, 22
  defective immune suppression in, 41
  development of tissue damage in, 43
  diagnosis, 28
  familial and racial susceptibility, 32
  future approaches to treatment, 54
  geographical distribution, 33
  histopathology, 35
  HLA association, 33
  inflammatory demyelinating lesions in, 21
  pathogenesis, 53
  polygenic inheritance, 33
  relapsing pattern, 74
  similarities with ADEM, 84
  treatment, 93
    antibodies, monoclonal, 103
    anti-CD4 monoclonal antibody, 103
    azathioprine, disappointing, 97
    bone marrow transplantation, 99
    Campath-1, 102
    copolymer-1, 102
    corticosteroids, 98
    cyclophosphamide, 96
    cyclosporin A, 98
    experimental, 103
    glatirimer acetate, 102
    interferons, 100
    intravenous immunoglobulin, 99
    metalloproteinase inhibitors, 106
    methotrexate, 98
    plasma exchange, 99
    symptomatic, 29
Muscle stiffness, differential diagnosis, 140
Myasthenia gravis, paraneoplastic, 119
Myelin basic protein, *see* MBP
Myelin, phagocytosis of, 51
Myelin-associated glycoprotein (MAG), 42
Myelinoligodendrocyte glycoprotein (MOG), 15
Myelitis:
  necrotising, 81, 121
  transverse, 77
Myelopathy:
  in inflammatory bowel disease, 184
  in SLE, 78, 161, 163
Myoclonus, 123
Myxoedema encephalopathy, 189

N-acetylaspartate, axon-specific, 27
Neuromyelitis optica, 80
Neuromyotonia, 140
Neuronopathy, subacute sensory, 121
Neuropathy:
  inflammatory peripheral; in rheumatoid arthritis, 148
  paraneoplastic motor, 122
  paraneoplastic sensory, 121
Neurosarcoidosis, *see* Sarcoidosis
Nitric oxide oligodendrocytes, 48
Nova, 129
Numb chin syndrome, 123

Oligoclonal bands of immunoglobulin in spinal fluid:
  electrophoretic examination, 29
  in cerebral vasculitis, 221
  in multiple sclerosis, 76
  in paraneoplastic disorders, 120
  in stiff man syndrome, 141
Oligodendrocyte myelin damage
  complement, 48
  MOG and MAG antibodies, 49
  reversible, 47
  TNF and nitric oxide, 48, 50
Oligodendrocytes:
  absence in chronic plaques, 35
  and multiple sclerosis, 24
  fas, 40, 50
  progenitor cells, 55
Ophthalmoplegia, Graves, 189
Oppenheim's useless limb, 22
Opsoclonus syndrome, 123
Optic neuritis:
  in giant cell arteritis, 238
  in multiple sclerosis, 22, 24, 74
  in sarcoidosis, 197
  in Sjögren's syndrome, 151

in SLE, 162
Oral antigens, 108

PACNS (primary angiitis of the central nervous system), 212, 226
Paraneoplastic disorders
central nervous system, 118
histology, 125
treatment, 131
vasculitis, 232
Paraplegia, transverse myelitis, 77
Pause cell, 126
Peptide antigens in treatment of multiple sclerosis, 110
Perforin, T cell-derived:
causes calcium flux, 47
causes reversible oligodendrocyte damage, 48
Pericytes, 44
Perivascular:
deposits of C9 and membrane attack complex in multiple sclerosis, 49
inflammatory lesions in multiple sclerosis, 36
PEWR, see Progressive encephalomyelitis with rigidity
Plasma cells, 3
Plasmapheresis in paraneoplastic disorders, 131
PLP (proteolipid protein), 42
Polyangiitis, microscopic, 228
Polyarteritis nodosa:
histology, 212
neurological complications, 228
Polymerase chain reaction to detect DNA of viruses in multiple sclerosis, 34
Poser committee diagnostic criteria for multiple sclerosis, 30
Prazocin, EAE, 44
Primary angiitis of the central nervous system (PACNS), 212, 226
Progressive encephalomyelitis with rigidity (PEWR), 144
Proteolipid protein (PLP), 42

Rabies virus vaccine:
encephalomyelitis, 1, 82
Ramsay–Hunt syndrome, 188
Ranvier nodes, 24
Rebif, see IFN-β
Recoverin antibodies, 130
Reiter's disease, neurological complications, 170
Remyelination, 55
Retinopathy, cancer-associated, 124
Rheopathy in SLE encephalopathy, 164
Rheumatoid arthritis:
association with HLA-DR1 and -DR4, 147
meningitis in, 149

Rheumatoid:
factor IgM, 148
nodules in central nervous system, 148
Rheumatological diseases, neurological complications, 147
Rolipram treatment of multiple sclerosis, 106

Saltatory conduction, 47
disrupted in demyelinating diseases, 24
Sarcoidosis, 193
Sarcoidosis:
cerebral:
clinical presentation, 196
criteria for diagnosis, 200
pathogenesis, 195
treatment:
corticosteroids, 206
other immunomodulatory, 207
(see specific drugs)
Schilder's diffuse sclerosis, 87
Schirmer's test, 150
Schwann cells to remyelinate, 56
Schwarz–Jampel disease, 139
Scleroderma and Raynaud's phenomenon, 152
Selectins, 217
and emigration of lymphocytes, 7
Semple rabies vaccine, encephalomyelitis following, 82
SHLE, see Subacute leukoencephalitis
Single photon emission computed tomography (SPECT) in cerebral vasculitis, 222
Sjögren's syndrome, 150
and multiple sclerosis, 151
optic neuropathy in, 151
SLE (systemic lupus erythematosus), 78, 153
ACA, in 158
American College of Rheumatology diagnostic criteria, 154
anti-brain antibodies, 166
anti-cardiolipin antibodies, 154
chorea, 161
encephalopathy, 158
diagnosis, 168
microinfarctions, 164
aspirin and warfarin, 169
rheopathy, 164
steroids and azathioprine, 170
ESR raised in, 163
genetic factors, 164
intravenous immunoglobulin for, 170
microvasculopathy, mechanisms, 165
myelopathy in, 161
neurological complications, 154
optic neuritis in, 162
psychiatric changes in, 157
seizures in, 157
thrombosis in, 158
Sneddon's syndrome, 159, 166

South Africa, multiple sclerosis rare in, 34

SPECT (single photon emission computed tomography) in cerebral vasculitis, 222

Spinal cord compression:
distinguished from transverse myelitis, 78
in rheumatoid arthritis, 148

Spinal cord ischaemia, distinguished from transverse myelitis, 78

Stiff man syndrome, 139
and diabetes mellitus, 141
paraneoplastic, 143
treatment, 142

Strokes in young people, differential diagnosis, 219

Subacute leukoencephalitis, multiple sclerosis, 96

Superantigens, TCR, 4, 12

Susac's syndrome, 219

Systemic lupus erythematosus, see SLE

Systemic sclerosis, 152
neurological complications, 152

T cells:
cerebrospinal fluid in multiple sclerosis, 41
and multiple sclerosis, 39
and paraneoplastic encephalitis, 130
blood–brain barrier, 7
depleting monoclonal antibody, see Campath-1H
maturation in thymus, 10
oligodendrocyte myelin antigen interaction is crucial, 46
receptor, see TCR
with $\gamma\delta$ chains:
are cytotoxic to oligodendrocytes, 40
release IFN-γ, 5

Takayasu's disease, 239

TCR (T cell receptor), 3
Vα and Vβ, biased engagement of in multiple sclerosis, 42
γ and δ chains recognize antigens without HLA class restriction, 5

Temporal arteritis, see Giant cell arteritis

Terminal membrane attack complex, 6

TGF-β (transforming growth factor-β) treatment of multiple sclerosis, 104

T_h0 (T helper cell 0) CD4$^+$ cells secrete few cytokines, 5

T_h1 (T helper cell 1) CD4$^+$ cells secrete IL-12, TNF-β, IFN-γ, 5

T_h1 CD4$^+$ -T_h2 CD4$^+$ cell:
balance is critical, 5
phenotype switching may be hazardous, 15

T_h2 (T helper cell 2) CD4$^+$ cells secrete IL-4 and IL-10, 5
treatment of multiple sclerosis, 109

Thalamotomy for multiple sclerosis treatment, 32

Thalidomide in Behçet's disease, 242

Theiler's murine encephalitis virus (TMEV) infection, 95
virus-induced demyelination, 9

Thymoma and myasthenia gravis, 119

Thyroid disease, neurological complications, 189

TMEV (Theiler's murine encephalitis virus), 95

TNF-α (tumour necrosis factor), 5
antibody treatment of multiple sclerosis, 105
and oligodendrocytes, 48, 50

TNF-β (lymphotoxin) causes oligodendrocyte myelin damage, 50

Tolerance, 13
antigen-specific, 10
to unknown autoantigens, 16

Transverse myelitis, 77
MRI in, 79
pathology, 79

Trigeminal neuropathy in systemic sclerosis, 152

Trimolecular complex is HLA-antigen-TCR, 4

Tropheryma whippelii, 184

Tumour necrosis factor, see TNF

Twins, multiple sclerosis, 32

Uhtoff phenomenon, 26

Ulcers, aphthous, in Behçet's disease, 240

Uveitis in Behçet's disease, 240

Vascular:
cell adhesion molecule-1, see VCAM-1
leak, retinal, in optic neuritis, 76

Vasculitis:
aetiology unknown, 214
anti-neutrophil cytoplasmic antibodies-related, 215
cell-mediated, 217
cerebral, 210
classification, 211
clinical manifestation, 218
differential diagnosis, 219
in rheumatoid arthritis, 149
investigations, 220
treatment by:
Campath-1H, 237
intravenous immunoglobulin, 237
methotrexate, 236
pentoxifylline, dapsone, thalidomide, 237
plasmapheresis, 237
steroids and cyclophosphamide, 234
direct antibody attack against endothelium, 215
from amphetamines, 231
histology, 212

immune complex-mediated, 214
infective, 232
in inflammatory bowel disease, 183
VCAM-1 (vascular cell adhesion molecule),
    46, 217
Very late antigen-6 (VLA-6), 45
Viruses, in multiple sclerosis, 34
Visual evoked potential abnormal in multiple
    sclerosis, 28
VLA-4 antibodies treatment of multiple
    sclerosis, 106
VLA-6 (very late antigen-6), 45
Vogt–Koyanagi–Harada syndrome, 243

Wegener's granuloma:
    ANCA in, 216
    diagnostic criteria, 227
    histology, 212
    ICAM-1 in, 217
    LFA-3 in, 217
    neurological complications, 227
Weston–Hurst disease, 85
Whipple's disease, 184
    cerebral, 186
    neurological complications, 184
Witebsky's postulates, 10